THE NUTRITION
SUPERBOOK

1

THE ANTIOXIDANTS

KEATS TITLES OF RELATED INTEREST

The Big Family Guide to All the Minerals
Frank Murray

The Big Family Guide to All the Vitamins
Ruth Adams

Maximize Your Health-Span with Antioxidants
Carmia Borek, Ph.D.

Dr. Wright's Guide to Healing with Nutrition
Jonathan V. Wright, M.D.

Mental and Elemental Nutrients
Carl C. Pfeiffer, M.D., Ph.D.

The Nutrition Desk Reference
Robert H. Garrison, Jr., M.A.,R.Ph. and
Elizabeth Somer, M.A.,R.D.

Nutritional Influences on Illness
Melvyn R. Werbach, M.D.

Pycnogenol: The Super "Protector" Nutrient
Richard A. Passwater, Ph.D. and
Chithan Kandaswami, Ph.D.

Vitamin C: The Master Nutrient
Sandra Goodman, Ph.D.

Wellness Medicine
Robert A. Anderson, M.D.

THE NUTRITION SUPERBOOK

1

THE ANTIOXIDANTS

EDITED BY

Jean Barilla, M.S.

Keats Publishing, Inc.

NEW CANAAN, CONNECTICUT

The information contained in this book is not intended as medical advice. Its intention is solely informational and educational. Please consult a medical or health professional should the need for one be indicated.

THE NUTRITION SUPERBOOK:
VOLUME I: THE ANTIOXDANTS

Library of Congress Cataloging-in-Publication Data
The Nutrition superbook / edited by Jean Barilla.
     p.   cm.
  Includes bibliographical references and index.
  Contents: v. 1. The antioxidants.
  ISBN 0-87983-671-7
  1. Vitamins in human nutrition. 2. Antioxidants. I. Barrila,
Jean.
  QP771.N88 1995
  612.3'99—dc20   95-11419
                                            CIP

Printed in the United States of America

Published by Keats Publishing, Inc.
27 Pine Street, Box 876
New Canaan, Connecticut 06840-0876

10 9 8 7 6 5 4 3 2

To

LINUS PAULING

*whose pursuit of knowledge and revelations in molecular biology
made the world a healthier place for all of us.*

CONTENTS

Foreword   WILLIAM A. PRYOR, PH.D.   xiii

PART ONE: THE BASICS   1

The Antioxidants. The Nutrients
That Guard the Body Against Cancer, Heart Disease, Arthritis
and Allergies—and Even Slow the Aging Process
                  RICHARD A. PASSWATER, PH.D.   5

    The Protectors   5
    Cancer   8
    The Immune System and Vitamin A   9
    The Key Antioxidants—an Overview   14
    Antioxidant Combinations Are Better   25
    What Is Aging?   25
    Antioxidants and Disease   27
    How Much?   32
    Bibliography   33

Health News: World Conference on Antioxidants Shows Many
Preventive Functions   34

Health News: Antioxidants Are Crucial for Heart Health; They
Protect Against Stroke, Heart Attack   39

Health News: How Antioxidant Nutrients Form First Line of
Cancer Defense   42

PART TWO: THE KEY ANTIOXIDANTS   47

Beta-Carotene. The Backstage Nutrient Now Universally
Recognized for Cancer Prevention
                  RICHARD A. PASSWATER, PH.D.   49

    Beta-Carotene and Vitamin A   50
    Cancer: 50 Years of Research   53
    Sources and Daily Requirement   64

Health News: Beyond Beta: Alpha and Other Carotenes Shown
to Have Up to 100 Times More Antioxidant Power   69

Vitamin C. The Great Vitamin That Provides Optimum
Health and Immunity   JACK JOSEPH CHALLEM   73
    The Discovery and Rediscovery of Vitamin C   75
    What Happens When You "Catch" a Cold?   77
    Vitamin C Reverses Degenerative Diseases   84
    Vitamin C in the Prevention and Control of Cancer   86
    Vitamin C Relieves Periodontal Disease   89
    Vitamin C Lowers Cholesterol, Strengthens Heart Muscle 90
    Vitamin C Prevents Sudden Infant Death Syndrome   91
    Other Benefits of Vitamin C   92
    Vitamin C Is for Everyone   94
    References   95

Health News: The Absolute Latest on Vitamin C from Its
Foremost Advocate   98

Vitamin E. New Roles for the Vitamin That Preserves the
Health and Integrity of Body Cells   LEN MERVYN, PH.D.   100
    How Vitamin E Functions and Protects   102
    Vitamin E as a Therapeutic Agent   114
    New Insight into Vitamin E Potency   122
    References   125

Health News: Vitamin E Pioneers Were Right: E Fights Heart
Disease & More   127

Health News: Research Shows Roles for Vitamin E in Ills from
Cataracts to Cancer   130

Health News: Vitamin E Is for Elephants   134

Selenium. How It Protects
Against Cancer, Heart Disease, Arthritis and Aging
    RICHARD A. PASSWATER, PH.D.   136
    Cancer   140
    Heart Disease   153
    Arthritis   159

Health News: Why Selenium May Be the Secret of Your
Longer Life   163

Health News: Garlic . . . Ancients' Answer to Poison Now
Modern Remedy for Blood Clotting and Variety of Human Ills 165

Health News: Folklore, Old Wives Were Right   168

PART THREE: MORE ANTIOXIDANTS   173

The New Superantioxidant—Plus. The Amazing Story of
Pycnogenol, Free-Radical Antagonist and Vitamin C Potentiator
                          RICHARD A. PASSWATER, PH.D.   175
    The Discovery of Pycnogenol   178
    Pycnogenol, the Powerful Antioxidant   183
    Preventing Heart Disease   190
    Blood Vessel Health and Circulation   196
    The Skin Cosmetic in a Capsule   201
    Other Important Relationships   204
    Pycnogenol's Outstanding Safety   209

Health News: Amazing Antioxidant Derived from Plants Has
Triple Action Against Free Radicals   212

Coenzyme Q-10. Is It Our New Fountain of Youth?
                          WILLIAM H. LEE, R.PH., PH.D.   215
    Enzymes and Coenzymes   217
    Coenzyme Q-10, Medicine and Longevity   222
    Periodontal Disease   234
    Diabetes Mellitus   235
    Coenzyme Q-10 and the Cardiotoxicity of Adriamycin 237
    Weight Loss   238
    Athletic Performance   239
    Coenzyme Q-10 and the Immune System   239
    Antioxidant Power   241
    Safety   241
    Bibliography   242

Bioflavonoids. The Friends and Helpers of Vitamin C in
Many Hard-to-Treat Ailments   JEFFREY BLAND, PH.D.   244
    Bioflavonoids—What and Where?   246
    Biological and Clinical Investigations   248
    Recent Discoveries about the Bioflavonoids   249
    Uses of Bioflavonoids   252
    Bioflavonoids as Nutritional Supplements:
    The Controversy   254
    Vitamin C Metabolites and Bioflavonoids   258

Conclusion   261
References   261

Health News: The Bioflavonoids–Vitamin C Partnership—
How They Work to Promote, Improve Your Health   263

A New Generation of Phytomedicines—Plant Antioxidants
                        J. AUGUSTE MOCKLE, D. PHARM.   267
Phytomedicines   266
Ginkgo   269
Bilberry   272
Garlic   273
Conclusion   276
References   277

Ginkgo Biloba. The Amazing 200 Million-Year-Old
Healer   FRANK MURRAY
Foreword by   STEPHEN E. LANGER, M.D.   281
The "Living Fossil"   283
Alzheimer's Disease   288
Headaches   295
Organ Transplants   296
Asthma   297
Tinnitus and Hearing Loss   299
Impotence   302
Circulatory Disorders   303
Eye Disorders   308
Hemorrhoids   309
Free-Radical Scavenger   311
Dosage and Side Effects   313
Conclusion   314
References   315

PART FOUR: SUMMARY: AS WE LIVE AND BREATHE   323

Health News: How Young Are You? Good Habits, Nutrition &
Antioxidants Can Slow Down Biological Aging   338

Health News: Smog Peril Grows, Seniors at High Risk;
Antioxidants Help   341

GLOSSARY   347

BIBLIOGRAPHY 352

APPENDICES 353

A. More about Free Radicals 355

Health News: Free Radicals Shouldn't Be Free! 357

Health News: Antioxidant Nutrients May Act As Armor Against
Free-Radical Damage, Cancer 359

B. Free Radical-Fighting Foods 361

C. Diseases Associated with Free Radical Damage 363

D. Recommended Amounts of Antioxidants 364

E. Antioxidant Food Values 365

ABOUT THE AUTHORS 369

INDEX 371

An eight-page photographic section follows page 158.

FOREWORD

WILLIAM A. PRYOR, PH.D.

*Director of the Biodynamics Institute
and Thomas & David Boyd Professor
Louisiana State University, Baton Rouge, LA*

In the 1930s and 1940s the effects of ionizing radiation received intense scrutiny because of the interest of governments in the effects of X rays and nuclear radiation. Since almost all of the damage caused to animals by radiation occurs through free-radical[1] pathways, the field of radiation biology developed insights into the harmful effects of radicals on living systems. In this period, radicals were viewed as arising from external sources (such as radiation or toxins like carbon tetrachloride or ethanol) and were always regarded as pathological agents that caused damage to cells.

In 1967, Joe McCord and Irwin Fridovich discovered the enzyme superoxide dismutase (SOD). Since SOD can easily be obtained in pure form, laboratories all over the world began studying the extent to which superoxide[2] was involved in the chemistry that occurs inside cells. To the surprise of almost everybody, research with SOD showed conclusively that superoxide is produced continuously in all cells that use oxygen to burn food and produce energy (a process called respiration).

Thus, the discovery of SOD changed a field that had been largely dominated by radiation biologists to an area of science of interest to biochemists and physicians who were studying how cells produce en-

---

1. A radical is a chemical species with an odd number of electrons.
2. Superoxide is produced when oxygen (O_2) adds a single electron to form the species $O_2{}^{\bullet}-$.

ergy, metabolize food, detoxify toxins and, in general, simply "live." The field of free-radical biology was born!

In the late 1970s and 1980s, biochemists and physiologists began studying a hormone of unknown structure that was called the endothelium-dependent relaxation factor (EDRF). This hormone was found to relax smooth muscles, including the muscles in the lining of blood vessels (the endothelium), and therefore lower blood pressure. In the 1980s Steven Tannenbaum and others showed that mammals excrete large amounts of sodium nitrite and sodium nitrate in their urine, and later Michael Marletta and others showed that white blood cells and other related cells produce nitrate and nitrite when they defend the cell against invaders. In 1986, Robert Furchgott and Louis Ignarro suggested that EDRF is nitric oxide. This remarkable suggestion has revolutionized the study of hormones, since nitric oxide is a simple gas with the chemical structure •NO. All other hormones are complex organic molecules that contain a large number of carbon atoms, whereas nitric oxide contains none. As shown from its structure (with the odd electron shown as a dot), nitric oxide is a free radical.

Thus, free radical biology has come of age. Cells produce not one but two radicals: superoxide and nitric oxide. Furthermore, these two radicals can react in the cell to form a nonradical product, peroxynitrous acid (equation 1), which is a potent and destructive oxidant of biomolecules.

Equation 1. $O_2^{•-} + •NO + H_+ \rightarrow H\text{-}OO\text{-}N=O$

As free-radical biology was coming to maturity, Denham Harman was postulating that the pathological effects of free radicals on tissue could be prevented by radical scavengers. Harman believed that drugs that protected cells against radiation damage should also protect cells against random free-radical damage. After testing a number of the best-known radiation protectant drugs on small rodents, he found that the average life span of a colony of rodents was increased if they were fed a radiation-protectant drug over the course of their lives.

Other scientists rapidly confirmed Harman's findings and extended them to antioxidants, in addition to the radiation drugs. One of the first antioxidants tested in this way was vitamin E, the most important naturally occurring antioxidant. Vitamin E has the role of protecting our cells against damage from radicals.

Scientists rapidly began to discover that when animals were subjected to unusually high oxidative stress, which produces greater-than-normal amounts of free radicals, the antioxidant vitamins markedly protected both against pathological changes and against death. For example, both vitamin E and vitamin C protect animals against ozone, the principal oxidant in smog. In addition, both of these antioxidants protect against damage from cigarette smoke, which contains large numbers of free radicals.

During the 1970s and 1980s, the evidence for protection of animals against oxidative stress by antioxidants became so strong that a number of groups proposed human studies in which the protective effects of antioxidants against life-shortening diseases such as cancer and heart disease would be studied. In the last several years, a number of these studies have been reported in the literature, and almost all of them have shown an impressive protective effect from antioxidant vitamins.

For example, the group at Harvard that is directing the U.S. Nurses Study (of women) and the Allied Health Professional Study (of men) reported that heart disease is reduced by almost half in persons whose diet includes more than 100 International Units (IU) of vitamin E for at least two years. Since this amount of vitamin E cannot be obtained from foods, supplemental vitamin E tablets must be taken.

Antioxidants are thought to protect against heart disease because the fatty deposits in arteries (that cause atherosclerosis) build up when fatty droplets in our blood (called low-density lipoproteins, LDL) become oxidized. The most important antioxidant in LDL that protects it against oxidation is known to be vitamin E. Thus, theory suggests that vitamin E should prevent LDL oxidation, and thus help prevent atherosclerosis; both animal and human data suggest that this theory is correct.

Antioxidant vitamins also should help prevent certain types of cancer. Most chemicals that are carcinogens (i.e., cause cancer) must be oxidized to become active, and antioxidants should help prevent that oxidation. In fact, recently a group at the National Cancer Institute, working with a group of scientists in China, studied a number of populations in that country and found that antioxidant supplements also provide striking protection against a number of types of cancer.

Despite the large number of studies in animals and man that have now been reported, many scientists regard the idea that antioxidants protect humans against heart disease and cancer as a hypothesis that has not yet been conclusively established. However, the evidence is increasing with each passing year, as you will learn when you read this book. It is my belief that studies published in the coming years will increasingly demonstrate the correctness of this idea.

PART ONE

—•—

THE BASICS

Antioxidants! Oxidants! Free radicals! What have we here? Biology and chemistry (biochemistry) have come out of the laboratory, and here they are, front and center, bringing you the knowledge to improve your health. This book will show you how to use this information in the most important way possible—to enhance the quality of your life. Our goal is not only to live longer lives, but also to be healthy enough to enjoy those extra years! This is the place to start.

We need oxygen to live; that is a fact. But as our body uses oxygen, free radicals are produced—and that's bad. Before you finish this book, you will know intimately just what a free radical is and know what to do about it.

Free radicals are also produced in our bodies by environmental insults—from the toxic substances we breathe, smoke, eat and touch. However, free radicals do have some redeeming qualities. Cells in our immune system purposely make free radicals and use them to kill bacteria or viruses—and that's good. But if the free radicals run amok, if they are unchecked, they damage healthy body cells and injure genetic material—and that's bad. We do have natural defenses against free radicals—and that's good. But these defenses, cellular enzymes that we make from nutrients in our diets, often get overwhelmed—and that's bad. But that's where antioxidants, the superstars of nutritional biochemistry, come to the rescue! Here's where vitamins C, E, beta-carotene, selenium, coenzyme-Q and other antioxidants do their job. They prevent or stop free-radical damage. Just how well, you will now learn.

This book will
• Explain just what an antioxidant is, what it is "anti-" to and why it is important for you to know the difference.
• Tell the "free-radical" story. You will learn what these dangerous entities are, where they come from, how they threaten the cells in our bodies and accelerate aging and how to stop the damage they produce.
• Introduce you to the key antioxidants—Vitamin E, Vitamin C, beta-carotene, selenium, pycnogenol, coenzyme Q-10, and the bio-

flavonoids—all in one volume. There is no need to read a dozen different books; all the information is here at your fingertips.

• Tell you what diseases are linked to free-radical destruction, and show you how to prevent these diseases or reduce their effects.

• Explain how antioxidants can prevent or slow down some types of cancers.

• Discuss the studies that prove the benefits of antioxidants and give you a "Who's Who" in antioxidant research.

• Preview the future of antioxidant research—discuss the newly discovered antioxidants and what they will do to improve your life.

If the failed attempt at health care reform has taught us anything, it is that we should do our best to avoid having to use such a chaotic and expensive system. And the best way to be healthy and prevent illness is to learn how to properly nourish and protect your body. This means more than just putting food in your mouth. Your body is ultimately a collection of cells. In order for these cells to work properly, and the organs they comprise to do the same, the cells must get the nutrients they need for fuel and protection.

Antioxidants, as you will see, play a key role as cell protectors. In doing so, they allow the cells to reach the full life span programmed into the DNA (deoxyribonucleic acid), the genetic material. When your cells live longer, so do the organs, and so do you.

Aging is inevitable, but medical problems such as heart disease, stroke and cancer, as well as conditions such as cataracts and senility, are not a part of normal aging. They are a result of deficiencies in the key defense mechanisms of our body. Antioxidants are a major part of that defense—they are the cellular police. We can see that there are enough of these amazing nutrients to ensure the longevity that is rightfully ours.

ANTIOXIDANTS

The Nutrients That Guard the Body Against Cancer,
Heart Disease, Arthritis and Allergies
—and Even Slow the Aging Process

RICHARD A. PASSWATER, PH.D.

FOUR HEALTH GUARDIANS

The major antioxidant nutrients—vitamins A, C and E and the trace mineral selenium—act as a quadruple-threat defense against many of the diseases we dread most, and even have been shown to avert some of the "inevitable" effects of aging. This essay details the fascinating research behind these discoveries, the remarkable clinical results they have led to, the varied ways in which antioxidants work in the body, and, most important, how you can use them to maintain and enhance your most important possession, your health.

THE PROTECTORS

Studies over the last 20 years have shown that a group of nutrients called antioxidants can protect against cancer, heart disease, arthritis, cataracts and allergies, and at the same time slow the aging process. Some of the most important of these nutrients are vitamins A, C and E, and the trace mineral selenium.

We are still learning ways in which these common nutrients protect us from, control or even help us overcome an increasing number of seemingly totally unrelated diseases, and we are beginning to understand the common factors linking them. They are not caused by germs—bacteria or viruses—but by deleterious biochemical reactions with molecular fragments called free radicals. The process that causes these diseases, often considered to be a normal part of the aging process, is called free-radical pathology. The antioxidant nutrients block the deleterious free-radical reactions and thus protect the body.

Antioxidants are compounds that sacrifice themselves to oxygen, thus preventing it from reacting with other compounds. Antioxidant compounds have chemistries that allow them to react readily with oxygen. This ease of reaction enables antioxidant compounds to interact with free-radical generators and quench free-radical production.

The antioxidants do more than protect; they also stimulate the immune response to help fight already existing disease, and they normalize the balance of hormone-like chemicals in the body that control pain, inflammation and fever.

If you did not understand that an antibiotic such as penicillin cured a great number of diseases by destroying the bacteria that cause those diseases, you would find it difficult to believe that one drug could work against so many diseases; it's much the same with antioxidants. So let's take a brief look at the common free radical-initiated diseases: cancer, heart disease, aging, arthritis and cataracts, and then take up the role of the antioxidant nutrients in preventing or controlling those diseases.

WHAT IS A FREE RADICAL?

A free radical is an incomplete molecule, highly reactive because its electron arrangement is out of "spin" balance. Atoms, molecules and ions are more stable entities because they have more balanced electron arrangements. (See Appendix A for more about free radicals.)

The highly reactive free radicals do more damage than does a one molecule-to-one molecule reaction. Each free radical is capable of destroying an enzyme or protein molecule or even an entire cell. The damage is actually much more extensive than that because each free radical usually generates a chain of free-radical reactions, resulting in thousands of free radicals being released to destroy body components. This process is called biological magnification.

Dr. William Pryor of Louisiana State University points out several ways in which free radicals do extensive damage to our bodies. "This biological magnification occurs for two reasons. The first, and most important, is the enormous sensitivity of the cell to modifications in its heredity apparatus such as its DNA. The chromosomes, which control the reproduction of the cell, are extremely radiation-sensitive; the cytoplasm is much less so. Largely because of the sensitivity of DNA, radiation that destroys only one molecule in one million or ten million in the cell can be lethal."

"The second cause of biological magnification is that any polymeric system [one involving large numbers of similar molecules joined together] is sensitive to small chemical changes, and many important biomolecules are polymers."

Free-radical reactions leading to cell membrane damage can cause cancer, heart disease or accelerated aging.

These are five basic types of damage caused by free radicals:

1. Lipid peroxidation, in which free radicals initiate damage to fat compounds in the body, causing them to turn rancid and release more free radicals.
2. Cross-linking, in which free-radical reactions cause proteins and/ or DNA molecules to fuse together.
3. Membrane damage, in which free-radical reactions destroy the integrity of the cell membrane, which in turn interferes with the cell's ability to take in nutrients and expel wastes.
4. Lysosome damage, in which free-radical reactions rupture lysosome (cell digestive particle) membranes; these then spill into the cell and digest critical cell compounds.
5. Accumulation of the age pigment (lipofuscin), which may interfere with cell chemistry.

The most damaging agents of free-radical reactions include the superoxide, hydroxyl and lipid peroxide radicals and hydrogen peroxide.

The body defends itself against these agents with vitamin E (a general antiradical), superoxide dismutase (an enzyme that destroys the superoxide radical), catalase (an enzyme that converts hydrogen peroxide to water) and glutathione peroxidase (a selenium-containing enzyme that deactivates lipid peroxides). Each molecule of glutathione peroxidase contains four atoms of selenium. Thus selenium is a key component of the body's defense against free radicals.

CANCER

It seems that nearly every week we read that scientists have found that yet another widely encountered chemical causes cancer. But there is some good news. A moderate lifestyle and good nutrition are protective against cancer, and it's *not* true that everything causes cancer. In fact, many of the cancer-causing chemicals that we read of aren't worth worrying about. Normally, you won't eat, drink or breathe in enough of them to cause cancer. Yet if you are malnourished, your chances of getting all types of cancer increase.

Some more good news is that several vitamins and minerals have special protective properties.

• **Vitamin A and beta-carotene,** shown for forty years to be effective in treating and preventing cancers of the lung, breast and skin.

• **Vitamin C,** estimated by one researcher to have the potential of cutting the cancer death rate by 75 percent.

• **Vitamin E** combats cancer-causing pollution and works with anti-cancer drugs.

• **Selenium,** the missing mineral—where it is absent, cancer rates soar.

A healthy body can overcome cancer, just as it can ward off cancer. Those who disagree with this statement don't fully understand what a *healthy* body is. As our understanding of nutrition and health has advanced beyond the obvious relationship of vitamin C to scurvy or vitamin B1 and beriberi, there have been many experiments that demonstrate the role of vitamins and minerals in protecting the cells against the agents that cause cancer and in stimulating the immune response to destroy cancers.

Nutritional therapy, which brings the body to its peak of immune response, in no way conflicts with surgery, radiation or chemotherapy.

Cancer is often described as a disease of civilization, but it will strike only when the body's defenses are down or when the cancer-causing agent is abnormally strong and its presence prolonged. Our strategy should be to keep our defenses up and to prevent unnecessary exposure to cancer-causing agents.

We can accomplish this by following a few simple guidelines, and by using common sense and avoiding extremes or fanaticism. The Bible summarized the wisdom thus: "Let your moderation be known unto all men" (Philippians 4:5).

Many scientists believe that cancer occurs only when the body's immune system fails. There is evidence that cells regularly grow wildly, but are detected and destroyed by the immune system.

Defective cells can grow uncontrollably. As long as nutrients are available, these cells will continue to grow and divide irregularly. Normally, antibodies are summoned which surround and isolate the premalignant cells and, with the help of macrophages (large scavenger cells), destroy them. If the body does not detect the premalignant cells as foreign, or cannot produce adequate antibodies, or if the antibodies are blocked before they do their job, then the cells develop their own blood supply and become malignant tissue.

THE IMMUNE SYSTEM AND VITAMIN A

The stimulation of the immune system is receiving increasing interest as a cure for cancer. The immune system is a complicated and poorly understood defense mechanism. It can destroy cancer unless it is weakened by poor nutrition, emotional strain or "blocking factors" formed in advanced cancers.

Researchers first noticed in 1925 that there was a relationship between a deficiency in vitamin A and cancer. Several experiments from the 1930s through the 1950s confirmed this relationship, and since then we have learned that cancer-causing chemicals can react strongly with DNA in vitamin A-deficient cells, that cancers are hard to transplant into animals adequately nourished with vitamin A and that vitamin A is therapeutic in dealing with precancerous cells.

Scientific optimism about the effectiveness of vitamin A increased in 1974. At that time Dr. Frank Chytill of Vanderbilt University remarked, "Recent dramatic findings about vitamin A and its effects on cancer have opened up a whole new approach to cancer therapy. With vitamin A therapy, doctors may some day have a way to restore body cells to normal—rather than destroy them with surgery, chemotherapy or radiation. We now have laboratory evidence that, under certain laboratory conditions, cancers such as breast, lung, and skin tumors can be cured by treatment with vitamin A. . . . People can certainly cut their chances of getting cancer by making sure they are not deficient in vitamin A."

Dr. David Ong, a co-researcher of Dr. Chytill's at Vanderbilt, says: "We know that lack of vitamin A retards normal growth, weakens the mucous linings of the body and causes night blindness. But when the proper level of vitamin A is restored, the body returns to normal. Preliminary evidence from Europe strongly indicates that vitamin A works the same way with cancer."

Dr. George Plotkin of the Massachusetts Institute of Technology adds, "A deficiency of vitamin A prevents a mucous coating from forming on the trachea, lungs, rectum, digestive system and on the inside of the skin. The vitamin A deficiency doesn't cause cancer, but it makes these areas less able to resist cancer."

Dr. Plotkin and his colleague Dr. Paul Newberne reported that giving rats ten times their usual vitamin A intake dramatically slashed their susceptibility to lung cancer.

In one of Dr. Umberto Saffioti's experiments when he was at the Chicago Medical School (he later joined the National Cancer Institute), 113 hamsters were dosed with the cigarette smoke carcinogen benzopyrene. In the 53 control animals not given extra vitamin A protection, 16 developed lung cancer. However, in the 60 vitamin A-treated animals, only one developed lung cancer and four developed benign tumors. Dr. Saffiotti had similar results with carcinogens that cause cancer in the stomach, gastrointestinal tract and uterine cervix.

Dr. E. Bjelke of the Cancer Registry of Norway found that 74 percent of the men with lung cancer were in the lowest third of the population, ranked by vitamin A intake. He also found that vitamin A especially helped smokers living in cities. Vitamin A-deficient city dwellers have three times the lung cancer rate of better nourished city dwellers.

In a December 1977 interview, Dr. Sporn discussed with me the effects of vitamin A deficiency and his tests of more efficient vitamin A derivatives. "If you are vitamin A-deficient, there is no question that you may be more susceptible to development of cancer, but you do not need to take a lot of vitamin A to correct a deficiency. Any sort of multivitamin tablet will alleviate a deficiency state. That includes keeping your mucous membranes and respiratory tract in proper working order.

"I am not recommending that anybody take megadoses of vitamin A, but probably one of the best investments you can make in your food budget is to spend a few cents a day for that multivitamin capsule."

Dr. Sporn pointed out, "Well over half of all human cancer starts in epithelial tissue, the tissue that forms the lining of organs, forms glands such as mammary glands, skin, and passages in the body. The respiratory tract, the digestive tract, the urinary tract and the reproductive tract are all lined with epithelial tissue. And all of the specialized cells that form epithelial tissue depend on vitamin A for their normal development.

"But as far as vitamin A deficiency is concerned, there is work way back in the 1920s by D. S. B. Wolbach of Harvard which suggests a relationship between vitamin A deficiency and cancer. Dr. Wolbach pointed out that there were similarities between the cancerous process and what goes on in tissues that are vitamin A-deficient in terms of loss of control in cell differentiation. The problem that exists in cancer was pointed out over sixty years ago."

There is a debate over how vitamin A and its derivatives control early precancerous stages to prevent the development of cancer.

I asked Dr. Sporn if the retinoids (vitamin A and similar compounds) destroy a precancerous cell or just keep it from spreading.

Dr. Sporn's answer not only sheds light on how vitamin A works, but strengthens the contention that cancer can be prevented or slowed with vitamins.

"We don't have all the answers to that question, so a lot of research is being done in that area now. None of the retinoids, if used appropriately, are cytotoxic [cell-killing] agents. You can kill a cell or a person with too much of anything—even salt or water. But one does not think of salt and water as toxic agents. Similarly, if used in sensible amounts, the retinoids are not toxic agents.

"They are hormone-like controllers of cell differentiation. The approach that we are trying to develop is to use them not to kill cancer cells but to control the differentiation of precancerous cells."

What Dr. Sporn means by cell differentiation is that the cells stay in a mature differentiated state, rather than reverting to the undifferentiated condition that is characteristic of cancer.

Dr. Sporn further explained, "Now whether this actually arrests the process of development of cancer or whether this causes the precancerous cells to disappear from tissue is a topic of current research.

"If all you do is just slow down this process of development of cancer so that instead of the typical twenty-year latent period from the time people may be first exposed to a carcinogen and the time that they develop cancer, you double that latent period, then there would be twenty additional years of good life that you would be offering people.

"Now in terms of modern surgery and chemotherapy, if they get an additional five years of survival, this is considered a very major achievement. So what we are really trying to do is to slow down or prevent the development of malignancy.

"If you slow it down enough, then for practical purposes it never occurs, although the basic process of development of cancer may still be going on, but at a very, very slow rate—such that it really never causes anyone any problems.

"The latent period is like a fire that is smoldering beneath the surface. It gives no symptoms; but, if one goes and looks for precancerous [premalignant] cells, you can find evidence of the chronic disease process. The object of the preventive approach as I see it is to do something about the disease process when it is in this early smoldering stage, before you have the fire. Once you have invasive cancer, then you can't do prevention any more. You have to change your approach.

"It's pretty clear that retinoids have a hormone-like action in controlling cell differentiation. Cancer would appear to be a disease in which the gene material, DNA, has been damaged by chemicals or radiation. Usually the damage will kill the cells, but sometimes the damage leads to cancer.

"Once DNA is damaged, cancer doesn't occur immediately. It can be twenty years after DNA damage occurs before malignancy develops.

"The word retinoid is just a generic word which describes a family of substances. Within this family there are hundreds of different individual compounds. Some of the individual compounds are the naturally-occurring forms of vitamin A such as those we eat in our diet or take in vitamin pills.

"These natural forms of vitamin A are largely stored in the liver and if taken in excess, they can cause very severe liver damage and also cause other undesirable toxic side effects. There have been cases of people who have symptoms resembling brain tumor due to excessive dosages of vitamin A. Some people believe that if some is good, then some more is better. With massive amounts of vitamin A, they can get themselves into rather severe side effects.

"Also," Dr. Sporn points out, "vitamin A does not get into all the body parts in high enough concentrations that we want for effectiveness. If you were worried about the development of bladder cancer and took a large amount of vitamin A, this would be mostly stored in the liver and would not be getting additional vitamin A to your bladder."

THE KEY ANTIOXIDANTS—AN OVERVIEW

BETA-CAROTENE

Dr. Sporn's recent interest has been in the natural nutrient that the body converts into vitamin A and other retinoids. This nutrient is beta-carotene, which is found in carrots and other yellow vegetables, and dark green leafy vegetables. All those vegetables said to contain vitamin A actually have not vitamin A but its precursor, beta-carotene.

The body can split a molecule of beta-carotene in half to form two molecules of vitamin A. But beta-carotene is more than just the precursor of vitamin A. Beta-carotene has its own chemistry independent of its vitamin A chemistry. Thus beta-carotene can give you all the protection of vitamin A and then some. Scientists have found that beta-carotene becomes a unique antioxidant under certain low-pressure conditions in the cell, and it is a quencher of the deleterious form of oxygen called singlet oxygen.

In February 1981, the doctor whose research first linked smoking to lung cancer reported that a diet heavy in carrots reduces the risk of lung cancer. Dr. Richard Doll, president of the British Association for Cancer Research, found that beta-carotene reduced cancer incidence in laboratory animals by 40 percent.

In April 1981, Dr. Eli Seifter of the Albert Einstein College of Medicine reported research with mice showing that beta-carotene could limit or prevent growth of cancer cells. Dr. Seifter found that from two to five times as many mice not given beta-carotene developed cancer when inoculated with breast cancer cells, as did the beta-carotene fed cells. When the mice were given radiation therapy plus beta-carotene, the tumors regressed completely.

SELENIUM

The trace mineral selenium may be an even more powerful protector against cancer. Hundreds of animal tests plus several epidemiological studies provide evidence of selenium's effectiveness and safety. Only a few will be cited here, but many more can be found in my book on the subject, *Selenium as Food and Medicine* (Keats Publishing, 1980).

Dr. Gerhard Schrauzer of the University of California at San Diego found that dietary selenium reduced the incidence of cancer in a strain of mice that normally have an 80–85 percent incidence of breast cancer, due to a virus that they ingest with their mother's milk, to only 10 percent. The eightfold-reduced incidence of cancer in Dr. Schrauzer's study is striking, but it is important to note as well that even among the 10 percent of the selenium-supplemented mice that did develop cancer, the disease did not appear until 50 percent later than among the control animals, the tumors were less malignant and the control animals' survival time was 50 percent longer. In a less cancer-prone strain of mice, the breast cancer might have been totally prevented. Many studies have led to a growing conviction of the importance of selenium in preventing and controlling cancer.

Dr. Schrauzer firmly states: "We now think that if a breast cancer patient has especially low selenium blood levels, her tendency to develop metastases is increased, her possibility for survival is diminished, and her outlook in general is poorer than if she has normal levels. The key to cancer prevention lies in assuring the adequate intake of selenium, as well as of other essential trace elements."

In 1969, Dr. Raymond Shamberger of the Cleveland Clinic and Dr. Doug Frost of Brattleboro, Vermont, noticed an inverse relationship between the incidence of cancer and the amount of selenium in patients' blood samples. Also, the lower the level of selenium in locally grown crops, the higher the incidence of cancer.

Let's look at some of the epidemiological data. Rapid City, South Dakota, has the lowest cancer rate of any city in the United States, according to one survey. The citizens of Rapid City also have the highest measured blood selenium levels in the nation. But in Lima, Ohio, which has twice the cancer rate of Rapid City, the citizens have only 60 percent of the blood selenium levels of those in Rapid City.

In another study, Drs. Shamberger and Willis found healthy persons between the ages of 50 and 71 to average 21.7 micrograms of selenium per 100 milliliters of blood, whereas cancer patients of the same age range averaged only 16.2 micrograms per 100 milliliters. The worst cancer cases had the lowest selenium levels, 13.7, 13.9 and 14.3.

The association between high selenium levels in the diet and a lower-than-average cancer rate was suggested in a paper delivered by Dr. Christine S. Wilson, a nutritionist at the University of California, San Francisco. At the FASEB meeting she told the participants that high selenium levels in the diet may explain why the breast cancer rate is substantially lower in Asian women then in women from Western countries.

After comparing the nutrient content of an average non-Western diet supplying 2500 calories to that of a typical American diet providing the same number of calories, Wilson determined that the Western diets contained about a fourth of the selenium of the Asian diets. She says that it is also significant that the Asian diets contained much less "easily oxidizable" polyunsaturated fats (7.5 to 8.7 grams a day) than the Western diets (10 to 30 grams).

Dr. Wilson hypothesizes that it is the dietary combination of high selenium and low polyunsaturated fatty acids that may be protecting the Asian women against breast cancer. She notes that selenium is a component of the glutathione peroxidase system. Because the enzyme acts to inhibit the oxidation of unsaturated fats, it blocks the formation of peroxides and free radicals, both of which are believed to trigger various forms of cancer. The connection between a low cancer rate and high-selenium diet was reinforced by Shamberger, who says that another Cleveland Clinic survey suggests that high selenium levels appear to be associated with a corresponding decrease in deaths from cancer of the colon.

In Venezuela, the death rate from cancer of the large intestine is 3.06 per 100,000, while in the United States it is 13.69 per 100,000. Venezuela has a high selenium content in its soils compared to U.S. levels. Japan, another high-selenium country, has less breast cancer, as already mentioned, and also has a lower lung cancer death rate—12.65 per 100,000 compared to our 38.86 per 100,000.

There is even stronger evidence that selenium protects against cancer. So far, we have learned that extra selenium has reduced spontaneous cancer in mice and that epidemiological studies associate low selenium levels with high incidence of cancer.

Dr. Shamberger had also shown that painting selenium on the skin of mice near areas that had been painted with the carcinogen DMBA reduced the number of tumors normally obtained with DMBA. The selenium was neither mixed with nor painted on the same spot as the DMBA.

In one series of such nondietary experiments, the incidence of tumors dropped by 43 percent with the nonselenium-treated mice to 17 percent with the selenium-treated mice. A second part of the experiment involved different timing of the selenium application, and the incidence dropped from 89 percent in the controls to 45 percent among the selenium-treated.

In still another nondietary series, this time using the carcinogen MCA instead of DMBA, the incidence dropped from 87 percent in the controls to 68 percent in the selenium-treated mice.

In another series of experiments, the selenium was added in the diet rather than being painted on the skin. This approximates the human experience of environmental exposure to carcinogens being contained by dietary supplementation more nearly than do the painted tests.

Dr. Shamberger tested several timing schedules for beginning the diet supplementation after painting the carcinogen on the skin of the mice. The two-week delay experiment described typical results.

In one experiment testing a selenium-fortified diet against the effects of DMBA-croton oil, 14 of 35 mice on the selenium-fortified diet had tumors after 20 weeks, compared to 26 of 36 mice on the selenium-deficient diet. Those mice on the selenium-fortified diet that did get tumors took longer to develop them.

A similar experiment with the carcinogen benzopyrene showed 31 of 36 mice on a selenium-deficient diet developing cancer, as opposed to only 16 of 36 mice on the selenium-fortified diet.

To more nearly simulate the ingesting of carcinogens in food or water, carcinogens can be added to the diet, and comparisons made between normal diets and selenium-fortified diets. This has been done by Drs. C. G. Clayton and C. A. Baumann with azo dyes, by

Dr. J. R. Harr et al. with the carcinogen FAA (1972), and by myself with DMBA (1969–1972). Dr. Lee Wattenberg has done similar experiments with other antioxidants besides selenium.

My experiments were conducted with several antioxidants used in synergistic combination to provide animal protection at the lowest total dosage of antioxidants possible. The incidence of stomach cancer to be expected in mice given DMBA is 85 to 90 percent. That can be reduced to 5 to 15 percent with mixtures of water- and fat-soluble natural and synthetic antioxidants, including selenium.

In my experiments, the mice were all given the same dose of the carcinogen continually in their diets. Subgroups of the animals were then fed one of three different amounts of antioxidants as a percentage of their total diet throughout their life spans.

Dr. Harr's group fed the animals the FAA continually as a part of their diet, during the entire experiment. Various amounts of selenium were also added to the diet and were thus fed concomitantly with the carcinogen.

They used groups of 20 mice. Group one received 150 parts per million (ppm) FAA and 2.5 ppm added selenium; group two received 150 ppm FAA and 0.5 ppm added selenium; group three received 150 ppm FAA and 0.1 ppm added selenium; and group four received 150 ppm FFA and no added selenium.

After 210 days, 80 percent of groups three and four had cancer, compared to 10 percent of group two and 3 percent of group one. The selenium had a definite protective effect.

At a February 1978 conference on preventing cancer, held at the National Cancer Institute in Bethesda, Maryland, considerable emphasis was given to the role of selenium in preventing cancer. In addition to the updates on the research conducted by Drs. Shamberger and Schrauzer, Dr. A. Clark Griffin, of the M.D. Anderson Hospital and Tumor Institute in Houston, reported that selenium added to drinking water, or selenium fed in the form of high-selenium yeast, can protect rats exposed to three different kinds of cancer-causing chemicals from developing colon and liver cancer. Dr. Griffin's group has also shown that selenium can prevent the conversion of potentially cancer-causing chemicals into other harmful forms. Experiments by Dr. Charles R. Shaw, also of M.D. Anderson Hospital, show that selenium cuts the bowel cancer rate from 87 percent down to 40 percent in animals fed carcinogens.

Many different types of laboratory experiments have been conducted, and they all show that selenium is protective against cancer. Tumor cells injected into animals grow when the animals are selenium-deficient, but do not survive in selenium-fortified animals; these animals are protected against both carcinogen-induced cancer and virus-induced cancer. The research has been examined by many scientists and is considered meaningful.

VITAMIN E

Vitamin E has been shown to help prevent cancers caused by many chemicals in our environment. This is important because scientists estimate that 80 to 95 percent of human cancers are caused by environmental carcinogens.

Vitamin E also appears to lessen the harmful effects of the anti-cancer drug Adriamycin. The drug had limited usage because of its harmful side effects, but in combination with vitamin E, more effective dosages were safely be given to more people.

Additional vitamin E is also required by those who overconsume polyunsaturated oils on many low-cholesterol diets. These oils have been shown to be cofactors in protentiating the effect of other cancer-causing chemicals.

Vitamin E gives us a second chance by stimulating our immune response, which can destroy precancerous cells before they turn into a malignancy.

VITAMIN C

Vitamin C has several modes of action useful for preventing or controlling cancer. It strengthens the body's defenses against cancer by increasing the effectiveness of the immune system that destroys cancer cells, and it makes it more difficult for cancer cells to reproduce and spread by strengthening an intercellular material called "ground substance." Vitamin C also protects us by preventing the formation of cancer-causing chemicals called nitrosamines from nitrites, and directly detoxifies still other carcinogens. Vitamin C also stimulates the production of interferon.

Not many people are familiar with the clinical evidence that caused Dr. Linus Pauling, two-time Nobel laureate, to conclude that "a high intake of vitamin C is beneficial to all patients with cancer."

Drs. Pauling and Ewan Cameron jointly published a report on the beneficial effects of vitamin C on terminal cancer patients in 1976 in the *Proceedings of the National Academy of Science*.

The Cameron-Pauling study compared 100 terminally ill patients given 10 grams (10,000 milligrams) of vitamin C per day to 1000 other such patients. Both groups were treated identically in all ways— by the same physicians in the same hospital—except one was not given the vitamin C.

At the time the study report was prepared, those patients given vitamin C had lived more than four times longer than the matched "control" patients. The patient survival rate continued to improve long after the report was published.

Sixteen of the 100 in the vitamin C group lived more than a year as opposed to only three of the 1000 patients not given vitamin C.

These patients, now apparently healthy, were once considered terminal. The progress of their disease was such that in the considered opinion of at least two independent physicians, the continuance of any conventional form of treatment would offer no further benefit.

At the time of the 1976 report, 13 vitamin C-treated colon cancer patients had lived more than seven times as long as the 130 matched control patients, with improved quality of life and lessened pain.

The 1976 report also indicated that the vitamin C-treated breast cancer patients lived six times longer than their matched control group, and vitamin C-treated kidney cancer patients lived five times longer.

Drs. Cameron and Pauling also noted that survival time was increased by a factor of at least 20 for some 10 percent of the patients.

This caused them to wonder what the results would be if treatment were started earlier and if larger amounts of vitamin C were used.

In 1983, the Mayo Clinic ran a similar test on cancer patients who had had chemotherapy and reported no benefit from the use of vitamin C. Dr. Pauling has since explained to them that vitamin C could not work in those cases because the drugs had destroyed the patients' immune systems. Mayo repeated the test, using patients not given the drugs, again with negative results. However, the patients received vitamin C for only a short time while Dr. Cameron's patients continued the vitamin.

When asked how many lives could be saved with the use of vitamin C in cancer treatment, Dr. Pauling replied, "In 1971 when I first suggested that vitamin C might be of use against cancer, I estimated that it might save 10 percent of the people who die of cancer. The reason that I was saying that was, although there are some very good arguments why vitamin C might be effective, there was very little direct evidence. There was only some epidemiological evidence at that point. Now 10 percent is 36,000 Americans a year, kept from dying of cancer. That's about a hundred a day. Today I'm around to saying that with proper use of vitamin C for cancer, we could cut the death rate by 75 percent. This would be 75 percent of 360,000 people who die every year of cancer. These are people whose lives could have been extended with the use of vitamin C."

Why did Dr. Cameron try vitamin C? What indications did Dr. Pauling have that vitamin C would help cancer survival?

In 1951 it was established that cancer patients have lower than average amounts of vitamin C in their blood plasma and white blood corpuscles; therefore, their weakened immune systems can't destroy cancer cells.

In 1948, epidemiologists Drs. A. C. Chope and Lester Breslow interviewed 577 older residents of San Mateo Country, California. When they followed up the interviews eight years later, they found the death rate for those with the highest amounts of dietary vitamin C was less than half (40 percent) of those getting lesser amounts of vitamin C. This was true for the cancer death rate as well.

Irwin Stone reported that German physicians W. G. Deucher

(1940), Von Wendt (1949) and L. Huber (1953) used 1 and 2 gram doses of vitamin C (with and without vitamin A) with good results.

Stone also reported that in 1954 Dr. W. J. McCormick found that "the degree of malignancy is determined inversely by the degree of connective tissue resistance which in turn is dependent upon the adequacy of vitamin C status."

Earlier, in 1948, Drs. Goth and Littman found that "cancers most frequently originate in organs whose vitamin C levels are below 4.5 mg percent and rarely grow in organs containing vitamin C above this concentration."

In 1966, Dr. Cameron had published his book *Hyaluronidase and Cancer* (Pergamon Press, 1966) outlining his views that strengthening the intercellular ground substance (the material that holds tissue cells together and is often called cellular cement) would prevent infiltration of cancer cells. He had noticed that cancer cells produced an enzyme, hyaluronidase, that attacked this intercellular cement and allowed the cancer to invade surrounding tissues.

In 1971 Dr. Cameron read of Dr. Pauling's comments that vitamin C increased the rate of collagen production, which strengthened the intercellular cement. This stimulated Dr. Cameron to begin cautious treatment of cancer patients with vitamin C, and the two researchers joined on some projects. One of Dr. Cameron's first observations was that vitamin C reduced the patients' pain and improved their sense of well-being, appetite and mental alertness. Patients who had been receiving large doses of morphine or diamorphine no longer needed the painkilling drugs.

In 1973, the Norwegian Cancer Registry's researcher, Dr. Bjelke, surveyed 30,000 people and found that the greater the intake of vitamin C, the smaller the incidence of cancer—as Drs. Chope and Breslow had found in 1948.

In 1969, Dr. Dean Burk of the National Cancer Institute found that vitamin C caused changes in cultures of cancer cells that destroyed them while being harmless to normal cells. Dr. Burk concluded, "The future of effective cancer chemotherapy will not rest on the use of host-toxic compounds now so widely employed, but upon virtually host-nontoxic compounds that are lethal to cancer cells, of which vitamin C represents an excellent prototype example."

Later that year, Dr. J. U. Schlegel of the Tulane University School of Medicine showed that bladder cancer due to smoking could be prevented by vitamin C.

In response to questions about the Cameron-Pauling report, Dr. Paul Chretien, Chief of Tumor Immunology in the Surgical branch of the National Cancer Institute, said, "It is possible they did arrest the progress of tumor growth with massive doses of vitamin C. National Cancer Institute research has shown that vitamin C given to healthy patients stimulates the body's defense system and this usually means an increased immune response."

The immune system defends the body against bacteria, viruses and other foreign invaders, as well as misformed materials in the body. It quickly recognizes, attacks and destroys all foreign bodies that can do harm.

Lymphocytes are a particular variety of white blood cell that typically make up 25 to 30 percent of all white blood cells. Some lymphocytes are made in the thymus, a small gland in the neck and upper part of the chest behind the breastbone, but they are primarily made in the bone marrow. After their formation, lymphocytes are transported to the lymph nodes and spleen for lifetime storage to be used when needed. Major lymph nodes are under the arms, in the groin, behind the ears, and in the abdominal cavity and a few other places. These white blood cells are released in response to infection.

But even before the supply of lymphocytes is released in the body to fight infection, the available lymphocytes react immediately to any threat by releasing proteins called antibodies. After antibodies attack the invader, larger cells called macrophages are summoned to "chew up" the invader. Both antibodies and lymphocytes are released in response to the presence of cancerous cells.

Dr. Chretien's comment on the immune system referred to research he conducted with his NCI colleague Dr. T. F. Tehniger and Dr. Robert Yonemoto, Director of Surgical Laboratories at the City of Hope National Medical Center in Duarte, California. The researchers were looking for a solution to a perplexing problem of cancer surgery.

Immediately after the surgical removal of malignant tumors, the immune system is very weak. Often cancer cells spill into the bloodstream during surgery, and when the immune response is weak the spilled cancer cells spread secondary cancers—metastases—throughout the body.

The group published a study in 1976 showing that 5 grams of vitamin C daily increased the production of lymphocytes when the body was threatened by a foreign substance, and that 10 grams daily produced an even greater effect. Cancer patients have a poor capacity for making new lymphocytes, yet their ability to survive relates strongly to their lymphocyte production.

The study subjects were healthy volunteers, and the researchers are now studying cancer patients to see if the same results can be observed.

All studies discussed so far have been with people. Preliminary cancer research is normally carried out with laboratory animals such as rats and mice, but there is a great difference with respect to vitamin C between humans and most animals. Most animals make their own vitamin C or at least make most of what they need. Man, primates, guinea pigs and a few other animals cannot produce vitamin C because of the lack of a required enzyme, believed to be caused by a genetic abnormality developed during evolution.

The guinea pig is a suitable experimental animal for vitamin C research, but not much is known about cancer in guinea pigs, although Dr. George Feigen, professor of physiology at Stanford University, in studying the effects of vitamin C on their immune systems, has observed a large increase in the production of one of the components of the immune response.

Previously, researchers at the Bowman Gray School of Medicine in Winston-Salem, North Carolina, reported that vitamin C activated the immune response. At the June 1971 meeting of the American Society of Biological Chemists in San Francisco, Drs. Lawrence R. DeChatelet, Charles E. McCall and M. Robert Cooper reported that adding vitamin C to test-tube mixtures of white cells and bacteria stimulated increased activity of the white blood cells. Without the added vitamin C, the cells can engulf the bacteria, but they cannot break them down.

All these reports illustrate the fact that vitamin C boosts immunity, which is the body's most important line of defense against cancer.

In 1983, Dr. Bernard Kennes of the Université Libre de Bruxelles in Belgium, reported that the immune system of elderly persons could be significantly enhanced with 500 milligrams of vitamin C daily. In *Gerontology* (29:305–310, 1983) he concludes, "vitamin C should be considered as a possible successful, nontoxic and inexpensive substance that improves the immune competence of the aging."

ANTIOXIDANT COMBINATIONS ARE BETTER

Combinations of antioxidants provide better protection than might be expected when considering each antioxidant individually; the effect is synergistic, an example of the whole being greater than the sum of its parts. In my experiments I found that combinations of vitamins A, C and E plus the trace mineral selenium were more effective than larger amounts of the individual antioxidant nutrients. This observation was the basis of several worldwide patents that I applied for in the early 1970s. This research and much more about the role of antioxidants against cancer, along with the evidence, is described in my book *Cancer and Its Nutritional Therapies* (Keats Publishing, 1978, 1983).

The importance of the antioxidant nutrients has recently been recognized by the National Cancer Institute and the American Cancer Society. Studies are now under way to explore further the roles of selenium and beta-carotene in countering cancer in humans.

WHAT IS AGING?

The American Medical Association's Committee on Aging has studied the problem of human aging for more than three decades. The committee has so far not found one physical or mental condition that can be directly attributed simply to the passage of time. Some of the alleged diseases of aging—such as high blood pressure and arthritis—are prevalent in the very young as well as the very old. What exactly *is* aging, then, and what are its causes?

Aging can be described as the process that reduces the number of healthy cells in the body. Although we have noted the increase of some enzymes in the body and the decrease of others, the most striking factor in the aging process is the body's loss of reserve due to the decreasing amount of cells in each organ. For example, fasting blood glucose levels remain fairly constant throughout life, but the glucose tolerance measurement, which measures the reserve capacity of this system to respond to the stress of the glucose load, shows a loss of response with aging. The same holds true concerning the recovery mechanisms of other parameters.

Cellular aging actually begins before birth and is the one factor underlying the aging process of the entire body. The stability of the living system becomes progressively impaired by chemical reactions, not the passage of time.

If we can control the rate of these deleterious reactions, then we can control the advance of physiological aging.

Free-radical reactions, discussed earlier, result in the loss of active cells. The cumulative effect of billions of cellular free-radical reactions is to add to the body's loss of reserve. Again, that is what the aging process is—the loss of reserve function.

Not only are antioxidant nutrients protective against cancer, they can slow the aging process or at least slow its acceleration. This is not to suggest that antioxidants will rejuvenate you. It means that they will help protect you against the damage that adds signs of aging to your body.

My experiments have shown that certain combinations of antioxidant nutrients can extend the average life span of laboratory animals by 20 to 30 percent, and the maximum life span by 5 to 10 percent. In experiments in which laboratory conditions were designed to accelerate the aging process, the antioxidants increased the life spans of the animals by as much as 175 percent.

Other researchers such as Dr. Denham Harman of the University of Nebraska School of Medicine, England's Dr. Alex Comfort and Dr. Al Tappel of the University of California at Davis have found that individual antioxidant nutrients produce significant lifespan increases, though less than that of the synergistic combinations.

ANTIOXIDANTS AND DISEASE

HEART DISEASE

Antioxidant nutrients help prevent heart disease by protecting the arteries against the damage that leads to the cholesterol deposits called plaque, but the risk of heart attacks is more significantly decreased by the nutrients' ability to keep fatal blood clots from forming in the coronary arteries.

Let's consider both these roles of the antioxidant nutrients. Dr. Earl Benditt of the University of Washington discovered that the cholesterol-containing plaque in the lining of arteries actually begins as a mutated muscle cell in the middle layer of the artery.

In my view, the mutation described by Dr. Benditt is caused by free radicals. My research centers on free radicals and their involvement in accelerating aging and initiating cancer and heart disease. Dr. Benditt's observations explain the link between free-radical production and heart disease found in experiments.

The overall process in plaque formation then is as follows: The initial plaque formed is due to a mutation of a cell in the artery wall. Certain chemicals in the bloodstream, including pollutants, smoke components and free radicals, cause a normal smooth muscle cell in the arterial walls to go haywire (mutate).

The cell that mutated because of the reactive chemicals reproduced itself (proliferates) precisely. All derived cells are exact replicas (monoclonal) and form a growth differing from normal artery tissue. This growth, the first step in plaque formation, has been missed by other researchers.

The plaque now develops in stages. In stage one, the proliferating smooth muscle cells spread through the artery wall, causing the production of extracellular substances including collagen (a structural protein) and glycosaminoglycans (carbohydrates).

Monoclonal proliferation continues at a fast rate until cell crowding results. At this stage, cholesterol is manufactured by the crowded cell as a result of cellular injury from the overcrowding of monoclonal cells. This second stage produces the uncomplicated plaque that for a century has been wrongly considered characteristic of the first stage.

The third stage is a complication of the second stage; in it, the fibrous mass protrudes through the arterial wall where it comes into contact with the flowing blood; calcium and additional cholesterol from the bloodstream can now add to the fibrous plaque. This third stage is independent of blood cholesterol level, but may be related to the concentration of low-density lipoprotein (LDL) in the blood.

In 1974, Swedish researcher, Dr. K. Korsan-Bengsten, of the medical department of the Sahlgrens Hospital in Göteborg, reported that vitamin E returns abnormal platelets to normal.

Brown University researchers Drs. Manfred Steiner and John Anastasi reported in the *Journal of Clinical Investigation* (March 1976) that platelet adhesion was reduced as the dosage of tocopherol was increased to a level of 1800 International Units (IU). In the men and women tested, platelet adhesion was lowered by as much as 50 percent.

The mechanism by which vitamin E normalized blood platelets to reduce their stickiness involves the production of prostaglandin X. Prostaglandins are hormone-like compounds that control many body functions (sometimes banefully, as with arthritis). Prostaglandin X is manufactured in the artery linings and converts damaged platelets back to normal. Vitamin E increases prostaglandin X production, while the peroxidized polyunsaturated fats inhibit it (Moncade et al., *Lancet*, 1977).

The action of vitamin E in keeping blood free-flowing so that coronaries are reduced explains why vitamin E lowers the incidence of heart disease in long-term users. In *Supernutrition for Healthy Hearts* (1977) I report the results of my study of 17,894 people showing that the amount of heart disease in any age group decreased proportionally with the length of time the participants took vitamin E.

Two groups in the survey well illustrate this point. One group consisted of those who had taken 400 IU or more of vitamin E daily for ten years or more. The study included 2508 such people between the ages of 50 and 98. Based on Department of Health, Education and Welfare figures (HRS 74-1222, 1976), normally 836 of the 2508 would be expected to have heart disease. Instead there were only four. This is less than 2 percent of the expected number.

A second group of 1038 had taken 1200 IU or more of vitamin E daily for four years or more. In this group (differing slightly from the first in age-group composition), normally there would be 323 suffering from heart disease rather than the seven actually found.

Vitamin E has been found to greatly increase the beneficial blood component high-density lipoprotein (HDL). We owe this most important discovery to the alertness of Dr. W. J. Hermann of Memorial City General Hospital in Houston.

Dr. Hermann found that his HDL ratio increased from 9 percent to 40 percent after taking 600 IU of vitamin E for one month. Realizing the importance of this observation, he recruited ten volunteers for a clinical trial to see if the incredible improvement was a general response to vitamin E.

Five of the volunteers had normal HDL levels prior to taking vitamin E and five had low HDL levels. Thirty days of taking 600 IU of vitamin E brought about significant improvement in HDL levels in both groups. Those having normal HDL levels averaged a 50 percent improvement, while those with low HDL levels averaged a whopping 200 percent increase.

The results were published by Dr. Hermann and his colleagues, Drs. K. Ward and J. Faucett, in the *American Journal of Clinical Pathology* in late 1979.

Drs. Evan and Wilfrid Shute taught for 30 years that vitamin E was helpful to those with heart disease because it was anti-clotting, improved oxygen utilization, controlled the patch-scar that replaces damaged heart tissue, and improved capillary permeability. Some physicians found similar results in their practices; others did not. Perhaps those that did not have success with vitamin E did not use it long enough for the platelet normalization effect to occur. The new findings about prostaglandin X and platelets should end the confusion.

However, pounds of vitamin E will not protect you if you are deficient in other nutrients or fail to follow the ideal lifestyle of moderation. The antioxidant mineral selenium is required as a partner for vitamin E. Reasonable amounts of vitamin E for those seeking protection are 400 IU daily and up to 800 IU daily for control. Reasonable recommendations for selenium are 50 micrograms daily for protection and 100 mcg daily for control. These are only general recommendations. Because of the individual variations in diet, lifestyle and genetic background, the optimum level will differ for each individual. Several nutrients help control blood pressure. Selenium and vitamin E are especially important. A selenium deficiency causes a harmful compound to build up in the blood that increases blood pressure. Selenium is involved in the production of several prostaglandins which regulate blood pressure. When there is a selenium deficiency, a critical enzyme that contains selenium is not produced, and as a result an intermediate compound in the production of prostaglandin accumulates. When this intermediate compound is in excess, blood pressure is increased.

ARTHRITIS

The pain, swelling and inflammation of arthritis are also caused by free radicals. Human studies in Great Britain have found that approximately 80 percent of arthritis sufferers found significant relief from pain and reduced swelling and inflammation by taking the combination of antioxidant nutrients, vitamins A, C, and E, plus the trace mineral selenium. This study was undertaken when the head of a British arthritis group noticed that his arthritis symptoms disappeared after he had been taking the antioxidants for a time for another reason. The placebo effect can be discounted because the person was not taking the antioxidant nutrients in an effort to control his arthritis.

One hundred other members of the British Arthritic Association were asked to try the antioxidant nutrients, and after initial success, a larger study involving 418 members was undertaken.

In Israel, a double-blind crossover study in which 600 milligrams of vitamin E or placebo were given for ten days to osteoarthritis patients found that more than 50 percent of the patients had significant relief from pain during the vitamin E period compared to only 4 percent during the placebo period.

At the May 1980 meeting of selenium researchers, Norwegian scientists reported the beneficial results of selenium in arthritis patients. The researchers found that the rheumatoid arthritis patients had lower-than-normal levels of selenium in their blood. Supplementation with selenium and vitamin E brought about significant reduction in symptoms.

Another physician at this conference, Dr. E. Crary of Smyrna, Georgia, had also treated patients having traumatic arthritis with selenium and the vitamins A, C and E, successfully relieving the pain in their traumatized joints.

These favorable results could have been predicted from the knowledge that the free-radical scavenger superoxide dismutase has been proven highly successful against arthritis. In tissues, free radicals generate superoxide radicals and lipoperoxides that promote the release of the deleterious prostaglandins that cause pain, inflammation, and swelling. Selenium (in the enzyme glutathione peroxidase) protects against this damage, as do other antioxidants. In addition, vitamin E directly decreases the output of the deleterious postaglandins.

The anti-inflammatory action of selenium has been widely accepted in animal treatment. Injectable and oral veterinary formulations of vitamin E and selenium have been used for years. Several such preparations are FDA-approved for symptomatic relief of arthritic inflammation in dogs. Topical vitamin E has been shown to have anti-inflammatory action in rats and rabbits.

CATARACTS

Recent research has linked antioxidant deficiencies to cataract development. The antioxidants normally protect the sensitive proteins in the eye lens. When there isn't sufficient antioxidant protection, the proteins can oxidize in the lens, causing it to cloud and scatter light.

Antioxidant levels in a cataracted lens are a fraction of those in a healthy lens. Several researchers have found that they can slow or halt the growth of cataracts by having their patients take supplements of the antioxidant nutrients, thus normalizing the antioxidant levels of the lens.

Dr. Alex Duarte of the Cataract Control Center in Huntington
Beach, California, has written a book describing the role of free radicals in the production of cataracts and how the antioxidant nutrients
are protective. His book *Cataract Breakthrough* (International Institute
of Natural Health Sciences, Inc. P.O. Box 5550, Huntington Beach,
California) also describes the treatment for the cure of cataracts.

ALLERGIES

Chemical hypersensitivities are often caused by free-radical reactions. Some seemingly inert chemicals can be converted into potent
free-radical generators by the actions of body enzymes as they metabolize the foreign chemicals in an attempt to remove them from the
body. Many people who are allergic (sensitive) to various chemicals
have found that their allergies disappeared soon after taking antioxidant nutrients for some other reason such as protection against cancer
or heart disease.

Dr. Stephen A. Levine of the Allergy Research Group in Pleasant
Hill, California, is one such individual. He suffered considerably until
he started taking antioxidants in 1980. Now he has studied the mechanisms fully and has published his clinical observations in the *Journal
of Orthomolecular Psychiatry* and the *Allergy Research Review.*

HOW MUCH?

The amount of each antioxidant required for protection against the
various free-radical pathologies varies from individual to individual
and with the total nutrition and lifestyle of the individual. The first
consideration is whether a deficiency does exist. The following table
lists the Recommended Dietary Allowance (to determine deficiency)
and a safe and effective range to consider for therapeutic supplementation.

Nutrient Range	RDA	Supplementation
Vitamin A	5,000 IU (RE)	5,000–25,000 IU
Beta-carotene	(included in the above for vitamin A)	10,000–20,000 IU
Vitamin C	60 mg.	500–2,000 mg
Vitamin E	15 IU	50–600 IU
Selenium	50–200 mcg	100–200 mcg

BIBLIOGRAPHY

Hailey, Herbert. *E, the Essential Vitamin*. New York: Bantam Books, 1983.

Cameron, Ewan and Linus Pauling. *Cancer and Vitamin C*. New York: Warner Books, 1981.

Hoffer, Abram and Morton Walker. *Orthomolecular Nutrition*. New Canaan, Conn.: Keats Publishing, 1978.

Kugler, Hans. *Seven Keys to a Longer Life*. Briarcliff Manor, N.Y.: Stein & Day, 1978.

Passwater, Richard A. *Cancer and Its Nutritional Therapies*. New Canaan, Conn.: Keats Publishing, 1983.

———. *EPA—Marine Lipids*. New Canaan, Conn.: Keats Publishing, 1982.

———. *Selenium as Food and Medicine*. New Canaan, Conn.: Keats Publishing, 1980.

———. *Supernutrition for Healthy Hearts*. New York: Dial Press, 1977.

Pryor, W. *Free Radicals*. New York: McGraw-Hill Publishing Co., 1966.

Spallholz, Martin and Ganther, eds. *Selenium in Biology and Medicine*. Westport, Conn.: AVI Press, 1981.

World Conference on Antioxidants Shows Many Preventive Functions

Beta-Carotene Fights Lung Cancer; Cell Fats, Fluids Protected by Vitamins E, C

At the three-day conference on Antioxidants Vitamins and Beta-Carotene in Disease Prevention held in London, England in the fall of 1989, 36 scientists from around the world discussed the roles of vitamin C, vitamin E and beta-carotene (provitamin A) in preventing a variety of degenerative diseases. The meeting was sponsored by the World Health Organization, the British Nutrition Foundation and other institutions.

Scientists from the United States, the United Kingdom, France, Germany, Italy, Switzerland, Canada, Austria, Finland, Japan and South Africa described the protective role of the antioxidants, which block or retard cell damage from the oxidative reactions that are a normal part of metabolism.

GOING RANCID

Oxidative damage produces highly reactive fragments of molecules—free radicals—which roam at will inside the body. These unstable compounds react with fats in cell membranes and destroy them through peroxidation, which is a process similar to what turns butter rancid. This damage is thought to contribute to such degenerative conditions as cancer, heart disease, cataracts, rheumatoid arthritis, Parkinson's disease and aging.

The brain and nervous system are rich in lipids, so that the nervous system is especially vulnerable to free-radical attack. Vitamin E, a fat-soluble vitamin, acts as a free-radical scavenger and protects the fats in cell membranes. Vitamin C, which is water-soluble, serves a similar function in cellular fluids.

George W. Comstock, Ph.D., of the Johns Hopkins University, Baltimore, Maryland, discussed a new analysis of data from a Maryland study in which, in 1974, some 26,000 people donated blood samples for a blood bank. The samples were stored at -70°. until they could be analyzed for nutrients, hormones, antibodies, etc.

When a sufficient number of cancers of various types were reported to a cancer registry, blood from the volunteers who had developed cancer was withdrawn from the bank, along with blood from matched controls. The data showed a strong inverse association between the amount of beta-carotene in the blood and the risk of squamous-cell carcinoma of the lung, as well as an association between low levels of vitamin E and lung cancer.

CAROTENOIDS AND CANCER

In both prospective and retrospective epidemiologic studies, low dietary intake of fruits and vegetables (carotenoids) is associated with an increased risk of lung cancer, according to Regina G. Ziegler, Ph.D., M.P.H., of the National Cancer Institute, Bethesda, Maryland. Diet does not necessarily eliminate the risk of lung cancer attributable to smoking, she said, but the levels of carotenoid intake characteristic of about 30 percent of a typical community may be sufficient for a noticeable reduction—25 to 55 percent—in lung cancer risk.

MAJOR ANTIOXIDANTS
AND SOME DISEASES
THEY FIGHT

VITAMIN C
High Blood Pressure

VITAMIN E
Lung Cancer, Heart Disease

CAROTENOIDS
Lung Cancer, Cataracts

"Since preformed vitamin A (retinol), found in animal foods, is not related in a similar manner to lung cancer risk, beta-carotene appears to function through a mechanism that does not require its conversion to vitamin A," Dr. Ziegler explained.

There is evidence of a possible protective role for vitamin E in various cancers which affect women, Paul Knekt, Ph.D., of the Social Insurance

Institution, Helsinki, Finland, told the conference. Analysis of stored blood samples from cancer patients and controls revealed that women with the lowest levels of vitamin E in their blood had 1.6 times the risk of cancer of those with higher levels. Women with low levels of vitamin E and selenium, the mineral that is also an antioxidant, had 10 times the breast cancer risk.

Vitamin C is useful in lowering blood pressure, according to two intervention studies by David Trout, Ph.D., of the U.S. Department of Agriculture, Beltsville, Maryland, and Eunsook Koh, Ph.D., and Odutola Osileski, Ph.D., of the Alcorn State University, Lorman, Mississippi. In a placebo-controlled, double-blind study involving 20 female volunteers with moderately high blood pressure, one gram (1000 mg) of vitamin C daily for six weeks reduced systolic (beating) and pulse pressure but not diastolic (resting) pressure.

C AND BLOOD PRESSURE

Dr. Trout reported that, in the Kuopio Heart Disease Risk Factor Study of 1984–1986 in Finland, there was a clear inverse association between vitamin C and blood pressure. The study involved 722 men, all 54 years old. The volunteers with higher blood levels of vitamin C had lower disastolic and systolic blood pressure. An inverse correlation was also found with selenium, which led investigators to conclude that the antioxidants play a significant role in the development of hypertension.

"Plasma ascorbic acid has also been associated with other factors that correlate with blood pressure, such as smoking, blood levels of selenium, and intakes of potassium," Dr. Trout continued. "However, the connection between blood pressure and vitamin C persists after controlling for all the other variables."

Low-density lipoprotein cholesterol (LDL), which is most often associated with an increased risk for heart disease, may become potentially harmful only after it is no longer protected by vitamin E, according to Hermann Esterbauer, Ph.D., of the University of Graz, Austria. In test-tube experiments, he was able to show that LDL cholesterol attacked by free radicals rapidly loses its antioxidants, with vitamin E depleted first.

This supposition was confirmed by Professor J.C. Fruchart of the Pasteur Institute, Paris, France, who reported the biochemical changes in LDL that occur as it becomes oxidized.

"A high inverse correlation was found between the age-specific mortality from ischemic heart disease and plasma vitamin E," said K. Friedrich Gey, M.D., of the University of Bern, Switzerland.

PARKINSONISM DELAYED

Vitamins C and E possibly can reduce the severity, and delay the progression of symptoms of Parkinson's disease. Stanley Fahn, M.D., director of Parkinsonism and Movement Disorder Research at Columbia University's College of Physicians and Surgeons, New York, pointed out.

"Beginning in June 1979, I recommended to all Parkinson's disease patients who were not yet receiving levodopa therapy [a drug], that they take high doses of vitamins E and C at 3200 IU and 3000 mg per daily, respectively. Of the patients I have followed continuously, those taking the vitamins went two and a half years longer before needing levodopa to treat their symptoms, compared to patients followed elsewhere without antioxidants."

Dr. Fahn suggested that the two vitamins may slow the progression of Parkinson's disease by inactivating the free radicals which normal cause some degeneration of nerve cells in the brain.

Ronald Anderson, M.D., of the University of Pretoria, South Africa, told the meeting that cigarette smoke damages the lungs by inducing a flood of white blood cells (phagocytes) into the lungs. This initiates extensive free-radical production, which results in inflammation, tissue injury and probably the initiation of cancer. In his study, smokers who were supplemented with beta-carotene showed a gradual, cumulative inhibition of free-radical production to 30 percent after six weeks.

"It appears that supplementation with high levels of vitamin E and beta-carotene may regulate the production of toxic radicals, at least in the short term," Dr. Anderson noted.

Several researchers reported that preliminary evidence suggests that antioxidants can jump-start the immune system, prevent the development and/or cause regression of premalignant lesions and perhaps even retard aging.

ANTIOXIDANTS MAY SLOW AGING

"Oxidation may be a major cause of cell and tissue aging, no matter where it occurs in the body," said Richard G. Cutler, Ph.D., of the Gerontology Research Center, National Institute of Aging, Baltimore, Maryland. "We are in the exciting process of finding out where and to what degree antioxidants might be able to intervene. With more of our population living longer, it is critical that we find preventive techniques such as dietary alterations that will keep us healthier throughout our lifespan."

Since cataracts are caused in part by oxidation of the lens of the eye, several scientists have theorized that antioxidants may prevent this oxidative damage and thus forestall the development of cataracts.

Paul F. Jacques, Sc.D., of the USDA Human Nutrition Center at Tufts University, Boston, Massachusetts, reviewed the data from a study of 112 volunteers, aged 40 to 70. Seventy-seven of the people had cataracts, while the remaining 35, cataract free, served as controls.

Dr. Jacques reported that people with the lowest carotenoid levels had a seven-fold increase in risk of cataracts compared to those with high levels of carotenoids. And those with the lowest vitamin C levels were at 11 times the increased risk for the disorder.

A study by James McD. Robertson, D.V.M., M.Sc., of the University of Western Ontario, Canada, indicated that those who took only vitamin E supplements had an average 56 percent decrease in cataract risk when compared with nonsupplement users, and those who took only vitamin C had a 70 percent decrease in risk compared with nonsupplement takers.

With such strong evidence in favor of the antioxidants, it seems prudent to increase our intake of fruits and vegetables, as well as vitamin C, vitamin E, beta-carotene and selenium.

JOHN MITCHELL

Antioxidants Are Crucial for Heart Health; They Protect Against Stroke, Heart Attack

The Vitamins C, A, E and Beta-Carotene Can Also Help Protect Smokers and Even Guard Against Cancer, Cataracts, Viruses

The consumption of antioxidants such as beta-carotene, vitamin A and vitamin E reduces the risk of stroke by 40 percent in women and heart attack by 22 percent, according to JoAnn Manson, M.D., of Harvard University, Cambridge, Mass. The study, which was reported at the annual meeting of the American Heart Association in Anaheim, Calif., involved 87,245 nurses ranging in age from 34 to 59, reported the December 12, 1991 issue of *Medical Tribune.*

Women who consumed over 15 mg of beta-carotene, which is provitamin A, were offered protection against heart attack and stroke, when compared to controls who ingested only 6 mg daily, Dr. Manson said. This protection was provided by a daily one-quarter cup serving of carrots, spinach, sweet potatoes, apricots, etc., she added.

LESSENED CORONARY RISK

"Dr. Manson reported that women who took 100 mg supplements of vitamin E—three times the recommended daily allowance—lowered heart attack risks by 36 percent," *Medical Tribune* said. "Compared with women who had the lowest consumption of vitamins, the relative risks of coronary heart disease for those with the highest consumption were 0.78 for beta-carotene, 0.66 for vitamin E and 0.70 for vitamin A."

Those who are at risk for coronary heart disease or have a history of chest pain (angina) might benefit from diets rich in beta-carotene, vitamin C, vitamin E and other antioxidants, according to papers read at a symposium, "Antioxidant Vitamins: Good News for Healthy Hearts," held in May 1991 in New York. The conference was sponsored by the Vitamin Nutrition Information Service, of Nutley, New Jersey.

Michael F. Oliver, M.D., of the Wynn Institute, London, England, studied 110 angina patients and found that they had low levels of beta-carotene, vitamin C and vitamin E. He reported that the relative risk of developing angina was 2.7 times higher at the lowest plasma concentrations of vitamin E when compared to the highest readings.

Another speaker, Donald Mickle, M.D., of Toronto General Hospital in Canada, said that the antioxidants may be more important in the treatment of heart disease, and he presented evidence that vitamin E, regarded as the only membrane-soluble antioxidant, helped prevent or minimize the damage to heart tissues during bypass surgery and other medical procedures.

"When the heart is deprived of oxygen, then resupplied with oxygen-rich blood, a high concentration of damaging compounds called oxygen-free radicals is released, which overwhelm the tissues' defense system and cause severe damage," Dr. Mickle said. "Vitamin E is an excellent scavenger of free-radicals and thus mitigates some of this damage."

In three separate studies vitamin C seems to minimize certain cardiovascular risks associated with high blood pressure, elevated blood cholesterol and cigarette smoking, the conference was told.

"The risk reduction associated with vitamin C is of great potential significance, since it affects all three of the major risk factors for heart disease," said David Kritchevsky, Ph.D., associate director of the Wistar Institute of Anatomy and Biology in Philadelphia, Pennsylvania, chairman of the conference.

VITAMIN C IS VITAL

At the USDA Human Nutrition Research Center on Aging at Tufts University in Boston, Paul F. Jacques, Ph.D., and his colleagues have found that diet is believed to play an important role in the increase in blood pressure as we age. Sodium, potassium, calcium, magnesium, fatty acids and alcohol consumption have long been associated with fluctuations in blood pressure, and now vitamin C has been added to the list.

"Observational studies consistently demonstrate decreasing blood pressure with increasing blood levels of vitamin C," Dr. Jacques told in the meeting. "Systolic [beating] and diastolic [resting] blood pressure levels are approximately 5 to 10 percent lower in subjects with high vitamin C, vitamin A, beta-carotene and selenium. However, our studies have indicated that smokers have significantly depressed blood and white blood cell levels of vitamin C and depressed plasma levels of total carotenes vitamin A, compared to nonsmokers. Plasma vitamin E and selenium levels were not significantly different."

At another international seminar, "Vitamin E in Modern Medicine," held on October 16, 1991, in La Grange, Illinois, researchers from around the world reported on the benefits of vitamin E in stimulating the immune system of senior citizens, and in dealing with hardening of the arteries, diabetes, arthritis, acute pancreatitis, wound healing, and epilepsy.

C VERSUS VIRUSES

In the August 1991 issue of *Current Eye Research*, Allen Taylor, M.D., of the USDA Human Nutrition Research Center on Aging at Tufts University in Boston, and his colleagues have found that vitamin C helps protect against cataracts. They reported that higher intakes of this antioxidant vitamin provide higher levels in the eyes' lenses, where cataracts form, and in the fluid that nourishes the lens.

Vitamin C attacks viruses, such as HIV, the AIDS virus, and it offers protection against many types of cancer, heart disease, arthritis, and many other health conditions, according to Sandra Goodman, Ph.D. in *Vitamin C: The Master Nutrient* (Keats Publishing, Inc., New Canaan, Conn.).

Scientific literature is brimming over with evidence that many of us may need to increase the antioxidants in our diet and supplement programs

---

Since the scientific literature is brimming over with evidence that many of us may need to increase the antioxidants in our diet and supplement programs, it would make sense to pay attention to these important nutrients.

SHELBY TYSON

How Antioxidant Nutrients Form First Line of Cancer Defense

It seems that nearly every week we read that scientists have found that yet another widely encountered chemical causes cancer. But there is some good news. A moderate lifestyle and good nutrition are protective against cancer, and it's *not* true that everything causes cancer. In fact, many of the cancer-causing chemicals that we read of aren't worth worrying about. Normally, you won't eat, drink or breathe in enough of them to cause cancer. Yet if you are malnourished, your chances of getting all types of cancer increase.

Some more good news is that several vitamins and minerals have special protective properties.

• *Vitamin A and beta-carotene*, shown for forty years to be effective in treating and preventing cancers of the lung, breast and skin.

• *Vitamin C*, estimated by one researcher to have the potential of cutting the cancer death rate by 75 percent.

• *Vitamin E* combats cancer-causing pollution and works with anti-cancer drugs.

• *Selenium*, the missing mineral—where it is absent, cancer rates soar.

THE ANTIOXIDANTS

Studies over the last 20 years have shown that a group of nutrients called antioxidants can protect against cancer, heart disease, arthritis, cataracts and allergies, and at the same time slow the aging process. Some of the most important of these nutrients are vitamins A, C and E, and the trace mineral selenium.

We are still learning ways in which these common nutrients protect us from, control or even help us overcome an increasing number of seemingly totally unrelated diseases, and we are beginning to understand the common factors linking them. They are not caused by germs—bacteria or viruses— but by deleterious biochemical reactions with molecular fragments called free radicals. The process that causes these diseases, often considered to be a normal part of the aging process, is called free-radical pathology. The antioxidant nutrients block the deleterious free-radical reactions and thus protect the body.

Antioxidants are compounds that sacrifice themselves to oxygen, thus preventing it from reacting with other compounds. Antioxidant compounds have chemistries that allow them to react readily with oxygen. This ease of reaction enables antioxidant compounds to interact with free-radical generators and quench free-radical production.

The antioxidants do more than protect; they also stimulate the immune response to help fight already existing disease, and they normalize the balance of hormone-like chemicals in the body that control pain, inflammation and fever.

THE A TEAM

The stimulation of the immune system is receiving increasing interest as a cure for cancer. The immune system is a complicated and poorly understood defense mechanism. It can destroy cancer unless it is weakened by poor nutrition, emotional strain or "blocking factors" formed in advanced cancers.

Researchers first noticed in 1925 that there was a relationship between a deficiency in vitamin A and cancer. Several experiments from the 1930s through the 1950s confirmed this relationship, and since then we have learned that cancer-causing chemicals can react strongly with DNA and vitamin A-deficient cells, that cancers are hard to transplant into animals adequately nourished with vitamin A, and that vitamin A is therapeutic in dealing with precancerous cells.

Researchers for the Cancer Registry of Norway found that 74 percent of the men with lung cancer were in the lowest third of the population, ranked by vitamin A intake. They also found that vitamin A especially helped smokers living in cities. Vitamin A-deficient city dwellers have three times the lung cancer rate of better-nourished city dwellers. Major research interest has recently developed in the natural nutrient that the body converts into vitamin A and other retinoids. This nutrient is beta-carotene, which is found in carrots and other yellow vegetables, and dark green leafy vegetables. All those vegetables said to contain vitamin A actually have not vitamin A but its precursor, beta-carotene.

The body can split a molecule of beta-carotene in half to form two molecules of vitamin A. But beta-carotene is more than just a precursor of vitamin A. Beta-carotene has its own chemistry independent of its vitamin A chemistry. Thus beta-carotene can give you all the protection of vitamin A and then some. Scientists have found that beta-carotene becomes a unique antioxidant under certain low-pressure conditions in the cell, and it is a quencher of the deleterious form of oxygen called singlet oxygen.

In February 1981 the doctor whose research first linked smoking to lung cancer reported that a diet heavy in carrots reduces the risk of lung cancer. Dr. Richard Doll, president of the British Association for Cancer Research, found that beta-carotene reduced cancer incidence in laboratory animals by 40 percent.

SELENIUM'S PROTECTIVE ROLE

The trace mineral selenium may be an even more powerful protector against cancer. Hundreds of animal tests plus several epidemiological studies provide evidence of selenium's effectiveness and safety. Only a few will be cited here, but many more can be found in my book on the subject, *Selenium as Food & Medicine* (Keats Publishing, 1980).

Let's look at some of the epidemiological data. Rapid City, South Dakota, has the lowest cancer rate of any city in the United States, according to one survey. The citizens of Rapid City also have the highest measured blood selenium levels in the nation. But in Lima, Ohio, which has twice the cancer rate of Rapid City, the citizens have only 60 percent of the blood selenium levels of those in Rapid City.

In another study, it was found that healthy persons between the ages of 50 and 71 averaged 21.7 micrograms of selenium per 100 milliliters of blood, whereas cancer patients of the same age range averaged only 16.2 micrograms per 100 milliliters. The worst cancer cases had the lowest selenium levels, 13.7, 13.9 and 14.3.

The association between high selenium levels in the diet and a lower-than-average cancer rate was suggested in a paper delivered by Dr. Christine S. Wilson, a nutritionist at the University of California, San Francisco. She told a meeting of scientists that high selenium levels in the diet may explain why the breast cancer rate is substantially lower in Asian women than in women from Western countries.

Vitamin E has been shown to help prevent cancers caused by many chemicals in our environment. This is important because scientists estimate that 80 to 95 percent of human cancers are caused by environmental carcinogens.

Vitamin E also appears to lessen the harmful effects of the anti-cancer drug Adriamycin. The drug had limited usage because of its harmful side effects, but in combination with vitamin E, more effective dosages were safely given to more people.

C FOR CANCER CONTROL

Vitamin C has several modes of action useful for preventing or controlling cancer. It strengthens the body's defenses against cancer by increasing the effectiveness of the immune system that destroys cancer cells, and makes it more difficult for cancer cells to reproduce and spread by strengthening an intercellular material called "ground substance." Vitamin C also protects us by preventing the formation of cancer-causing chemicals called nitrosamines from nitrites, and directly detoxifies still other carcinogens. Vitamin C also stimulates the production of interferon.

Linus Pauling and Ewan Cameron jointly published a report on the beneficial effects of vitamin C on terminal cancer patients in 1976 in the *Proceedings of the National Academy of Science*. The Cameron-Pauling study compared 100 terminally ill patients given 10 grams (10,000 milligrams) of vitamin C per day to 1000 other such patients. Both groups were treated identically in all ways—by the same physicians in the same hospital—except one was not given the vitamin C.

At the time the study report was prepared, those patients given vitamin C had lived more than four times longer than the matched "control" patients. The patient survival rate continued to improve long after the report was published.

Sixteen of the 100 in the vitamin C group lived more than a year as opposed to only three of the 1000 patients not given vitamin C.

These patients, now apparently healthy, were once considered terminal. The progress of their disease was such that in the considered opinion of at least two independent physicians, the continuance of any conventional form of treatment would offer no further benefit.

At the time of the 1976 report, 13 vitamin C-treated colon cancer patients had lived more than seven times as long as the 130 matched control patients, with improved quality of life and lessened pain.

When asked how many lives could be saved with the use of vitamin C in cancer treatment, Dr. Pauling replied, "In 1971 when I first suggested that vitamin C might be used against cancer, I estimated that it might save 10 percent of the people who die of cancer. The reason that I was saying that was, although there are some very good arguments why vitamin C might be effective, there was very little direct evidence. There was only some epidemiological evidence at that point. Now 10 percent is 36,000 Americans a year, kept from dying of cancer. That's about a hundred a day. Today I'm around to saying that with proper use of vitamin C for cancer, we could cut the death rate by 75 percent. This would be 75 percent of 360,000 people who die every year of cancer. These are people whose lives could have been extended with the use of vitamin C."

Though this article has dealt with cancer, I want to emphasize that the antioxidants' protective effect against the ravages of free radicals is also significant in other degenerative diseases, from arthritis to cataracts, and in many symptoms of aging. Making sure of an adequate intake—in general, substantially more than the officially recommended amounts, which are pegged to prevention of outright deficiency diseases—of these nutrients is one of the most effective forms of health insurance you can take out.

RICHARD A. PASSWATER, PH.D.

PART TWO

—◆—

THE KEY ANTIOXIDANTS

BETA-CAROTENE

The Backstage Nutrient Now Universally
Recognized for Cancer Prevention

RICHARD A. PASSWATER, PH.D.

THE ELUSIVE FACTOR

For years, beta-carotene was looked on only as one of a number of sources of vitamin A—and as the substance that made carrots and sweet potatoes yellow. Now it has been established that this disregarded vitamin precursor has unique health benefits of its own, protecting the individual from many harmful conditions, possibly including cancer—and may be used in almost any amount with complete freedom from toxic effects associated with excess vitamin A. This chapter presents the background, preventive-health effects and best sources of this remarkable natural nutrient.

Much excitement has been generated among nutritionists and health care professionals by a substance called beta-carotene, because of the extensive evidence that it appears to reduce the risk of contracting cancer. Many studies have strongly indicated that a dietary deficiency of beta-carotene greatly increases susceptibility to cancer. Not long ago, few people had ever heard of beta-carotene. Even nutritionists didn't pay much attention to it, thinking of it merely as a precursor of vitamin A—that is, one of a group of substances which is converted to vitamin A in the body. Beta-carotene was discussed, if at all, in conjunction with vitamin A, as if the two were interchangeable. Recent discoveries of the important differences between the vitamin and

its precursor have changed the thinking—and even the research inter-
ests and strategies—involving beta-carotene.

Yes—beta-carotene can become vitamin A, but it can do more than
that, and do it more safely. The safety feature makes beta-carotene pref-
erable to vitamin A for cancer prevention, but it has other advantages
as well. Beta-carotene reaches more areas of the body for longer periods of time than vitamin A, and thus offers greater protection. Another advantage is that it protects against a toxic form of oxygen
produced in our bodies called "singlet oxygen." Both of these characteristics will be discussed later in this chapter.

Decades of research linking a deficiency in beta-carotene or vitamin A with increased risk of cancer have been acknowledged by the
National Academy of Sciences and the National Cancer Institute, and
there are several large-scale clinical studies now under way or planned
to begin in the near future that will scientifically test the ability of
beta-carotene to prevent cancer. I propose to examine the role of
beta-carotene in health and nutrition, particularly its anti-cancer
properties. Topics to be discussed include basic facts about beta-
carotene, the recommended daily amounts to include in your diet,
sources, safety, comparisons with vitamin A, the evidence that beta-
carotene prevents cancer and the clinical studies now being conducted of its protective effect.

BETA-CAROTENE AND VITAMIN A

Beta-carotene is a yellowish compound found in most yellow, orange
or dark green vegetables; it is converted in the body into vitamin A.
In 1928, Dr. B. von Euler discovered that beta-carotene was the
precursor or pro-vitamin for the "real" or active form of vitamin A.
Beta-carotene is one of a family of similar compounds called carotenoids. Other carotenoids—such as alpha-carotene, gamma-carotene,
and cryptoxanthin—occur naturally in these same foods but do not
produce nearly as much vitamin A. You will sometimes see the carotenoids referred to as α-carotene (alpha), β-carotene (beta) and γ-

carotene (gamma), as chemists have the custom of using the Greek letters for this purpose.

The reason that beta-carotene is such an efficient producer of vitamin A is that the body splits a molecule of it exactly in half to produce two molecules of vitamin A. The other carotenoids yield at most only one molecule of vitamin A, and not all carotenoids can be converted to vitamin A because of differences in chemical structure.

Beta-carotene is converted into vitamin A in the body by the enzyme beta-carotene-15,15'-dioxygenase. An enzyme is a compound that helps reactions occur without entering into the reaction itself— a reusable catalyst that controls a reaction. When vitamin A levels in the body fall, more dioxygenase is produced to increase the conversion of beta-carotene into vitamin A. When vitamin A levels in the body are restored, the amount of dioxygenase is diminished. Excess beta-carotene does not produce vitamin A toxicity, because no more of it is converted to vitamin A than the body requires at the moment. Excess vitamin A in the bloodstream (as from animal sources or excessive supplementation) is eventually stored in the liver, with potential toxic effects.

The conversion of beta-carotene into vitamin A occurs in two known sites in the body, the mucosa of the small intestine and the liver. The intestines do most of this conversion during the absorption process, while the liver converts circulating beta-carotene. The enzyme exists also in the kidneys and perhaps in other tissues. (Another mechanism exists in the body that nonenzymatically converts beta-carotene into vitamin A in a five-step process.)

Some individuals appear to have reduced ability to convert beta-carotene into vitamin A, and genetic differences and chronic conditions such as diabetes or thyroid disease may impair the conversion.

Beta-carotene not converted into vitamin A during absorption is stored until needed. The principal storage site for beta-carotene is fat tissue, but significant quantities circulate in the blood and are present in fatty areas of all cells. An excess of beta-carotene—which, as I mentioned, is not harmful—can be recognized by a yellowish cast to the skin, especially in the palms of the hands, resulting from its storage in fat just beneath the skin.

There in fact are two vitamin A's. Vitamin A-1, retinol, is produced from beta-carotene by most animals including humans. Freshwater fish produce a slightly different form called vitamin A-2 or 3-dehydroretinol, which is only about 40 percent as active as vitamin A-1.

There are several chemical forms, or vitamers, of vitamin A-1. The body converts beta-carotene into retinol, which is the alcohol form. New vitamers are being identified all the time. There are only a few vitamers for most vitamins; vitamin B-6, for example, has six known vitamers at this writing. However, vitamin A has over one hundred vitamers.

Vitamers of vitamin A include the carotenoid and retinoid families of compounds. Significant vitamers of the retinoid family other than retinol include retinal (vitamin A aldehyde), retinoic acid (vitamin A acid), vitamin A acetate, and vitamin A palmitate.

All forms of vitamin A have vitamin A activity and should be considered essentially the same. The differences in activity of the various vitamers are compensated for by describing the "vitamin A" content in standard units of activity.

Thus 5,000 International Units of vitamin A palmitate designates the same vitamin A activity as 5,000 International Units of vitamin A-2 or retinol—even though the quantity required to produce that activity will be different for each vitamer. Vitamin A units will be discussed later.

Vitamin A is required for the normal differentiation and maintenance of the epithelial cells, which form the tissues of the outer layer of skin and mucous membranes that line the mouth and other cavities, including the digestive, respiratory and genitourinary tracts. This function is of special interest in view of research indicating that adequate amounts of vitamin A maintain cell normality in the presence of chemicals that have the capability of mutating normal cells into cancerous ones. The mucous membranes are barriers against invasion by bacteria, viruses and carcinogens. Impairment of their structure and function by a vitamin A deficiency lowers resistance to diseases of all types.

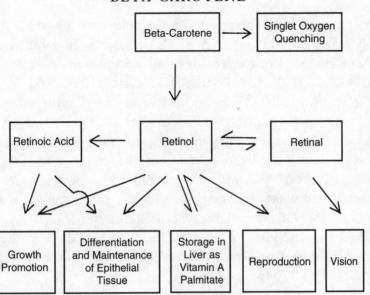

**THE VARIOUS FORMS OF VITAMIN A AND
THEIR BIOLOGICAL ROLES**

Vitamin A also functions to protect the thymus gland from atrophy and to maintain night vision. It is required for ribonucleic acid (RNA) and protein synthesis and is thus essential for growth. Vitamin A is an antioxidant which helps protect cell membranes against undesirable oxidation, and also has significant antiradical activity which helps quell many undesirable reactions. It is required for adrenal cortex function and steroid hormone synthesis, gluconeogenesis, mucopolysaccharide synthesis, bone development and maintenance of myelin and membranes. Vitamin A deficiency signs are discussed later.

CANCER: 50 YEARS OF RESEARCH

Although there have been numerous reports on it both in the mass media and in professional journals, the research linking a beta-carotene or vitamin A deficiency with cancer was not taken very seriously by the majority of medical practitioners until the National Academy of Sciences' 1982 report, "Diet and Cancer."

Evidence had been presented in the scientific literature for more than 60 years, but was ignored by all but a few. In 1928, Drs. Erdmann and Haagen concluded that the lack of vitamin A was an important factor in the development of cancer (reported in *Ger. J. Cancer Res.* 1928). Dr. Y. Fujimaki had reported earlier that laboratory animals on a vitamin A-deficient diet were more susceptible to cancer than animals receiving the recommended amounts of vitamin A (*J. of Cancer Res.*, 1926). At about the same time, Dr. D.S.B. Wolbach of Harvard pointed out the similarities between the cancerous process and what goes on in tissues that are vitamin A-deficient in terms of loss of control in cell differentiation (*J. Exp. Med* 42, 753-778, 1925 and *Arch. Pathol.* 5, 239, 1928). Clues to the role of vitamin A in preventing metaplastic changes in epithelial cells were reported by Dr. S. Mori in 1922.

Drs. A. Goerner and M. Goerner reported in 1939 on the relationship between a vitamin A deficiency and increased incidence of cancer (*J. Biological Chem.*, 1939). Other investigators soon confirmed this relationship (P. G. Seeger, *Arch. Exptl. Zellforsch.* 24, 59, 1940; C. P. Rhoads et al., *Trans. Assoc. Amer. Physicians* 56, 173, 1941; R. W. Swick and C. A. Baumann. *Cancer Research* 11, 948, 1951; and J. C. Radice and S. Kaplan, *Semana Med.* 114, 432, 1959).

A deficiency of vitamin A was shown to make animals more susceptible to carcinogens (cancer-causing agents) as early as 1944 by Nobel prize-winner E. v. Euler of Sweden (E. v. Euler et. al., *Arkiv Kemi, Mineral Geol.* 17A, 29, 1949).

Vitamin A was shown to potentiate cancer drugs such as Urethan as early as 1948 (E. Morelli and G. Misler, *Farm. Sci. e Tec.* [Pavia] 3, 307, 1948).

A study of the relationship of vitamin A in protecting against experimentally induced cancer was published in 1959 (N. H. Rowe and R. J. Corlin, *J. Dental Research* 38:72-83, 1959; N. H. Rowe et al., *Cancer* 26, 436–444, 1970). The researchers studied oral cancer in hamsters given chemicals known to produce oral cancers. Five groups of hamsters were given different levels of vitamin A supplementation, but the same level of carcinogen. The cancer incidence was greatest in the least supplemented groups. The investigators concluded:

"These data suggest that vitamin A deficiency increased the susceptibility of hamsters to carcinogen-induced benign and malignant tumors."

Besides affording protection against carcinogen-induced oral cancer, vitamin A was shown in 1963 to cure and prevent leukoplakia— whitish warty patches in the mouth which may become cancerous (J. E. Johnson et al., *Arch. Dermatology* 88:607, 1963). In the same year, Dr. I. Lasnitzki showed that vitamin A prevented cell changes normally induced by chemical carcinogens.

In 1965, vitamin A palmitate—the salt of a saturated fatty acid, palmitic acid—was shown to reduce greatly the number of cancers in various epithelial tissues (surface cells of skin and mucous membranes) of hamsters caused by a carcinogen (E. W. Chu and R. A. Malmgren, *Cancer Res.* 25:884–895, 1965) and to reduce the number of cancers in the trachea and bronchi caused by a different carcinogen (U. Saffiotti et al., *Cancer* 20:857–864, 1967). Vitamin A palmitate also reduced skin cancer incidence in mice given a carcinogen (R. E. Davies, *Cancer Res.* 27:237–241, 1967).

In one of Dr. Umberto Saffiotti's experiments at the Chicago Medical School (he later joined the National Cancer Institute), 113 hamsters were dosed with the cigarette smoke carcinogen benzopyrene. In the 53 control animals not given extra vitamin A protection, 16 developed lung cancer. However, in the 60 vitamin A-treated animals, only one developed lung cancer and four developed benign tumors. Dr. Saffiotti had similar results with carcinogens that cause cancer in the stomach, gastrointestinal tract and uterine cervix.

Vitamin A was shown to have a therapeutic effect on premalignant lesions (W. Bollag, *Intern. J. Vitamin Res.* 40:299–313, 1970).

Thus vitamin A has been shown in animal studies to be protective against some carcinogens whether a deficiency exists or not, and to have a therapeutic effect on precancerous cells. It has not been demonstrated to be effective in any fully developed invasive cancer.

Dr. Raymond Shamberger of the Cleveland Clinic performed a series of animal tests which led him to conclude that "Vitamin A retards the growth and inhibits the induction of benign and malignant tumors." (*J. Nat. Cancer Inst.*, September 1971). In several series of tests, Dr. Shamberger painted carcinogens on the skins of mice. When vitamin A was added to the carcinogen, the tumor incidence was reduced by up to 76 percent.

In 1974, Drs. Donald Hill and Tzu-Wen Shih postulated that vitamin A acts as a specific antioxidant and inhibits the intermediate compound ordinarily formed in the body from the carcinogen. Thus the carcinogen is inactivated (*Cancer Res.* 34, 564-570, 1974).

Drs. Martin H. Cohen and Paul Carbone found that the protentiating effect of vitamin A (up to 100-fold) that had been reported for several antitumor drugs extended to the modern drug BCNU as well (*J. Nat. Cancer Inst.* 48:921–926, 1972).

Drs. Martin Zisblatt, Eli Seifter and their colleagues at the Albert Einstein College of Medicine in New York found that vitamin A was protective even in mice that develop tumors when injected with viral tumor extract. Typically, 40 to 50 percent tumor reduction was obtained with vitamin A supplementation.

When cancers were transplanted to other mice, vitamin A acetate inhibited the "taking" of the cancer transplant (M. T. Cone and P. Nettesheim, *J. Nat. Cancer Inst.* 50, 1599–1606, 1973).

The survival time for mice inoculated with a million breast tumor cells increased by 50 to 70 percent with vitamin A. In animals inoculated with ten thousand cells, 50 percent normally develop cancer, but only 10 percent of the mice on vitamin A therapy developed tumors (M. Bricklin, *Prevention* 46, November 1975).

Scientific interest was sparked by these results and a conference sponsored by the National Cancer Institute (NCI) and Hoffman-LaRoche, Inc. was held in Bethesda, Maryland, in November 1974.

The interest in the conference was sufficient to warrant a full report in *Science* by T. H. Maugh (*Science* 186:4170, 1198, 1974). At the conference, Drs. Michael Sporn and David Kaufman of NCI discussed their work showing that carcinogens bind much more tightly to DNA from vitamin A-deficient animals, thus possibly increasing the odds of the vitamin A-deficient animal developing cancer. Dr. Kaufman also demonstrated that when vitamin A is administered at the same time as carcinogens, the carcinogens are inhibited from binding to DNA.

Colon cancer was observed to be greater in vitamin A-deficient rats exposed to a carcinogen by Drs. Paul Newberne and Adrianne Rogers of the Massachusetts Institute of Technology. They also reported that giving rats ten times their usual vitamin A intake dramatically slashed their susceptibility to lung cancer.

Vitamin A was reported to reverse the effects of carcinogens in tissue cultures from the prostates of mice by Dr. Dharam Chopra of the Southern Research Institute in Birmingham. His colleague, Dr. Donald Hill, informed the conference that vitamin A prevents the carcinogen benzopyrene from being converted in the liver to its damaging epoxide form.

The incidence of lung tumors in rats fed a carcinogen was reduced by vitamin A, according to Dr. Paul Nettesheim of the Oak Ridge National Laboratory.

Even more encouraging, Dr. Curtis Port of the Illinois Institute of Technology reported that vitamin A, given after exposure to carcinogens, inhibited the formation of lung cancer.

Confirmation that the transplant of cancer from one animal to another is virtually impossible if the second animal has adequate vitamin A levels was made by Hoffman-La Roche's Dr. Richard Swarm (T. H. Maugh, *Science* 186:4170,1198, 1974).

Also in 1974, Dr. Eli Seifter suggested to the National Cancer Institute that beta-carotene should be tested as a cancer preventive. In the following year, Dr. E. Bjelke of the Cancer Registry of Norway published his five-year study involving 8278 male smokers. Dr. Bjelke found that 74 percent of the men with lung cancer were in the lowest one-third of the group according to vitamin A intake. He also found that vitamin A especially helped smokers living in cities. Vitamin A-deficient city dwellers had three times the lung cancer rate of those with adequate vitamin A levels (E. Bjelke, *Internat. J. Cancer* 15, 1975).

In 1976, Dr. Alex Sakula of Redhill General Hospital in Surrey, England, observed that blood levels of vitamin A were lower than normal in all of his 28 bronchial cancer patients (*Brit. Med. J.*, July 31, 1976).

Dr. Bernard P. Lane of the State University of New York at Stony

Brook exposed tissues from 200 tracheae (windpipes) to a carcinogen for three weeks. The precancerous changes caused by the carcinogen were reversed with vitamin A treatment (*Proc. Amer. Assoc. for Cancer Res.*, March 1976).

In 1978, I summarized this half-century of evidence in my book *Cancer and Its Nutritional Therapies*, which was updated in 1983.

An editorial in the March 15, 1980, issue of the prestigious British medical journal *Lancet* remarked, "Several studies indicate that low intake or subnormal plasma content of vitamin A may be associated with an increased incidence of squamous carcinomas of the lung and oral cavity. . . . We must take seriously the notion that low vitamin A intake makes people susceptible to cancer."

Later that year, Dr. Nicholas Wald and his colleagues reported a prospective clinical study of vitamin A levels and cancer incidence in 16,000 men aged 35 to 64. Since 1975, there had been seven retrospective studies confirming the protective role of vitamin A, but this was the first prospective study attempted.

Dr. Wald and his colleagues reported that the average vitamin A level in the blood for subjects with all types of cancer—210 IU/dl— was significantly lower than in those subjects without cancer (231 IU/ dl). The difference was greatest for subjects with lung cancer (183 IU/dl). The researchers reported the risk of cancer at any site for men with retinol levels in the lowest quintile (fifth) was 2.2 times that for men in the highest quintile. The risk was independent of age, smoking habits and cholesterol levels (*Lancet*, October 18, 1980).

In 1981, a major change occurred in cancer research. The medical establishment accidentally found out for itself that there was a link between certain vitamin deficiencies and cancer risk. This delayed discovery is an example of the NIH syndrome (no, not the "National Institutes of Health" but "Not Invented Here"). The earlier research by vitamin-oriented biochemists and a few pioneer epidemiologists that had resulted in more than 325 published articles had been ignored—or perhaps those in other specialties had not even known they existed—but in 1981, important members of the cancer research establishment—and even the heart disease establishment—accidentally confirmed the vitamin A deficiency-increased risk of cancer link.

In February 1981 the doctor whose research first linked smoking to lung cancer reported to a conference of an antismoking group that a diet heavy in carrots might help reduce the risk of cancer. Sir Richard Doll, president of the British Association for Cancer Research, told the members of ASH that his latest research indicated that there is a connection between reduced cancer risk and beta-carotene intake. Laboratory experiments had shown that animals given beta-carotene had a 40 percent lower risk of contracting cancer than animals without carrots in their diets.

"I believe there is now a light at the end of the tunnel in our fight against this disease," Doll concluded. "All we can say at this stage is that current evidence suggests there is a 40 percent lower risk of cancer occurring among men who maintain above average consumption of vitamin A."

Doll, knighted and awarded the UN Prize for Cancer Research in 1962 for his earlier work linking smoking to lung cancer, cautioned that his conclusions were still tentative: "At the moment, our evidence remains a matter for further research. There is nothing proven as yet."

Shortly thereafter, a well-thought-out and well-written review article, co-authored by Drs. Doll, R. Petro, J. Buckley, and Michael Sporn, was published in *Nature*. Dr. Sporn, of the National Cancer Institute, had been an advocate of chemoprevention using retinoid (Petro et al., *Nature* 290, 201–208, March 19, 1981). This review is invaluable both for gaining information about beta-carotene and for understanding the scientific thought process.

It also called for researchers who had large numbers of stored blood samples or vitamin A analyses of patients' blood to consider matching them up with death certificates and cancer registries to gain further information on the relationship. The authors argued that many factors *could* account for the study conclusions linking reduced cancer risk with increased amounts of vitamin A or beta-carotene consumption, but pointed out that the inverse association between dietary beta-carotene and cancer incidence might just as well be due to a genuine protective effect of beta-carotene against the onset of cancer. More compelling evidence might take decades to emerge without controlled trials. Thus, the authors elegantly note, the perfect may well be the enemy of the relevant. Progress towards important preventive measures might be more rapid if, in addition to fundamental research, researchers take reasonably seriously the inevitably inconclusive leads provided by epidemiologists and vice versa. The authors hoped that their view provided enough detail to encourage large randomized clinical trials. As we will see later, it helped to do just that.

Dr. Petro remarked later that many of the studies he and his coworkers examined seemed to be designed for more general purposes, and yielded the link between beta-carotene and reduced risk of cancer almost by accident.

At about the same time as this review article appeared, Dr. B. Modan and his Israeli colleagues published an interesting study in the *International Journal of Cancer* (28, 421–424, 1981). They analyzed the diets of 406 patients with gastrointestinal cancer and 812 controls and found a highly significant correlation between the consumption of beta-carotene-containing foods and decreased risk of cancer.

In April 1981, Dr. Eli Seifter of the Albert Einstein College of Medicine brought scientists attending the annual meeting of the Federation of American Societies for Experimental Biology up to date on his continuing prevention. (Remember, it was Dr. Seifter who in 1974 tried to get the National Cancer Institute interested in testing beta-carotene.)

Dr. Seifter reported that he and his colleagues found through experiments with mice that beta-carotene could limit or prevent the growth of transplanted cancer cells in the animals, prolong life span even after a large number of cancer cells were present and increase the effectiveness of chemotherapy and radiation treatment.

Researchers in Dr. Seifter's laboratory had been studying the antitumor actions of vitamin A for more than 15 years. They said they found that supplementary vitamin A slowed the growth of a certain type of breast tumor in mice given tumor cell transplants and inhibited the growth of tumors in mice inoculated with a tumor-promoting virus.

However, after other scientists expressed concern about the possible toxicity of vitamin A, Dr. Seifter and his co-workers decided to test the relatively nontoxic beta-carotene. Experiments showed that from two to five times as many mice not given beta-carotene developed tumors when inoculated with breast tumor cells as did the beta-carotene-fed animals. The tumors that did develop in the beta-carotene-fed mice grew more slowly and the animals lived longer than their counterparts. All the mice developed tumors when they were inoculated with many more tumor cells, but it took longer for the tumors to show up in the beta-carotene-fed animals, the tumors grew more slowly and the animals' survival time was increased. When tumors were well established in the mice before feeding beta-carotene, the beta-carotene-fed animals lived longer with or without chemotherapy and radiation treatment.

Dr. Seifter said that their most exciting result occurred when mice were given radiation therapy along with carotene feeding. All of the tumors in these animals regressed *completely* with no evidence of regrowth for two months. Only one had tumor regrowth and died during the first year. In a second year of experimentation, the animals were divided into two groups, one group receiving the supplement (either vitamin A or beta-carotene, depending on the experiment), while the other did not receive the supplement. The groups that continued to receive the vitamin A or beta-carotene did not redevelop their tumors and lived their normal two-year life span. In those previously on vitamin A but discontinued, five out of six redeveloped their tumors in 66 days. Only two of the six previously on beta-carotene redeveloped their tumors, and then only after 204 days.

Dr. Seifter emphasized that beta-carotene was very effective in preventing both tumor growth and regrowth and enhanced the action of chemotherapy and radiation treatment.

Later in 1981, a study was reported in the *Proceedings of the American Association for Cancer Research* by researchers at the Wisconsin Cancer Center in Madison, showing that chemotherapy was least effective in patients with the lowest vitamin A levels in their blood. More (83 percent) of those with higher vitamin A levels improved with chemotherapy than those with low levels (36 percent). None of the patients with the higher vitamin A levels worsened, but 40 percent in the low-vitamin A group did so.

The study that had the most impact on contemporary medicine was that published in *Lancet* (8257, 1185–1189, November 18, 1981). The impact was largely due to the prestige and "press relationships" of the research team leaders, Dr. Richard B. Shekelle of Chicago's Rush-Presbyterian-St. Luke's Medical Center and Dr. Jeremiah Stamler of the Northwestern University School of Medicine.

The researchers responded to the request made earlier in the year by Dr. Petro and his colleagues. They were able to do this study because they had assessed the dietary intake of both carotenoids and retinoids in a large group of Western Electric employees at the start of the study in 1957, after one year, and after 19 years. Having followed a group of 1954 middle-aged men for such a long period, they were able to show that a below-average intake of beta-carotene *preceded* the development of cancer and that low blood levels of vitamin A were therefore not a consequence of cancer.

At a press conference following the publication of the article. Dr. Shekelle said, "We were able to show, particularly among men who had smoked cigarettes for a number of years, that men with low levels of beta-carotene had higher risks than the ones with high levels of beta-carotene in the diet."

Of particular interest is his remark, "The men who had relatively high levels of beta-carotene in the diet had a risk of lung cancer that was very similar to that of men who had reportedly never smoked cigarettes but had low levels of beta-carotene in the diet."

During the 19 years of the Western Electric study, 33 of the workers developed lung cancer. Among the 488 men who had the lowest levels of beta-carotene consumption, there were 14 cases; among the 488 men who had the highest levels of beta-carotene in their diets, there were only two. Among the 978 men in middle-range beta-carotene consumption, 17 cases of lung cancer were reported.

Dietary vitamin A itself did not appear to prevent lung cancer. Perhaps cigarette smoke in the lungs immediately destroys vitamin A, whereas beta-carotene is converted to vitamin A over a period of time and so constantly replenishes vitamin A in the lung tissues.

Almost a year later, the conservative *Nutrition Reviews* (September 1982) published a review article by Dr. George Wolf of M.I.T. and an anonymous article discussing the Western Electric study just described. Both articles called for clinical trials before spreading word that beta-carotene might help prevent lung cancer.

The clinching factor in contemporary scientific and medical opinion was the 1982 National Academy of Sciences report on diet and cancer that acknowledged the beta-carotene link to cancer protection.

The 1981 series of reports did have their effect. During 1981, National Cancer Institute and Harvard Medical School researchers agreed that beta-carotene was worth testing in a double-blind prospective trial. The Harvard researchers already were planning a trial of aspirin to see if it could reduce heart attacks or strokes. It was relatively easy to add beta-carotene to the study.

In 1982, the combined research team, led by Dr. Charles H. Hennekens of Harvard, asked 200,000 male physicians to volunteer for the study. About 22,000 male physicians between the ages of 45 and 75 volunteered. On even days, they were taking either 325 milligrams of aspirin or a placebo. On odd days, they were taking either 30 milligrams of beta-carotene or a placebo. The health of the physicians has been monitored since then. The study should produce a clearer picture of the beta-carotene link to cancer protection. (See Summary for additional study results.)

Beta-carotene was chosen over retinoids for the Harvard–NCI study because it is less toxic and because there is some evidence that beta-carotene may be more protective against lung cancer than vitamin A. There is also evidence that beta-carotene may be more protective against skin cancer.

Dr. Albert Padwa of Emory University states that beta-carotene may help protect skin from damage caused by a special form of oxygen containing excess energy, called "singlet oxygen." Singlet oxygen is formed in the body as a toxic byproduct of many metabolic reactions, but smoking and sun exposure stimulate its formation.

There are no known enzymes in the body which deactivate singlet oxygen, but both vitamin E and beta-carotene can do so. However, when vitamin E deactivates singlet oxygen, the vitamin E is destroyed. Beta-carotene can "quench" the singlet oxygen without damage to itself and can thus be used over and over again. Beta-carotene is among the most efficient substances known for converting singlet oxygen back to normal oxygen without damage to the body, and also for trapping certain organic free radicals which are believed to cause cancer. Beta-carotene may break down singlet oxygen before it can cause damage that leads to skin cancer or lung cancer—perhaps even to uterine or other mucous-tissue cancers.

SOURCES AND DAILY REQUIREMENT

Beta-carotene is not itself considered an essential nutrient, but as just one source of vitamin A, which *is* an essential nutrient. However, our thinking may change if it is definitely established that beta-carotene has unique cancer-preventing properties separate from those of vitamin A. Or it may be found that certain diseases or abnormalities diminish the absorption of retinoids, in which circumstances vitamin A needs would be met only by carotenoid absorption.

Because of its "nonessential" character, there is no official RDA for beta-carotene, but the vitamin A RDA of 5000 IU in effect up until 1980 was composed half of retinol and half of beta-carotene; that is, approximately half from animal sources such as fish, liver or butter, and half from fruits and vegetables. Nutritionists now prefer to measure vitamin A activity in terms of Retinol Equivalents (RE); the daily requirement translates into 100 RE. Ten International Units of vitamin A activity *from beta-carotene* equals one Retinol Equivalent. One Retinol Equivalent is obtained from 0.6 microgram (0.0006 milligram) of beta-carotene, or one microgram of retinol. Or expressed another way, one milligram of beta-carotene provides 1667 IU of vitamin A activity, or 167 RE. This recast RDA works out to 750 micrograms of retinol, which equals 750 RE, and about 1500 micrograms of beta-carotene, for 250 RE.

If we want to know how much of a vitamin is in a particular food, we would ordinarily consult a food table. Almost any such table printed before 1983 would report how much vitamin A there was in carrots and so on, but there is a problem. Carrots and other vegetables, fruits and grains do not contain vitamin A as such; they contain carotenoids, and so simple listing of vitamin A content is misleading. It is also not necessarily consistently accurate even so, as the variety of the plant, its nutrition and planting time affect the beta-carotene content. Table 1 lists the approximate beta-carotene contents of 43 vegetables, fruits and grains expressed in International Units of vitamin A activity. A rough estimate of the weights of beta-carotene in these foods can be arrived at by multiplying the IU of vitamin A by 0.03, which gives the approximate number of micrograms of beta carotene. For beta-carotene supplements, the conversion factor is 0.06, but 0.03 is used for endogenous beta-carotene because of its lessened bioavailability in a complex-carbohydrate or protein matrix. The Food and Nutrition Board has been asked by the Food and Drug Administration to study the matter further. USDA Handbook No. 456 states that it is not now feasible to give a single factor for converting vitamin A values in food tables to their equivalent weights in micrograms of retinol. Values for foods of plant origin are based on averages that may not always accurately indicate the contribution to total vitamin A value of each precursor that may be present.

An approximation of the RE content of plant foods can be obtained by dividing the number of IU of vitamin A activity by ten; this can't be done with animal products, which contain varying mixtures of retinoids and carotenoids.

The National Academy of Sciences suggests that 500 to 600 micrograms of retinol, or twice as much beta-carotene, is a minimum requirement for adults if they are to maintain an adequate blood concentration and prevent all deficiency symptoms. An intake above this level is considered to be required for beta-carotene storage in the liver; and liver storage is apparently a necessary condition for the protective effects discussed earlier.

If the Harvard-NCI beta-carotene study shows a proven cancer-preventing quality in beta-carotene, the NAS recommendations should be revised to the levels used in the study, approximately 15 milligrams a day, or 2500 RE—the amount you would get from eating half a cup of carrot slices, one sweet potato and a good portion of spinach.

TABLE 1

BETA-CAROTENE CONTENT OF FOODS

Food	Serving Size	IU
Apple	1 small raw	120
Apricots	3 raw	2,890
Asparagus	1 cup	1,220
Banana	1 medium	230
Beans, green	½ cup	340
Beet greens	½ cup	3,700
Bran cereal	½ cup	1,410
Bread, whole wheat	2 slices	Trace
Broccoli	½ cup	1,940
Brussels sprouts	½ cup	405
Bulgur	½ cup	0
Cabbage, shredded	1 cup raw	90
Cantaloupe	1 cup cubes	2,720
Carrots	½ cup slices	8,140
Cauliflower	1 cup	80
Collard greens	½ cup	7,410
Corn kernels	½ cup	330
Cranberry juice cocktail	6 ounces	Trace
Grapefruit	½ medium	80
Grits (corn)	1 cup	150
Kale	½ cup	4,565
Kidney beans	1 cup	10
Lentils	½ cup	20
Oatmeal	1 cup	0
Orange	1 medium	400
Orange juice	4 ounces	250
Peach	1 large	2,030
Peas, green	½ cup	430
Pepper, green	½ cup strips	210
Pepper, red	½ cup strips	2,225
Potato, baked	1 large	Trace
Prunes, stewed	½ cup	1,065
Shredded wheat	2 biscuits or 1 cup bite-sized	2,590
Spinach	½ cup	7,290
Squash, winter	½ cup mashed	6,560
Strawberries	1 cup	90
Sweet potato	1 5-inch	9,230
Tangerine	1 medium	360
Tomato	1 medium	1,110
Tomato juice	6 ounces	1,460
Turnip greens	½ cup	4,570
Watermelon	1 cup diced	940
Zucchini	½ cup slices	270

IU = International Units of vitamin A activity from carotenes. For approximate Retinol Equivalents (RE), divide by 10.

(Source USDA Handbook No. 456)

The toxicity of excessive amounts of vitamin A has been widely discussed in the literature. Excellent reviews are given in *Nutrition Reviews* (40,9,272–274, September 1982), "The Safe Use of Vitamin A," A Report of the International Vitamin A Consultative Group (IVACG) September 1980 and *Osteopathic Medicine* (3,10,31–42, October 1978). The Recommended Dietary Allowance is 5000 IU or 1000 Retinol Equivalents daily for adult males, with toxicity normally not a problem unless 100,000 IU or more have been consumed for a long period of time. However, there are reports of a few individuals who have shown reversible toxicity symptoms at lower dosages. Vitamin A deficiency and toxicity signs are given in Table 2.

TABLE 2

VITAMIN A DEFICIENCY AND TOXICITY SIGNS

Deficiency Signs	Toxicity Signs
Night blindness	Painful joint swellings
Dry, rough skin	Nausea
Corneal thickening	Dry skin
Itching	Elevated spinal fluid pressure
Loss of sense of taste	

Beta-carotene, however, is free from toxicity according to all reports published so far. The joint Food and Agriculture Organization/World Health Organization Expert Committee on Food Additives (1975) reported that a daily intake of beta-carotene for a 150-pound person of 350 milligrams (583,000 IU) per day was not toxic. See Appendix D for recommended amounts. Physicians routinely prescribe 100 to 200 milligrams (170,000–333,000 IU) of beta-carotene per day for the treatment of erythropoietic protoporphyria (a photosensitivity skin disease) without any apparent ill effects. *Excessive* beta-carotene intake can cause a yellowing of the skin (carotenemia), which can be reversed by descreasing the dose.

Leukopenia, the reduction of a type of white blood cells called neutrophils, has been reported in patients who ingested large amounts of carrots, but this is now believed to have been due to other substances in the carrots, as it is not observed when pure beta-carotene supplements are taken. Medical researchers using large amounts of beta-carotene report that their patients do not develop vitamin A toxicity (hypervitaminosis A).

Given the half-century of evidence showing the inverse correlation between beta-carotene/vitamin A intake and cancer incidence, and the demonstrated safety of even large dosages of beta-carotene—and the fact that, in ingesting it from natural sources, you are also taking in a variety of complex carbohydrates with their multiple health benefits—it seems worthwhile for the nutrition-conscious individual to assure a generous supply of this nutrient in his or her diet, by supplementation, or a combination of both.

Beyond Beta: Alpha and Other Carotenes Shown to Have Up to 100 Times More Antioxidant Power

Step aside, beta-carotene. The new nutritional star is your closest relative: *alpha*-carotene.

Beta-carotene may be the most abundant carotene in fruits and vegetables, but it's hardly the only one. Scientists have identified more than 600 of these plant pigments—which do double duty as natural protectors against cancer.

About 50 to 60 of these carotenes are found in the typical U.S. diet. Among them are alpha-carotene, lutein, lycopene, gamma-carotene, zeaxanthin and beta-cryptoxanthin. Experts have discovered that some of these carotenes are anywhere from 10 to 100 times more powerful than beta-carotene and other antioxidant nutrients.

Research on alpha-carotene gained momentum in Japan during the mid-1980s. Over the past couple of years, researchers at the U.S. Department of Agriculture and the National Cancer Institute have been playing catch-up. They're now researching the health benefits of the carotenes as well.

Michiaki Murakoshi, Ph.D., and his colleagues at the Kyoto Prefectural University, Japan, are credited with sparking interest in alpha-carotene. Originally studying beta-carotene, Murakoshi became curious about the health benefits of other carotenoids. He turned his attention to alpha-carotene, which accounts for one-third of the carotenes in carrots.

POWERFUL CANCER FIGHTER

In the November 1, 1989, *Journal of the National Cancer Institute*, he became the first scientist to report that alpha-carotene suppressed the growth of several types of malignant tumors, including neuroblastomas, pancreatic cancer, glioblastoma and gastric cancer.

To his amazement, Murakoshi discovered that alpha-carotene was 10 times more effective than beta-carotene in suppressing the growth of neuroblastoma cells, a type of childhood cancer. Alpha-carotene began suppressing cancer growth after just 18 hours. The higher the dose, the greater the benefits, and many of the cancer cells even resumed normal behavior.

He then decided to see what effect alpha-carotene would have on liver cancer, since the organ both stores the nutrient and detoxifies carcinogens. Murakoshi found that mice getting abundant alpha-carotene in the diet developed fewer and smaller tumors than did mice receiving beta-carotene or no additional carotenes at all.

"The present findings clearly demonstrate that alpha-carotene has a potent inhibitory effect on spontaneous liver carcinogensis," he wrote in the December 1, 1992, *Cancer Research.* "It is noteworthy that alpha- but not beta-carotene showed potent inhibitory activity against liver carcinogenesis."

Murakoshi later discovered that alpha-carotene was also more effective than beta-carotene in preventing liver, lung, and skin cancers. For example, mice consuming alpha-carotene had one-third the incidence of lung cancer of animals that did not receive a supplement.

Alpha-carotene and related substances appear to work as antioxidants, which mop up free radicals. Free radicals are damaged molecules known to cause aging and degenerative diseases.

But the carotene revolution doesn't stop with alpha-carotene. Lycopene, a carotene abundant in tomato and guava, is 100 times more powerful as a "singlet oxygen" scavenger than vitamin E, perhaps the best known antioxidant nutrient. Perhaps not surprisingly, researchers have found that high lycopene intake can lower the risk of developing lung, pancreatic and bladder cancer.

In addition, gamma-carotene is 83 times more powerful than vitamin E, according to research by Paolo DiMascio, Ph.D., of the University of Düsseldorf. He also reported that zeaxanthin was 10 times more powerful and lutein 8 times more powerful as antioxidants than vitamin E.

BETA-CAROTENE REVISITED

The research on alpha and other carotenes comes at a time of increased confusion about beta-carotene. After more than a decade of headlines touting the benefits of beta-carotene, confidence in the vitamin was shaken in 1994.

The April 14, 1994, *New England Journal of Medicine* reported a Finnish study in which smokers taking beta-carotene had an *increased* risk of developing lung cancer. The study was a puzzler to scientists, because of more than 200 studies on beta-carotene, this was the first to show any potential hazard.

While some researchers suddenly urged caution about taking beta-carotene supplements, others roundly dismissed the study as a fluke. There were many reasons for doing so.

For example, the typical subject was a Finnish man who had smoked cigarettes for more than 35 years. Researchers did not encourage the men to stop smoking, which would have done more than anything else to reduce their risk of lung cancer.

Jeffrey Blumberg, Ph.D., of Tufts University, explained that the damage from smoking had already been done—cancers often take 20 years to develop—and that no vitamin should be viewed as a magic bullet after years of abusing the body.

Another problem is that the Finns have an extremely high incidence of cancer and heart disease compared with other Europeans. One recent study by William Connor, M.D., of Oregon Health Sciences University, found that the high incidence of disease may be the result of the Finns' low consumption of fruits and vegetables—and carotenes in general.

Yet another confounding factor may be that the beta-carotene used in the study was synthetic, not natural. It was also colored with quinoline yellow, a known carcinogen, according to herb writer and medical botanist Michael Weiner, Ph.D.

For hundreds of years, folk traditions have recommended that people "have a lot of color on the plate." People knew intuitively that colorful fruits and vegetables were good for health, but until recently they didn't understand that the colors of fruits and vegetables and many of their health benefits were the results of carotenes.

Because of the recent research on alpha and other carotenes, it doesn't make sense to depend just on beta-carotene. Scientists believe that they work at different sites in the body—the lungs, eyes, skin, etc. That means we may need all of the carotenes, not just the best-known one.

The lesson here is that some of the less common may even be better than the ones that have captured the headlines. In a sense, good things really do come in small carotenes.

JACK CHALLEM

FOOD SOURCES OF ALPHA-CAROTENE

Carrots are nature's richest source of both beta-carotene and alpha-carotene—63 and 32 percent, respectively. The remaining 2 percent consists of lycopene, gamma-carotene and lutein. But if you prefer jack-o'-lanterns to rabbit food, your next best source of alpha-carotene is pumpkins. Spinach, broccoli, turnips, mustard greens and collards are rich in lutein. Tomato products—even catsup—and guava are high in lycopene. Beta-cryptoxanthin is abundant in oranges, tangerines and peaches. If you want to go the supplemental route, you'll find that high alpha-carotene supplements are similar to carrots. Derived from palm oil, they contain 60 percent beta-carotene, 34 percent alpha-carotene and 6 percent of the other carotenes. Because of its cost, you won't find pure alpha-carotene outside a research laboratory.

VITAMIN C

*The Great Vitamin That Provides Optimum
Health and Immunity*

JACK JOSEPH CHALLEM

RECOGNITION COMES TO VITAMIN C

Vitamin C is becoming more respectable and respected every day as
its capacities are increasingly acknowledged. More than four thousand articles on this vitamin are now published each year in medical
journals. Controlled studies prove its contribution to the prevention
and treatment of infectious, degenerative and stress diseases, to resistance against pollution in air, water and food and to its supportive
role in the manufacture of white blood cells and interferon.

---

*If you are healthy, vitamin C can keep you that way. If you are sick,
vitamin C can help you feel better.*

With claims such as these, it's no wonder vitamin C has attracted
so much attention and controversy. Indeed, as claim after claim is
being proven, vitamin C is being propelled from virtual anonymity to
growing respectability. Many of the early skeptics have become vitamin C's strongest proponents. Within a few years, nearly everyone
will be taking vitamin C supplements.

It wasn't always this way.

In the not too distant past, we learned that vitamin C was an
important nutrient—but our needs for it could be satisfied with a
morning glass of orange juice and an occasional piece of fruit. That
comfortable view changed in 1970 with the publication of Dr. Linus

Pauling's book, *Vitamin C and the Common Cold.*[1] Linus Pauling, Ph.D., a two-time Nobel Laureate and an expert in molecular medicine, had become impressed by the effect of large doses of nutrients on health. His experience began as a personal one—as many medical breakthroughs do—and was continued by his remarkable work and that of his associates.[2] Pauling's stature in the scientific and medical worlds immediately forced attention to vitamin C. Pauling, his colleagues knew, was often controversial, but he was rarely wrong.

Now, in the 1990s, that controversy seems to be subsiding, and refinements in the early vitamin C research are being made at a breathtaking pace. In addition, new and important reports on the roles of vitamin C are being made daily; more than four thousand articles on this vitamin are being published each year in medical journals.

Evidence has mounted showing that vitamin C is valuable in the prevention and treatment of not just the common cold, but virtually all infectious diseases—the flu, mononucleosis, hepatitis, pneumonia, herpes—and many others. Vitamin C has a role in the prevention and treatment of cancer, perhaps the most feared disease we face. Vitamin C has also been found to help persons suffering from allergies, heart disease, periodontal disease, alcoholism and mental illness. It has been shown to increase our resistance to the pollutants in air and water as well as to the chemical additives in foods. Doctors have demonstrated that vitamin C can eliminate Sudden Infant Death Syndrome (SIDS), decrease the biological impact of x-rays and other types of radiation and slow the aging process.

These are not outlandish claims. Vitamin C is a substance so important to life that its absence can result in death, while small and inadequate amounts of it prevent us from reaching a state of optimal health.

In this chapter on vitamin C, you will read a short history of vitamin C and its amazing, but often ignored, *non*controversial roles in health. You will learn the rationale for its use in preventing and treating diseases in easily understood terms. Above all else, you will gain an understanding of how doctors are now using this remarkable vitamin to treat the diseases you suffer and fear the most.

THE DISCOVERY AND REDISCOVERY OF VITAMIN C

Until the end of the eighteenth century, most naval and other maritime pursuits were plagued by the death of sailors from scurvy. It was a terrible disease that claimed the lives of thousands each year. The sailors would be overcome by lethargy; their skin would spontaneously rupture and bleed. In 1751, the Royal British Navy's physician, Dr. James Lind, published *A Treatise of the Scurvy*. In it, Lind reported that this devastating disease could be prevented by giving its victims one fresh citrus fruit each day. The British sailors eventually became known as *limeys*, a reference to the dietary regimen Lind proposed.[3,4,5]

It was not until this century, however, that science gained an understanding of why citrus prevented and cured scurvy. During the late 1920s and early 1930s, several researchers, most notably Albert Szent-Györgyi, Ph.D., identified and then synthesized the antiscorbutic agent in citrus. It was called vitamin C or ascorbic acid, and it had the chemical formula $C_6H_8O_6$.[6]

The discovery of vitamin C prompted a tremendous amount of research on its role in health and disease in the 1930s and 1940s for vitamin C—but much of the work lay forgotten until the 1970s. Vitamin C, researchers found, is necessary for the growth of new tissue and the replacement of old tissue, as in wound healing. Vitamin C is necessary for the formation of collagen, a protein that acts as a biological cement holding the body cells together. The vitamin is also necessary for the formation of cartilage, dentine in teeth, and bone. Vitamin C maintains the integrity of our capillaries, the smallest of our blood vessels, and prevents them from bruising. It is a precursor to many hormones, such as adrenalin and cortisone, which are produced by the body as defenses. Vitamin C also protects vitamin A against oxidation, potentiates the benefits of vitamin B12, and partly compensates for deficiencies of pantothenic acid, another B vitamin.[3,6]

Vitamin C is found universally in the plant and animal kingdoms. Plants readily produce vitamin C, $C_6H_8O_6$, from the simple sugar glucose, $C_6H_{12}O_6$. Virtually all vertebrates and invertebrates produce vitamin C internally from glucose. Smaller animals characteristically manufacture it in the kidney, while larger animals manufacture it in the liver. One of the oddities is that a handful of animals do *not* manufacture their own vitamin C. Among them is the Anthropoidea suborder of primates, *which includes us*, the guinea pig, the fruit-eating bat of India and a songbird called the red-vented bulbul. We, the members of the *Homo sapiens* species, lack the fourth and last liver enzyme, L-gulonolactone oxidase, which is necessary to convert glucose to vitamin C.[3,6]

In the mid-1960s, Dr. Irwin Stone, a California biochemist, hypothesized that the ancestors of the human race lost the ability to manufacture vitamin C about sixty million years ago—but that the need for and ability to use the vitamin was retained. Dr. Stone contended that there was a freak genetic accident that selected against those who had the burdensome biochemical machinery to produce vitamin C and selected for those who could obtain vitamin C from food.

Dr. Stone reported in his book, *The Healing Factor: Vitamin C Against Disease*,[3] and numerous published papers, that the animals that produce their own vitamin C do so in amounts relatively consistent with body weight. The production of vitamin C increases relatively consistently with stress—and quite rapidly if the stress is severe.

As an illustration of this mechanism, and how it relates to people, Stone explains that a 150-pound goat produces 13,000 milligrams (13 grams) of vitamin C daily when unstressed. This unstressed rate of vitamin C production converts to about 86 milligrams per pound of body weight each day. Exposure to stress will double or triple the rate of glucose-to-vitamin C conversion.[3]

Contrast this with the official determination of what human needs are. The Recommended Daily Allowance (RDA), promulgated by the National Academy of Sciences and the Food and Drug Administration, is 45 milligrams of vitamin C *for an adult* (*not* per pound of body weight) to prevent scurvy. Converted to the amount needed per pound, the figure would be about one-third of a milligram. This is far from the 86 milligrams per pound the goat produces, and it is far

from the 20 milligram per pound amount recommended for laboratory monkeys, the closest of our biological relatives.

Because of the genetic accident preventing us from producing our
own vitamin C, Stone feels, we are all deficient in this vitamin from
birth. Many other scientists see scurvy, which the RDA is supposed
to protect us from, as not the first sign of vitamin C deficiency but
the last before death.[3]

Just as glucose seems a universal biological fuel, so vitamin C
appears to be necessary to maintain homeostasis, a state of equilib-
rium. Stresses necessitate a heightened production of vitamin C, because it is essential for the production of other biochemicals required
for normal and stressed metabolism. It doesn't matter whether the
stress is physical, such as an infection or cold weather exposure; psychological, as with anxiety or pressure at home and the office; or
attack—the so-called fight or flight syndrome in the animal world.
The body shifts into a defensive posture to meet and minimize the
effect of the stress. Vitamin C is necessary for the body to accomplish
this successfully.[1,3]

WHAT HAPPENS WHEN YOU "CATCH" A COLD?

A person can "catch" a cold in two ways, explains Sherry Lewin,
Ph.D., in *Vitamin C: Its Molecular Biology and Medical Potential.*[7] One
can occur when a person is exposed to low-temperature conditions.
There is good reason, besides not shivering, for adding clothing on
cold or windy days. Under such conditions (stresses), the respiratory
system becomes chilled, which, in turn, disturbs the delicate balance
of hormones in the body. Following this, the production of antibodies
and interferon is suppressed. This greatly reduces our ability to fight
infections and allows viruses or bacteria to gain a firm hold on tissues.
The second way a person can contract a cold is by exposure to active
viruses and bacteria, such as being in contact with a person who has
sneezed or by other means of transmitting the infection. This triggers

abnormal enzyme formation in respiratory tissues and other membranes, leading again to a disturbed hormone balance and depression of antibodies and interferon.

The human body has a magnificent array of immune system defenses to combat infections. They all, however, require large amounts of vitamin C to perform optimally—that is, to prevent an infection from taking hold or to fight an already existing infection. It is doubtful that the amount of vitamin C obtained from an ordinary diet is sufficient to support the immune system. Supplemental vitamin C is necessary.

The first line of defense consists of leukocytes, or white blood cells. These scavenge the bloodstream, searching for invasive microbes and, upon finding them, digest the foreign bodies. The white blood cells require vitamin C in order to perform efficiently. Another defender is the glycoprotein interferon, the production of which is increased to counter infectious microbes. In a study reported in *Medical World News*, researchers sprayed the noses of eleven volunteer subjects with interferon, then exposed the subject to a human virus. None of the subjects developed a cold, although three displayed mild symptoms. Given the same viral exposure without interferon, eight subjects developed clear infections, two had mild symptoms, and one remained without symptoms.[8]

While interferon has been promoted as a possible wonder drug, it remains exceedingly expensive and limited in quantity. Drs. Pauling and Stone insist there is little need to use it, because high doses of vitamin C—which is inexpensive and abundant—result in successful clinical responses that are almost identical with those obtained from interferon therapy. Dr. Stone has also observed that part of vitamin C's success in combating infections probably relates to the vitamin being an "interferon inducer." Interferon, normally produced by the body, can be enhanced by an increased intake of vitamin C—literally turning us into the excellent interferon factory our biology allows us to be.[9,10,11]

Still another immune system defense rests with antibodies. These are complex and tailor-made chemicals manufactured by the body to fight specific viruses or bacteria. Antibodies are formed during infections to seek out specific invasive microbes and distinguish them from normal substances in the body rather in the way sophisticated heat-seeking missiles distinguish enemy from friendly airplanes. Antibodies, like all of the immune system, require vitamin C to function at optimal levels.

BEATING THE COMMON COLD

In 1970, Dr. Linus Pauling recommended that most people could prevent colds by taking between 250 milligrams to 1000 milligrams (¼ to 1 gram) of vitamin C daily. To fight a cold, Pauling contended that most people could suppress symptoms with 1 or 2 grams daily, although he noted that some individuals might need 10 to 15 grams per day (averaging 1 to 2 grams per hour). He noted that low doses of vitamin C were virustatic and bacteriostatic; that is, the vitamin could halt the spread of infectious microbes. At higher doses, Pauling said, vitamin C became virucidal and bacteriocidal—it could kill the microorganisms. Dr. Pauling took 10 grams daily himself, and recommended this amount as a maintenance dose for most adults.[11]

These recommended doses seem conservative, however, when contrasted with those given patients by Dr. Robert Cathcart III, a physician practicing in San Mateo, California. Indeed, Dr. Cathcart believes that many of the mixed results scientists find while testing vitamin C efficacy relate to the fact that inadequate levels are used. Dr. Cathcart, one of the leading megavitamin doctors, has forged a unique approach to administering vitamin C in his clinical practice. He explains that taking two grams of vitamin C per hour would help a person with a very mild cold, but it would offer little benefit to one with a more severe cold. Ironically, he observes, most physicians don't see patients with mild colds; they see patients with severe colds. Treating these colds with only a couple of grams of vitamin C is unlikely to have a positive response in the patient, and the lack of results would be discouraging to both patient and physician.[12,13,14]

Dr. Cathcart startles many people when he characterizes colds as "25-gram colds," "50-gram colds," or "100-gram colds." His unusual prefix reflects the amount of vitamin C necessary to suppress symptoms at the peak of the infection. The prefix also indicates the severity of the infection, although when treated early less vitamin C may be necessary. Dr. Cathcart is fond of saying, "Don't send a boy to do a man's job." He means, clearly, don't settle for only a little vitamin C when a lot is needed.

TAILORING THE DOSE FOR COLDS
AND OTHER INFECTIONS

Behind Dr. Cathcart's extremely high doses of vitamin C for treating colds (and other infections to be discussed shortly) lies his concept of *bowel tolerance*. It has been known for many years that high doses of vitamin C cause diarrhea in many people. Through clinical observation, Dr. Cathcart has recognized that there is a methodology in what might otherwise appear as vitamin madness. Four out of five healthy patients could take 10 to 15 grams of vitamin C daily (as ascorbic acid crystals dissolved in water, spread across four doses) without developing diarrhea. Taking more than this amount would result in diarrhea. The same patients, when stressed by an infection, could dramatically increase their vitamin C intake without the onset of diarrhea. In other words, Dr. Cathcart found that the sicker a person was, the greater were his needs for and tolerance of vitamin C. He also noticed that patients do not benefit from the clinical effect of vitamin C (fighting an infection) until doses reach 80 to 90 percent of bowel tolerance.[12,13]

Dr. Cathcart describes this method of determining dosage "titrating to bowel tolerance." He has explained in *Medical Hypotheses*:

The maximum relief of symptoms which can be expected with oral doses of ascorbic acid is obtained at a point just short of the amount which produces diarrhea. This amount and the timing of the doses are usually sensed by the patient. The physician should not try to regulate exactly the amount and timing of these doses because the optimally effective dose will often change from dose to dose . . . the patient tries to titrate between that amount which begins to make him feel better and that amount which almost but not quite causes diarrhea.

Occasionally, a person will reach bowel tolerance without a significant relief of symptoms. For such intransigent infections, Dr. Cathcart recommends a buffered form of vitamin C.[12]

TABLE 3

USUAL BOWEL TOLERANCE DOSES OF VITAMIN C

Condition	Grams per 24 Hours	Number of Doses per 24 Hours
Normal	4–15	4
Mild cold	30–60	6–10
Severe cold	60–100	8–15
Influenza	100–150	8–20
ECHO, coxsackievirus	100–150	8–20
Mononucleosis	150–200+	12–25
Viral pneumonia	100–200+	12–25
Hay fever, asthma	15–50	4–8
Environmental and food allergy	0.5–50	4–8
Burn, injury, surgery	25–150	6–20
Anxiety, exercise and other mild stresses	15–25	4–6
Cancer	15–100	4–5
Ankylosing spondylitis	15–100	4–15
Reiter's syndrome	15–60	4–10
Acute anterior uveitis	30–100	4–15
Rheumatoid arthritis	15–100	4–15
Bacterial infections	30–200+	10–25
Infectious hepatitis	30–100	6–15
Candida infections	15–200+	6–25

Source: Robert F. Cathcart, III. 1981. *Medical Hypotheses* 7:1360–61.

The mechanisms by which a person contracts a severe infection are the same as the way common cold viruses are established in the body. The increased dangers of severe infections come from (1) a greater intensity of the infection-related symptoms; (2) the duration of those symptoms; and (3) an increase in secondary symptoms and infections that can, at times, be life threatening.

When an infection is contracted in local tissues, vitamin C is used to fight and contain the infection. Because tissue concentrations of the vitamin may be inadequate, vitamin C stores from the rest of the body are mobilized. Even these are usually limited because vitamin C is water soluble and quickly excreted from the body. If you ordinarily take 1 gram of vitamin C every day, how long would it last during a 100-gram cold? Not long. And without large quantities of vitamin C, a condition Dr. Cathcart describes as "acute induced scurvy" appears. This is a critical time for vitamin C needs.[12,13,14] Dr. Cathcart explains:

Some of this increased metabolic need for ascorbate undoubtedly occurs in areas of the body not primarily involved in the disease and can be accounted for by such functions as the adrenals producing more adrenaline and corticoids; the immune system producing more antibodies, interferon and other substances to fight the infection. . . . Also, there must be a tremendous draw on ascorbate locally by increased metabolic rates in the primarily infected tissues. The infecting organisms themselves liberate toxins which are neutralized by ascorbate, but in the process destroy ascorbate. The levels of ascorbate in the nose, throat, eustachian tubes and bronchial tubes locally infected by a 100-gram cold must be very low indeed. With this acute induced scurvy localized in these areas, it is small wonder that healing can be delayed and complications such as chronic sinusitis, otitis media and bronchitis, etc. develop.

This draw on ascorbate, from whatever source, lowers the blood level of ascorbate to a negligible level. I have coined the term *anascorbemia* for this condition. If this anascorbemia is not rapidly rectified by the oral administration of bowel tolerance doses of ascorbic acid or by intravenous administration of ascorbate, the remainder of the body is rapidly depleted of ascorbate and put at risk for disorders of the metabolic processes dependent upon vitamin C.[12]

These are some of the problems that could be expected with a severe depletion of vitamin C: immune system disorders, including secondary infections, rheumatoid arthritis, collagen diseases, allergies to drugs and foods and chronic herpes infections; cardiovascular and blood coagulation disorders, including hemorrhaging, heart attacks, elevated cholesterol, strokes and hemorrhoids; an impaired ability to cope with stresses, including poor healing of wounds, excessive scarring, bed sores and stretch marks; impaired nervous system function, such as malaise, lowered pain tolerance, muscle spasms, senility and other psychiatric disorders; and cancer from the suppressed immune system and carcinogens which have not been detoxified. "I am not saying that ascorbate depletion is the only cause of these disorders," explains Dr. Cathcart, "but I am pointing out that disorders of these systems would certainly predispose to these diseases, and that these systems are known to be dependent upon ascorbate for their proper function."[12]

Mononucleosis is an infection that can be positively diagnosed with a simple laboratory test; its course can be dramatically altered with supplemental vitamin C. Dr. Cathcart tells the story of a 23-year-old woman with severe mononucleosis who treated herself with two heaping tablespoons of vitamin C every two hours—consuming a full pound (454 grams) in two days. She felt almost completely well within three to four days, although she took 20 to 30 grams a day for two months. Most cases of mononucleosis, Dr. Cathcart notes, do not require maintenance doses for more than two to three weeks, and the tailoring of the dose can be sensed and adjusted by the patient.[12,13]

Surgery is a stress that indicates a need for additional vitamin C (see Table 3), but infectious hepatitis following surgery and blood transfusions is especially insidious. Fukumi Morishige, M.D., and Akira Murata, Ph.D., have conducted two studies that demonstrate that the incidence of hepatitis can be dramatically reduced when patients receive two grams of vitamin C daily during hospitalization. Dr. Cathcart recently treated two fellow orthopedic surgeons who contracted hepatitis by pricking their hands during surgery. One of the orthopedists treated had difficulty believing that vitamin C was responsible for his improvement, so he discontinued taking it. His condition deteriorated rapidly, but improved again when he resumed taking vitamin C.[12]

Herpes I and II, the simplex and genital varieties, are diseases nearly epidemic in scale. Both can be ameliorated by doses of vitamin C that approach bowel tolerance. If the herpes infection is recurrent or chronic, zinc supplements may be necessary as an adjunct. Dr. Cathcart recommends physician supervision for the therapeutic use of zinc, however, because high doses can upset mineral ratios within the body and lead to other problems.[7,12,13] Dr. Sherry Lewin found that 30 of 38 patients who regularly suffered from the "cold sore" variety of herpes remained free of the infection four years after beginning a 1 to 2 grams daily intake of vitamin C. The remaining eight patients were able to inhibit the infection with several grams of vitamin C at the first appearance of symptoms.[7]

Bacterial infections are commonly treated with penicillin or other antibiotics, but many patients react allergically to this treatment. Vitamin C is a powerful bacteriocide, and many such infections can be quickly controlled by administration to bowel tolerance levels. It is interesting that vitamin C seems to enhance the effect of antibiotics, while simultaneously reducing allergic reactions to them. The vitamin C and antibiotic should not be taken together, however. Allow at least one hour in between to prevent a decrease in antibiotic absorption. The combination of vitamin C and antibiotics is particularly effective against severe bacterial infections.[12,13]

VITAMIN C REVERSES
DEGENERATIVE DISEASES

One of the basic, and noncontroversial roles of vitamin C relates to its role in the formation of collagen protein. Collagen is an important component of what has been aptly described as our intercellular cement, the material that literally holds our bodies together. Intercellular cement consists of long molecular chains known as glycosaminoglycans, which are intertwined with fibrils of collagen protein. It is akin to a concrete wall reinforced by a network of steel rods. This makes surprising sense if you recall that victims of scurvy hemorrhaged spontaneously—their intercellular cement and collagen were so weakened by vitamin C deficiency that their bodies could no longer hold together.

This is elementary medicine. Somewhat more controversial is Dr. Linus Pauling's contention that supplemental vitamin C will increase the strength of collagen, fortifying the intercellular cement. This, in fact, is the rationale for much of vitamin C's beneficial effect in degenerative diseases. In simple terms, sufficient doses of vitamin C can reverse the degenerative process by strengthening tissue—that is, making it more resistant to degeneration.

Vitamin C accomplishes this, as we have seen, by stimulating many natural biological defense mechanisms within the body, as in the case of infectious diseases. In degenerative diseases, vitamin C counters a different kind of threat: the enzyme hyaluronidase. Hyaluronidase, which probably has a role in infections, is recognized as the "spreading factor" in many degenerative diseases. Hyaluronidase separates the long glycosaminoglycan chains into smaller molecules, thereby weakening the fabric of the intercellular cement. In tumors, and probably other diseases as well, the enzyme collagenase breaks down collagen protein. The action of these two destructive enzymes makes tissue susceptible to invasive diseases such as cancer, arthritis, infections or other diseases.[2,11,15]

The strength of collagen, however, can be dramatically increased through high doses of vitamin C. A study conducted at the Duke University Medical Center, and published in the *Proceedings of the National Academy of Sciences of the United States of America* (1981), demonstrates this. Dr. S. Murad and his colleagues added vitamin C to cultured human skin fibroblasts and found that collagen synthesis increased by eight times. Such an increase in collagen formation improves the strength of cellular cement. Vitamin C makes tissue more resistant to disease by establishing a barrier to disease expansion within the body.[16]

VITAMIN C IN THE PREVENTION AND CONTROL OF CANCER

In 1966, Dr. Ewan Cameron published *Hyaluronidase and Cancer*, proposing that any substance capable of strengthening the intercellular cement would have value in increasing a person's resistance to cancer. Dr. Cameron also felt there were other natural substances in the body that offered resistance to cancer. If these substances could be identified and enhanced, he thought our biological defenses against cancer could be dramatically improved.[17]

It is generally believed that cancer cells develop in persons at all times. Normally, when cells replicate, an exact copy is formed. We know, however, that this doesn't always happen. The body is composed of trillions of cells, and the odds are that something (such as a carcinogen or nutrient deficiency) will prevent exact replication in a certain number of cells. Often, those aberrant cells are cancer cells.

In individuals with well-tuned immune systems, cancer cells are identified and destroyed by antibodies and white blood cells. But in people with poor immune systems, the cancer cells are unchallenged; they are free to continue duplicating, enlarging the cancer from a cell to a mass that can take hold in tissues. As cancer cells proliferate, they become invasive—attacking specific organs and often the body as a whole. This is, admittedly, a simplified explanation of how cancers develop; but little more detail is really necessary, because the horrors of cancers are well known.

Vitamin C appears to improve resistance to cancer in two major ways: first, by stimulating the immune system; and second, by strengthening collagen and the intercellular cement. The first reduces the proliferation of cancer, whereas the second reduces its invasiveness.

Vitamin C stimulates the immune system against cancer cells in much the same way it does in combating infectious diseases. When saturated with vitamin C, white blood cells readily migrate to the sites of abnormalities in the bloodstream—in this case, cancer cells.

When saturated with vitamin C, white blood cells are also efficient in engulfing cancer cells. But low levels of vitamin C prevent white blood cells from functioning optimally. It should not be surprising, then, that cancer patients are typically low in vitamin C.

The invasiveness of cancer can be halted by vitamin C—both by strengthening collagen and intercellular cement and by inhibiting hyaluronidase formation. Cancers liberate the enzymes hyaluronidase and collagenase, which weaken the normal tissues surrounding cancer and permit the disease to spread. Increased collagen formation, by supplemental vitamin C, forms a stronger barrier to cancer. In addition, vitamin C seems to be a hyaluronidase and collagenase inhibitor. An established cancer is, in colloquial terms, cornered by the effect of vitamin C. It cannot invade because surrounding tissues are strengthened and spreading enzymes are inhibited. At the same time, the immune system is stimulated and attacks the cancer, reducing its mass.[11]

This, largely, was little more than theory in the late 1960s and early 1970s. But ten years of clinical trials by Dr. Cameron in Scotland showed that it works. Several hundred terminal cancer patients were treated by Dr. Cameron. (Since many other physicians have followed this course of treatment, the numbers are now in the thousands.) Matched against a control group consisting of patients of the same age, sex and type of cancer, Dr. Cameron's patients lived four times longer. Some of the patients had extremely long survival times, as much as twenty times the average. A handful of the patients, once considered terminal, were still alive and active many years after the treatment began.[11,18–21]

"In many cancer patients," explains Dr. Cameron, "the administration of ascorbate seems to improve the state of wellbeing, as measured by improved appetite, increased mental alertness, decreased requirement for pain-controlling drugs and other clinical criteria." In the clinical trials, conducted at the Vale of Leven Hospital (Scotland):

almost all patients received 10 grams of sodium ascorbate per day orally, some initially by intravenous solution. In one patient, recurrence of the cancer was observed to follow the cessation of intake of the vitamin, with a second regression when the intake was resumed. Larger amounts, up to 50 grams per day, both by intravenous infusion and orally, have been used in a few patients. The intake that is most effective in controlling cancer has still to be established. In the present state of our knowledge, it seems prudent to introduce supplemental ascorbate on a graduated scale, increasing intake by increments of 2 grams on successive days until a maintenance dose of around 10 grams is attained. Once such a regime has been established, it should be maintained indefinitely.

It is our opinion that supplemental vitamin C is of some benefit to patients with all forms of cancer, and it is our belief that, in time, this simple and safe form of supportive treatment will become an accepted part of all regimes for the treatment of cancer.[22]

The results obtained by Cameron and Pauling in using vitamin C to treat cancer patients have met with stiff criticism from the medical establishment. A skeptical reaction to something as cheap and abundant as vitamin C is to be expected; indeed, this was Dr. Cameron's first response to vitamin C. But this picture seems to be changing for the better. In February 1982, the University of Arizona hosted the First International Conference on the Modulation and Mediation of Cancer by Vitamins. Dr. Linus Pauling was the keynote speaker to an audience comprised of researchers studying the roles of vitamins in cancer prevention and control. The conference was followed by an announcement by the National Cancer Institute that a cancer prevention program, including broad support of vitamin research, was going to be funded. The research, according to a report in the *Journal of the American Medical Association*, "will seek to identify chemicals in food that inhibit development of cancers."[23,24]

VITAMIN C RELIEVES
PERIODONTAL DISEASE

Nutritionally oriented dentists such as Emanuel Cheraskin and Hal Huggins have long insisted that vitamin C was of utmost importance in the health of dental tissues. It is widely recognized that people who lose their teeth do so not because of poor teeth, but because of poor supporting structures. These supporting structures include the collagen protein that composes periodontal tissues.

Bleeding gums (periodontal tissues) are indicative of scurvy. Ironically, few physicians or dentists today recognize the symptoms of scurvy because they are taught that it no longer occurs. But this contrasts sharply with the incidence of people whose gums bleed when they brush their teeth.

The relationship between vitamin C deficiency and periodontal disease is attracting renewed attention. The *Journal of the American Medical Association* reported on findings by the National Institute of Dental Research. These studies "offer the first concrete evidence that subclinical vitamin C deficiency increases susceptibility to periodontal disease."

The *Journal of the American Medical Association* reported that "periodontal disease, a leading cause of tooth loss among adults after age thirty-five years, has long been thought to result primarily from the body's long-term reactions to certain bacteria and their products. However, scientists have long suspected that nutritional factors may also influence the maintenance and breakdown of periodontal tissues. For example, there is strong evidence that ascorbic acid (vitamin C) is necessary for adequate repair."

The study referred to, conducted by Dr. Olav Alvares and his colleagues at the University of Washington, "concludes that periodontal tissues of animals fed a diet marginally deficient in vitamin C are more susceptible to breakdown when challenged by experimentally induced plaque. . . . The protective functions of polymorphonuclear leukocytes (PMNs)—white blood cells normally rich in vitamin

C—were compared . . . at various points throughout the experiment. At the start of the experiment, PMN ability to engulf *Candida albicans*, a test organism, was equal in all the animals.

"However, at twenty-three weeks (namely, at the time of the experimentally induced periodontitis), PMNs of the marginally deficient animals showed a significant reduction in chemotaxis (the migration of leukocytes to antigen-containing sites) and in phagocytosis (the ability to engulf microorganisms) compared with PMN function in the pair-fed controls."[25]

Another study, by Drs. Olav Alvares and Ivens Siegel, published in the *Journal of Oral Pathology*, found that vitamin C deficiency increased permeability of the periodontal tissues, increasing the movement of antigenic and toxic substances from the surface of the underlying connective tissues. In healthy individuals, there is limited permeability of these tissues, preventing the passage of disease-causing microorganisms and other substances into periodontal tissues.[25,26]

VITAMIN C LOWERS CHOLESTEROL, STRENGTHENS HEART MUSCLE

Diseases of the heart and cardiovascular system are the major killers of Americans today, yet vitamin C supplementation could contribute to their eradication. Nearly twenty years ago, Dr. Constance Spittle-Leslie of England was one of the first to recognize that vitamin C could lower cholesterol levels in the bloodstream. She began her experiments, as many do, on herself. She placed herself on a high-cholesterol diet, but her serum cholesterol level dropped—apparently from her consumption of fresh fruits and vegetables rich in vitamin V. When Dr. Spittle-Leslie began cooking the fruits and vegetables, destroying the vitamin C, her cholesterol increased. This led to an experiment on 58 volunteer subjects. The results were the same. But when she gave the subjects an additional gram of vitamin C daily, according to a report in *Medical World News*, their cholesterol levels dropped.[27]

The benefits of vitamin C in cardiovascular disease have been confirmed in subsequent human and animal studies. An article in the *Journal of Human Nutrition* reported the results of another British study. Eleven elderly patients with coronary heart disease were given one gram of vitamin C daily. Within six weeks, their total blood cholesterol levels decreased. In conclusion, the researchers noted that "atherosclerosis and ischemic heart disease are not inevitable features of aging."[28]

An Australian study, published in *Nutrition Reports International*, placed mature male marmoset monkeys on a vitamin C-deficient diet. Within 30 days, blood tests showed the monkeys had a 17.5 percent increase in serum cholesterol levels. When vitamin C was returned to the diet, cholesterol levels returned to normal, indicating that the changes were related to vitamin C intake.[29]

Vitamin C is essential for the formation of collagen protein in heart muscle tissue, just as it is necessary in other tissues. Dr. Sherry Lewin has explained: "Damage to the collagen matrix of the muscles may readily be rectified when a plentiful supply of ascorbate is available. Heart muscle stores less ascorbate than other tissues except plasma—but the need for plentiful supply of ascorbate appears to be met by the leucocytes in the abundant blood vessel distribution which pervades the heart muscles."

When heart muscle is damaged after a heart attack, vitamin C stores in other parts of the body dropped to scorbutic levels within 12 hours. Dr. Lewin and others believe this is an attempt to mobilize vitamin C to damaged tissue in an effort to speed healing. But it is also a time during which supplemental vitamin C is extremely important. With all tissue and blood levels of vitamin C reduced to a deficiency state, infections and other complications dim the prospects for recovery.[7,13]

VITAMIN C PREVENTS
SUDDEN INFANT DEATH SYNDROME

Sudden Infant Death Syndrome (SIDS) is a disease that kills 8,000 to 10,000 babies in the United States every year. It is a mysterious disease, attacking with little warning. Many causes of sudden infant death have been suggested, but only the one associated with vitamin C deficiency seems to be clearly demonstrated.

Twenty years ago, Dr. Archie Kalokerinos began working at a rural hospital in an isolated area of Australia. More than half the infants born died, and many of these displayed the now known characteristics of SIDS. Over a ten-year period, Dr. Kalokerinos began administering vitamin C to the infants, and the rate of infant death dropped. Except for easily diagnosed causes, infant death has ceased at this hospital.[5,30,31]

OTHER BENEFITS OF VITAMIN C

Countless other benefits of vitamin C have been observed and reported in the medical literature. As I noted earlier, approximately four thousand articles are published on vitamin C in medical journals each year, making it impossible to do more than greatly condense available information for this booklet.

Presented so far have been reports on the role of vitamin C in major diseases affecting Americans. Any disease is a major disease to the person affected by it, and, for this reason, the following paragraphs are brief reports on other important vitamin C research:

• Vitamin C benefits individuals suffering from all manner of allergies. Hayfever and other pollen allergies are especially amenable to vitamin C supplementation, but the dosage often has to be tailored to bowel tolerance. Vitamin C won't always cure a person of allergies, but it is extremely effective in suppressing symptoms. The allergic symptoms are relieved partly by the vitamin's antihistamine effect (without the dangers of other antihistamines) and partly by improving the immune system's regulatory mechanisms.[12,13,32]

• Vitamin C helps wounds heal more rapidly than they would otherwise—and the more vitamin C taken after an injury, the faster it will heal. Vitamin C, combined with vitamin E, can speed the healing of burns without the formation of painful scar tissue. Used postoperatively, it can reduce the time needed to recover. Taken regularly, it is capable of preventing shock (depression of body processes) should an injury occur suddenly.[3,5,12]

• Vitamin C offers protection against air pollution. It has been shown to reduce the carcinogenicity of more than 50 pollutants found in the air and water. If it is combined with vitamins A and E, protection against the effects of air pollution is multiplied.[11]

• Vitamin C inhibits carcinogens and other toxins found in food or produced in the digestive tract from foods and food additives. Among the most powerful carcinogens are nitrosamines. These are formed in the stomach when we eat processed meats that contain nitrites or nitrates. If vitamin C is present in the digestive tract at the same time as the food, nitrosamine formation is blocked. Many studies have also shown that vitamin C can block the effects of poisons—especially if tissues are saturated prior to poisoning.[33]

• Vitamin C offers protection against radiation. Cells exposed to x rays do not become cancerous when vitamin C is present. Researchers believe this may be because vitamin C slows the rate of cell division.[33,34]

• Vitamin C may prevent cancer by a newly hypothesized mechanism. Cancer cells tend to be deficient in prostaglandin E1. Vitamin C is necessary for the conversion of dihomogammalinoleic acid to prostaglandin E1. By enhancing the conversion with a diet high in vitamin C, risk of cancer may be reduced.[35]

• Vitamin C, along with niacin (B3) and other B vitamins, may benefit schizophrenics and other psychiatrically ill persons. Drs. Abram Hoffer and Humphry Osmond hypothesized nearly 40 years ago that an oxidized form of adrenalin triggered hallucinations in some schizophrenics. Vitamin C prevents the oxidation of adrenaline to adrenochrome, which is the body-produced hallucinogen. Although this theory of schizophrenia is not new, more recent research has confirmed the biochemical basis—leading to growing acceptance of a megavitamin treatment modality.[36]

• Vitamin C, along with vitamin B6, is useful in treating arthritic symptoms. Both vitamins are precursors to body-produced adrenaline and cortisone, which reduce arthritic symptoms. The vitamins are far safer than taking the synthetic analogs of adrenaline or cortisone.[37]

• Using vitamin C to increase our own production of adrenaline helps us combat a variety of physical and psychological stresses. The production of adrenaline is a stress-induced reaction, and we are under so much stress that, without vitamin C supplementation, we may develop symptoms of adrenal exhaustion.[37]

• Vitamin C improves the condition of alcoholics and drug addicts and often helps wean them from the object of their addiction. It is believed that vitamin C and narcotics compete for the same receptor sites in individual cells. If vitamin C bonds with that site, the narcotic cannot.[38]

• Vitamin C can, in some individuals, reduce the pain and discomfort of hemorrhoids. Hemorrhoids are distended blood vessels that develop near the anus and lower rectum, often as a result of straining during bowel movements. A common treatment for hemorrhoids is to soften stools so the patient does not have to strain. Regular vitamin C intake—below bowel tolerance doses—can maintain soft stools, without the side effects of laxatives. In addition, vitamin C will strengthen the walls of the veins near the anus and thereby reduce the tendency toward distention and possible clotting.[20]

VITAMIN C IS FOR EVERYONE

Vitamin C is so important to so many different biochemical activities in the human body that some physicians and researchers now question whether it is truly a vitamin. They believe that vitamin C approaches a hormone in activity and diverse effects, although the amount required is far greater than the typical hormone. This scientific discussion will continue for many years and is probably unimportant for most of us.

What is important is what we have learned about vitamin C since its discovery 60 years ago. Research on vitamin C seems to continue at an ever-increasing pace. Major discoveries were made in the 1970s. More were made in the 1980s, and we are still gaining a better understanding of why vitamin C supplementation results in dramatic and beneficial changes in our health. Vitamin C is necessary, albeit in very small amounts, simply to stay alive. Larger quantities make us resistant to both infections and degenerative diseases. Large amounts also protect us from a range of hazardous substances found in our modern environment.

Perhaps the most remarkable qualities of vitamin C are its inherent safety and its nonspecific nature. The reports that claimed vitamin C destroys vitamin B12 and causes kidney stones have been found to be without scientific basis. The other problem, diarrhea, can be controlled simply by adjusting the dosage. This is no more difficult than determining how much water quenches thirst.

Although vitamin C is active against specific infections when a person is ill, its real benefit derives from it being nonspecific when we take it on a daily basis. That gives us general protection against disease, and this is the way most physicians recommend vitamin C be taken. It is always far better to prevent than to dislodge a disease.

The true test is to begin taking supplemental vitamin C in addition to eating more foods that contain the vitamin. You'll find that you feel better and, logically, you're likely to continue doing what makes you feel better.

REFERENCES

The author wishes to thank Robert F. Cathcart, III, M.D., Irwin Stone, D.Sc., and the staff of the Linus Pauling Institute of Science and Medicine for their help in providing the information for this chapter.

NOTED REFERENCES

1. Pauling, Linus. 1970. *Vitamin C and the Common Cold*. San Francisco: W. H. Freeman & Company.
2. Pauling, Linus. October 25, 1980. Personal conversation.
3. Stone, Irwin. 1972. *The Healing Factor: Vitamin C Against Disease*. New York: Grosset & Dunlap.
4. Stone, Irwin. June 15, 1980. Homo sapiens ascorbicus: the profile for health in the 21st century. Paper given at the International Symposium on the Conquest of Cancer, San Diego, CA.

5. Stone, Irwin. 1978. Sudden death: a look back from ascorbate's 50th anniversary. *Journal of the International Academy of Preventive Medicine* vol. 5, no. 1.

6. Kutsky, Roman J. 1973. *Handbook of Vitamins and Hormones.* New York: Van Nostrand Reinhold Company.

7. Lewin, Sherry. 1976. *Vitamin C: Its Molecular Biology and Medical Potential.* London: Academic Press.

8. *Medical World News*, November 23, 1981.

9. Stone, Irwin. 1980. The possible role of mega-ascorbate in the endogenous synthesis of interferon. *Medical Hypotheses*, vol. 6.

10. Stone, Irwin. November-December 1980. Inexpensive interferon therapy of cancer and the viral diseases now. *Nutritional Consultants*. December 1980.

11. Cameron, Ewan and Pauling, Linus. 1979. *Cancer and Vitamin C.* The Linus Pauling Institute.

12. Cathcart, Robert F., III. 1981. Vitamin C, titrating to bowel tolerance, anascorbemia, and acute induced scurvy. *Medical Hypotheses* vol. 7.

13. Cathcart, Robert F., III. February 13, 1982. Personal conversation.

14. Cathcart, Robert F., III. May 11, 1982. Personal conversation.

15. Cameron, Ewan and Pauling, Linus. 1973. Ascrobic acid and the glycosaminoglycans. *Oncology* vol. 27.

16. Murad, S. *et al.* 1981. Regulation of collagen synthesis by ascorbic acid. *Proceedings of the National Academy of Sciences of the United States of America.*

17. Cameron, Ewan. 1966. *Hyaluronidase and Cancer.* Elmsford, NY: Pergamon Press.

18. Cameron, Ewan and Pauling, Linus. 1974. The orthomolecular treatment of cancer. *Chem.-Biol. Interactions* vol. 9.

19. Pauling, Linus. 1980. Vitamin C and cancer. *The Linus Pauling Institute of Science Newsletter* vol. 1, no. 2.

20. Pauling, Linus. 1980. A Report on "Cancer Dialogue '80." *The Linus Pauling Institute of Science and Medicine Newsletter*, vol. 1, no. 10.

21. Challem, Jack J. March 1981. Recent developments on vitamin C: an exclusive interview with Dr. Linus Pauling. *Let's Live.*

22. Cameron, Ewan and Pauling, Linus. 1977. Vitamin C and cancer. *International Journal of Environmental Studies* vol. 10.

23. *Proceedings of the First International Conference on the Modulation and Mediation of Cancer by Vitamins.* University of Arizona, Tucson, February 23–26, 1982.

24. Research on vitamin-cancer relationship getting big boost. *Journal of the American Medical Association*, April 2, 1982.

25. Primate studies indicate that subclinical and acute vitamin C deficiency may lead to periodontal disease. *Journal of the American Medical Association*, August 14, 1982.

26. *Journal of Oral Pathology*. 1981. vol. 10.

27. *Medical World News*, September 13, 1974.

28. *Journal of Human Nutrition*. 1981. vol. 35, no. 1.

29. McIntosh, G. H. 1981. Vitamin C deficiency and hypercholesterolaemia in marmoset monkeys. *Nutrition Reports International*.

30. Kalokerinos, A. 1980. *Every Second Child*. New Canaan, Connecticut: Keats Publishing.

31. Stone, Irwin. September 1981. Personal conversation.

32. Kirschmann, John D. 1979. *Nutrition Almanac*. New York: McGraw-Hill Book Company.

33. Cameron, Ewan. March 1979. Ascrobic acid and cancer: a review. *Cancer Research* vol. 39.

34. *International Journal of Vitamin and Nutrition Research*. 1981. vol. 51, no. 2.

35. Horrobin, D. F. 1979. Vitamin C and prostaglandins. *Medical Hypotheses* vol. 5.

36. Hawkins, David and Pauling, Linus. 1973. *Orthomolecular Psychiatry*. San Francisco: W. H. Freeman and Company.

37. Atkins, Robert C. 1981. *Dr. Atkins' Nutrition Breakthrough: How to Treat Your Medical Condition Without Drugs*. New York: Bantam Books.

38. Libby, Alfred F. 1982. A study indicating a connection between paranoia, schizophrenia, perceptual disorders, and I.Q. in alcohol and drug abusers. *Journal of Orthomolecular Psychiatry* vol. 11, no. 1.

The Last Word on Vitamin C from Its Foremost Advocate

Vitamins C, E and beta-carotene decrease the probability of cancer.

For over twenty years the Linus Pauling Institute of Science and Medicine in Palo Alto, California has been studying the effect of vitamins upon illness and well-being.

"The whole idea that the optimum intake of vitamin C, perhaps 100 times the usually recommended intake (the RDA), might have great value in reducing the amount of human suffering was very appealing to me," Linus Pauling said, shortly before his death in 1994, about his decision to found the Institute in 1973.

LPI examined the effect of vitamin C in particular on a tremendous variety of conditions, from the common cold virus to cancer, and even its uses in preventing a paralyzing disease called neurolathyrism that is common in India, Bangladesh and Ethiopia.

"For many years one of our main efforts has been to get information about the value of vitamin C for preventing cancer and, as an adjunct to appropriate conventional therapy, in the treatment of cancer," Pauling continued.

"During the last few years it has been accepted generally that an intake of vitamin C, vitamin E and beta-carotene decreases the probability that cancer will strike. Moreover, valuable information about high-dose vitamin C in improving the well-being and increasing the survival time for patients with advanced cancer was obtained by our collaborator, Dr. Ewan Cameron in Vale of Leven Hospital, Scotland, later by Dr. Fukumi Morishige in Fukuoka, Japan, and Dr. Abram Hoffer in Victoria, British Columbia."

In recent years, Dr. Pauling added, another program utilizing vitamin C was begun, to determine the relationship between vitamin C intake and other substances in relation to heart disease, stroke and atherosclerosis.

In a study done by Dr. Matthias Rath in collaboration with Pauling, Dr. Rath discovered that one of the constituents of blood, lipoprotein (a), is the lipoprotein particle containing cholesterol that is deposited in the arteries, causing atherosclerosis and other forms of cardiovascular disease and strokes.

Furthermore, the scientists found that there is a relationship between vitamin C and lipoprotein (a), suggesting that an increased intake of vitamin C can "have great value in preventing atherosclerosis and controlling heart disease." This study is continuing.

What is the latest on vitamin C and that universal scourge, the cold? Vitamin C "has consistently decreased the duration of cold episode and the severity of symptoms," according to Professor Harri Hemila of the University of Helsinki in Finland.

Recommendations from the LPI are: "At the first sign of a cold, a person should take one or two grams of vitamin C, followed by similar doses every half hour or hour until symptoms disappear."

Pauling practiced what he preached, and now gerontologists are confirming that vitamin C can lengthen lives: "People who over the years have had large doses of vitamin C seem to live longer," said Ruth B. Weg, Ph.D. of the University of Southern California in Los Angeles.

"And Pauling also found that megadoses of vitamin C and other micronutrients improve the way people feel—which to me is much more significant than how long they're breathing," she concluded.

VITAMIN E

*New Roles for the Vitamin
That Preserves the Health and Integrity
of Body Cells*

LEN MERVYN, PH.D.

VITAMIN E—A PROTECTIVE FORCE

For decades accepted as merely an antioxidant, vitamin E's capacities has been increasingly recognized until it is now firmly established as a protective force in natural therapy. It is used by surgeons before and after operations to ensure against thrombosis and increase immunity to infection, by pediatricians to prevent blindness in premature babies and by other specialists to increase high-density lipoproteins. It decreases elevated hormone levels and prevents and treats anemias and cystic breast disease. Vitamin E has just begun to act.

It is not some 70 years since vitamin E was discovered and characterized, yet its functions, and even more its therapeutic uses, are still controversial in the scientific and medical fraternities. There are only three special situations where it is generally accepted that supplementary vitamin E has proved to be beneficial.

The first is in treating hemolytic anemia in newborn infants. Vitamin E is not actively transported from the maternal to the fetal circulation, and it is poorly absorbed by those infants whose gestational age is less than 36 weeks. A deficiency of tocopherol (vitamin E) causes hemolytic anemia and widespread edema, two conditions that are reversed by vitamin E treatment.

The second is in treating deficiencies caused by the malabsorption of fats and oils since vitamin E is an oil.

Cystic fibrosis is invariably associated with vitamin E deficiency. Di Sant'Agnese's group at Bethesda (Farrell, 1977) showed that most nonsupplemented patients suffering from cystic fibrosis are so deficient in vitamin E that their red blood cells are inadequately protected against oxidative stresses. Other conditions giving rise to malabsorption of fats and oils with subsequent vitamin E deficiency include liver cirrhosis, obstructive jaundice, pancreatic insufficiency and sprue. H. J. Binder and H. M. Shapiro (1967) studied patients with malabsorption problems and vitamin E deficiency and were able to relate this deficiency to the patients' long-term inability to absorb fats.

A study of any modern medical textbook will indicate that the only accepted therapy with vitamin E for a condition unrelated to fat absorption is for the treatment of intermittent claudication. This represents the third situation. Intermittent claudication is the term for calf pains when walking. It is caused by a narrowing of the arteries supplying blood to the leg muscles. The restricted blood supply gives rise to pain as the muscles become starved of oxygen. There are many publications in the world's medical press confirming the excellent response of this condition to vitamin E. Typical is that of K. Haeger (1974) who performed a double-blind study to show the benefits of vitamin E in this condition. The treatment requires 400 mg or more of vitamin E daily, and therapy must continue for at least three months.

Over the last few years we have become more aware of how vitamin E functions. This in turn has indicated how the vitamin might be used in treating certain clinical conditions whose etiology is related to abnormalities in those functions. The result is that it now looks likely that vitamin E may be beneficial in treating diseases in addition to those mentioned above. The evidence for such therapy will now be reviewed.

HOW VITAMIN E FUNCTIONS
AND PROTECTS

In humans, the only generally accepted role of vitamin E is a protective one, that of acting as an antioxidant in preserving the health and integrity of body cells and membranes. Biological membranes contain phospholipids, and degradation of these by oxygen can cause loss of cell integrity. Phospholipids contain high quantities of polyunsaturated fatty acids (PUFA) and the double bonds of these acids are easily attacked by oxygen to produce the toxic fatty peroxides The extent of formation of peroxides (i.e., peroxidation) increases with the number of double bonds in the fatty acids of the phospholipids, so membranes with a high PUFA content are especially likely to become oxidized. A common example of peroxidation is the rancidity of butter and vegetable oils. Vitamin E prevents this action of oxygen on the double bonds, possibly by inhibiting the enzyme catalyzing it, and so acts as a protective antioxidant.

Other agents produced both within and outside the body cells are the so-called free radicals. These substances are highly reactive because they are chemically incomplete and hence unstable, so they can latch onto other substances very readily. Some are known also as superoxide radicals, and they are produced within cells both by self-oxidation (as in peroxides) and by enzymatic processes. Their high intrinsic reactivity and their ability to generate even more potent oxidizing agents when combined with peroxides constitute a constant threat to cellular integrity. Free radicals do perform some useful functions, for example, during the bactericidal action of white blood cells and in mediating the inflammatory response.

However, it is when they are produced in large quantity and their metabolic products allowed to go unchecked that they can seriously damage membranes and even denature or disrupt DNA.

Since free radicals are continually being generated, the human body has developed a number of mechanisms to deal with their potentially damaging effects and those of their metabolites. The cellular

defense mechanisms involve various enzymes such as superoxide dismutase, glutathione synthetase, glutathione peroxidase, glutathione
reductase, glucose-6-phosphate dehydrogenase and catalase. Plasma
proteins with antioxidant potential include the copper-containing ce-
ruloplasmin and the iron-containing transferrin. Food constituents
that also contribute to protection include the sulphur-containing
amino acids, the minerals selenium, zinc and copper and the vitamins
riboflavin (vitamin B2) and tocopherol (vitamin E). The most widely
studied protective agent in recent years, however, is vitamin E, and
it now looks as if this vitamin plays this key role, either directly or
indirectly through the other agents. Ever since its discovery many
clinical claims have been attributed to vitamin E. Now these empiric
observations are finding a basis in sound biochemical functioning
that places vitamin E firmly in an essential and established protective role.

The susceptibility of any tissue to an oxidative stress induced by
free radicals or peroxide relates to the balance between the extent of
that stress and the antioxidant ability of the protective agents. Where
the tissue is genetically defective in its ability to provide protection,
giving extra quantities of the protective agents can go part of the way
in overcoming the defect. Hence, once we recognize the biological
antioxidant property of vitamin E, it is possible to equate the conditions where it is beneficial to the doses required for efficacy.

First, there are those conditions which relate to a simple deficiency
state. These include the hemolytic anemia of low-birthweight infants;
the shortening of red blood cell life in those suffering from cystic
fibrosis; the high tendency of blood platelets to aggregate in patients
with biliary atresia; the lack of growth and the brain dysfunctions that
occur in abetalipoproteinemia where essential plasma lipoproteins
are absent.

Second, there are those conditions where there is no evidence of
deficiency of the vitamin, but nevertheless large doses appear to prevent the effects of an oxidative assault. The prime example here is
the success of vitamin E in preventing or reducing the severity of
retrolental fibroplasia (producing blindness) in premature infants who

have been exposed to high oxygen intake for the treatment of respiratory distress.

The third category includes conditions where frank pharmacological doses of the vitamin have been employed. There is no sign of a deficiency, but there appears to be some preexisting defect in the body's defense mechanisms against free radicals. The diseases that respond are usually related to specific enzyme deficiencies, and the common factor is a hemolytic anemia or sickle-cell anemia.

All the above categories relate to the action of vitamin E in protecting against excessive oxidation stress or free-radical production. There are, however, also reports on how the vitamin has helped in overcoming blood vessel thromboses, blood platelet dysfunctions, atherosclerosis and breast tumors and cysts. It appears also to exert an influential effect upon the ability to resist infection (immune responses). Perhaps these benefits also relate to its antioxidant and protective role, but the evidence is not clearcut. What we shall do now is to review critically the evidence that once more puts vitamin E into the forefront of natural therapy. At the same time our increasing knowledge of how vitamin E functions indicates why it may help in therapy, and this too will be discussed.

THE PREVENTION OF THROMBOSIS

Thrombosis is the formation of a thrombus, defined in medical dictionaries as a clot of blood formed within the heart or blood vessels, usually due to a slowing of the circulation or to alteration of the blood or vessel walls. The coronary arteries supply blood and hence oxygen to the heart muscle itself, allowing the organ to function effectively. There are two types of coronary heart disease: (1) that due to partial or total blockage of the artery by a blood clot (coronary thrombosis); and (2) that due to deposition of fats onto the artery wall (atherosclerosis), which also leads to constriction of the blood flow. Research indicates that vitamin E can help prevent and in some cases reverse these two conditions.

During the 1940s, the Shute brothers, in their practice in Canada, noted that vitamin E both dissolved fresh preformed blood clots and prevented their formation. They believed the vitamin exerted its action by inhibiting the protein thrombin which normally functions as a blood clot inducer. Normally, this is a natural defense to prevent excessive bleeding when a blood vessel is damaged. However, sometimes the process gets out of hand, and a thrombus forms for no apparent reason, with serious manifestations.

During the 1950s further studies were published in the *Journal of the American Medical Association* on the importance of vitamin E in dissolving and preventing blood clots. In 1964 Dr. Alton Ochsner and his group published confirmatory studies in the *New England Journal of Medicine* and stated that "alpha tocopherol is a potent inhibitor of thrombin that does not produce excessive bleeding and is therefore a safe preventative agent against thrombosis."

Studies reported in the late 1970s gave a clearer insight into how a thrombus is formed, how platelets, the tiny white blood cells, contribute to this, and how the whole process may be controlled. It now seems as if vitamin E plays a prominent part in preventing platelet aggregation.

The first thing that happens when a blood vessel wall is damaged is that the blood platelets collect around the affected area, change shape and form aggregates. Red blood cells become enmeshed in the platelet aggregate and thicken it. The cell aggregates in turn are held together by the precipitation from the blood plasma of the protein fibrin which forms a network. The final result is a large, stable thrombus which may eventually occlude the blood vessel.

What makes platelets aggregate is their stickiness, and this in turn is controlled by certain hormones that are normally produced within the body. It is the production and balance of these hormones that determine the aggregation of platelets. They are known as prostaglandins, and they, in turn, are influenced by vitamin E.

The material from which prostaglandins are made is an essential polyunsaturated fatty acid called arachidonic, itself manufactured from linoleic acid. This gives rise to an important hormone called prostacyclin, produced by the blood vessel walls. It is also released by the lungs and other tissues and acts in the blood, constantly preventing platelets from sticking to vessel walls. Prostacyclin is the most potent inhibitor of platelet aggregation known and it also acts as a vasodilator, that is, keeps blood vessels open. However, from the same precursor, arachidonic acid, another hormone called thromboxane is produced. This is formed solely by the platelets, and it has an action directly opposite that of prostacyclin. It causes platelets to aggregate and blood vessels to narrow; in other words it is a vasoconstrictor. Hence the stickiness of the platelets and the ability to form blood clots or thrombi depends on the balance between the opposite effects of prostacyclin and thromboxane. Both hormones are unstable, breaking down into inert compounds. Prostacyclin is the "good" hormone, thromboxane the "bad" one, and an imbalance in favor of thromboxane could well contribute to a heart attack or stroke.

We have seen that arachidonic acid is the precursor of both prostacyclin and thromboxane, but at the same time there are alternative metabolic pathways for this highly unsaturated acid.

It can be oxidized by an enzyme called lipoxygenase to form hydroperoxy acids or peroxides. This process is similar to the oxidation that takes place to such acids left unprotected by antioxidants in the air outside the body. Hydroperoxy acids are highly undesirable since they are toxic to membranes and cells in a manner akin to rancidity in exposed fats. Hence any nutrient that prevents overproduction of hydroperoxy acids, either directly or through the enzyme that produces them, would be expected to be beneficial to health.

In two important papers from Ohio State University, D. Cornwell (1979) and E. T. Gwebu (1980) reported that vitamin E inhibits the platelet enzyme lipoxygenase in rabbits. Platelets from rabbits supplemented with vitamin E had much less lipoxygenase activity than platelets from vitamin E-deficient or normal rabbits. Extension of the studies to human platelets indicated that preincubation with the vitamin reduced the enzyme activity significantly. The importance of this finding was emphasized in Cornwell's paper; his studies suggested that the proliferation of smooth muscle cells of the aorta is controlled in part by the oxidant stress supplied by the hydroperoxy fatty acids produced by the enzyme lipoxygenase. Rapidly proliferating cells are resistant to peroxidation and hence desirable, and vitamin E stimulates cell proliferation by inhibiting the enzyme. This in turn prevents the formation of a fatty streak in the aorta which is a prerequisite of atherogenic plaque formation.

Hydroperoxy fatty acids are undesirable in other ways, according to publications by W. Forster (1980). These compounds actually inhibit the action of prostacyclin, the "good" hormone that prevents platelet aggregation. Hence any factor that reduces the level of hydroperoxy fatty acids will enable prostacyclin to function effectively. Forster was unable to show a direct effect of vitamin E on prostacyclin synthesis, but what he did demonstrate in his experimental rabbits was that pretreatment with vitamin E (1) inhibited the enzyme lipoxygenase and hence the formation of hydroperoxy acids and (2) inhibited the formation of the "bad" hormone thromboxane. Beneficial effects of vitamin E on inhibition of thrombus formation must therefore lie with its ability to prevent excessive production of the "bad" prostaglandin and its removal of the substances that inhibit the "good" prostaglandin.

Other reports have studied the effect of intravenous arachidonic acid on the blood of rabbits. This acid is a potent platelet aggregating agent, and when injected into the bloodstream of the rabbit it causes vasoconstriction and massive thrombus formations in the blood vessels and organs, killing the animal. Presumably the effect is due to a combination of overproduction of hydroperoxy acids which inhibit prostacyclin, and excessive synthesis of thromboxane. We thus have a useful test system to study the effect of antithrombotic drugs.

M. Barrett and S. O'Regan (1980) used this test system to study the effect of vitamin E. When the vitamin, at an intravenous dose of 150 mg/kg body weight, was given five minutes before the lethal dose of arachidonic acid, it prevented death of the rabbits. There was no deposition of thrombi or blood clots in the organs where they would be expected from injection of arachidonic acid alone. They suggest that "vitamin E succeeds in arresting and inhibiting completely the pathological cascade initiated by arachidonic acid infusion."

Much effort was put into ways of stabilizing prostacyclin so that it could be used as a drug to prevent and treat thrombosis and related diseases. Clinical reports indicated that prostacyclin was beneficial in the successful therapy of advanced arteriosclerosis. However, because of its instability the prostaglandin had to be infused into the blood-stream continuously for three days. Nevertheless, the patients involved continued to derive clinical benefit for a further six weeks (A. Szczeklik et al., 1979). All of the studies on vitamin E suggest that it is a natural substance that can exert the same beneficial effects as prostacyclin. How much simpler it is to ensure an adequate daily intake of the vitamin throughout life.

ATHEROSCLEROSIS

Atherosclerosis is a complex and multifactorial disorder which implies the presence of multiple risk factors. No matter what the cause, however, the end result is an invasion of the inner blood vessel wall by fats and cholesterol resulting in the deposition of atheromatous plaques. These plaques decrease the elasticity of the blood vessel wall and also thicken it, reducing the width of the blood vessel and restricting blood flow. Not all atheromatous plaques contain cholesterol but it is generally believed that a high blood cholesterol is more conducive to their development.

Before we look at the therapeutic role of vitamin E in preventing and treating atherosclerosis, it is necessary to review what we know about blood cholesterol. At a Washington symposium on March 24, 1981, Dr. Bryan Brewer of the National Heart, Lung and Blood Institute reported on the role of dietary cholesterol and fat in the development of heart disease. In the United States, heart attacks occur every 20 seconds and are a major cause of death. Factors in premature heart attack (before age 65) include high blood pressure, high blood cholesterol levels and smoking. Risk increases from low to high levels of these factors in a smooth progression.

Cholesterol is a fatty substance with distinct biochemical functions that are essential to the working of the body. Triglycerides are fats and oils containing three fatty acids, each of which may be saturated or unsaturated, combined with glycerol. Cholesterol and triglycerides cannot be dissolved or transported as such in plasma. They are carried by proteins and the protein-fat complex is called a lipoprotein. It is the way in which cholesterol and fats are carried in the plasma that determines to a large extent whether they are likely to be deposited on the blood vessel walls or not.

The four major groups of lipoproteins are characterized by density and size. They may be thought of as globules ranging from big light globules down to small heavy ones. The largest are called chylomicrons, and this is the form in which fat is absorbed from the diet. The next two smaller globules are known as Very Low Density Lipoproteins (VLDL) and Low Density Lipoproteins (LDL). The smallest and most dense globules are called High Density Lipoproteins (HDL). Each lipoprotein has a particular function, but the important feature is the proportion of each that is present in plasma.

When cholesterol and triglycerides are eaten, they are reduced to globule size (chylomicrons) and transported from the intestine to the liver. In the liver they are transferred to VLDL, then transported from that organ to other parts of the body. However, those destined for muscle cells are transported there by LDL. The reverse process from body cells back to the liver involves carriage by HDL. The only way excess cholesterol in the body can be disposed of is by the liver. This organ converts it to bile salts, which are eventually excreted via the bile and feces.

High plasma cholesterol is a risk factor for coronary heart disease, but the risk is primarily associated with LDL. In contrast, HDL has a protective effect against heart disease. Hence HDL is the "good" form of cholesterol, probably because high levels of it result in a more efficient removal of excess body cholesterol from body cells.

Vitamin E can influence cholesterol metabolism in two ways. First, it appears to actually decrease blood cholesterol levels. Second, it can alter the proportion of the various density lipoproteins to favor an increase in the good HDL. The animal model for studying cholesterol metabolism is usually the rabbit, and many studies have indicated a beneficial effect of vitamin E.

Typical is the report by R. B. Wilson et al. (1978), who compared vitamin E with synthetic antioxidants. Rabbits were fed an atherosclerosis-producing diet consisting of high butter intakes. There were three groups of animals on the diet: one group received supplementary vitamin E (equivalent to 400 IU per day in humans); a second group was given BHA (butylated hydroxyanisole), a synthetic antioxidant much used in foods and drugs; and the third group was fed the basal diet. After three years on the diets, it was found that aortic and coronary atherosclerosis were less frequent and less extensive in rabbits supplemented with vitamin E than in those fed the basal diet or the one supplemented with BHA. Measurement of blood levels of cholesterol over the three years indicated that these were lower in the vitamin E-treated animals. Prevention of hypercholesterolemia was regarded as the main factor in inhibiting atherosclerosis.

Human studies confirming the effect of vitamin E in reducing blood cholesterol levels were reported by M. Passeri and U. Butturini, of the University of Parma, Italy, in a 1981 international symposium in Madrid. They point out, however, that although vitamin E alone has this beneficial effect at the 300–400 IU per day intake, a synergistic action with adequate intakes of vitamin A and C is probably more efficient.

In a personal report Dr. W. J. Hermann (1979) claimed that when he took 600 IU of d-alpha tocopherol acetate (natural vitamin E) daily for 30 days, the proportion of HDL cholesterol in his blood plasma increased dramatically from 9 percent to 40 percent. He then repeated this dosage regime on ten volunteers, five of whom had normal blood plasma lipoprotein profiles and five who had low HDL cholesterol levels. After one month's supplementation with daily 600 IU of vitamin E, there was a change in the proportion of HDL cholesterol present. The normal group showed a 50 percent increase in HDL cholesterol, but most significant was the 200 percent increase in the proportion of HDL cholesterol in the other group. In no case was there a significant change in total plasma cholesterol.

These findings were not confirmed in another study, reported by L. Hatam and H. Kayden (1981). These researchers found no effect of vitamin E on the distribution of cholesterol in various lipoproteins, but they were using different analytical techniques. The main objection to this study was in the choice of subjects, over half of whom had higher than normal HDL cholesterol levels anyway, so that any increase in them would be minimal. Differences in subject age and the prevalence of obesity may also account for the variations in response in both studies.

Further studies from other groups that were reported in 1982 also give variable results, indicating that there was no clearcut conclusion at that time to be drawn about the beneficial effect of vitamin E on HDL cholesterol levels. (See summary for the latest research on vitamin E and cholesterol.) Joseph J. Barboriak (1982), from the Medical College of Wisconsin, gave 43 subjects a total of 800 IU of alpha tocopherol daily for four weeks. Male patients with spinal cord injuries were included, since as a group such patients have low HDL cholesterol levels. Some of the men who were joggers or long-distance runners had unusually high initial levels of HDL cholesterol, while others had low levels. Administration of vitamin E for four weeks "resulted in a statistically significant increase of plasma HDL cholesterol levels" in men who had low initial levels and in women. The levels decreased after vitamin E was discontinued. The results were claimed to have "confirmed the initial report by Hermann (1980) that the effect of alpha tocopherol is primarily seen in subjects with low initial HDL cholesterol levels."

Donald R. Howard (1982) from the Maine Medical Center claimed he was unable to repeat the beneficial effects of vitamin E reported by Hermann. A total of 39 normal volunteers were given 600 IU of dl-alpha tocopherol daily for 30 days. There was no significant change in HDL cholesterol. As in previous studies, it looks as if differences in response to vitamin E may be explained by variation in the choice of subjects for study. Normal, healthy subjects are likely to have the right proportion of HDL cholesterol in their plasma; therefore vitamin E is unlikely to change this significantly. It is only where there is a prevalence of the LDL cholesterol that the vitamin is likely to redress the balance in favor of HDL cholesterol.

It is highly probable that vitamin E is not the only factor that determines the proportion of the "good" HDL cholesterol in the blood. Other experiments (F. Yokata, 1981) indicate that in vitamin C deficiency, the level of HDL cholesterol is low. Once vitamin C is given there is a dramatic increase in HDL cholesterol. Hence any trial where only one factor is studied in isolation may give variable results. The moral of this work seems to ensure an adequate intake of vitamin E to keep HDL cholesterol levels up but at the same time make certain that vitamin C and vitamin A intakes are sufficient for complete inhibition of atherosclerosis.

Although we should therefore aim at increasing the proportion of HDL cholesterol in the blood, it must be remembered that low-density lipoproteins have other functions and that they are essential, albeit in lower concentration. When low-density lipoproteins are absent, the result is a rare hereditary disease called abetalipoproteinemia or acanthocytosis. This is related to very low levels of vitamin E in the blood, due mainly to malabsorption. Growth failure is prominent in childhood. In adolescence neurological abnormality results in progressive disability. Death may occur in early adult life, usually from cardiac involvement. There is no medical treatment available.

However, a report by E. Azizi et al. (1978) offers some hope to those suffering from the disease. An 11-year-old girl with the disease was treated with vitamins A and E via the intramuscular route, once a week for two and a half years. This was essential because of the inability of the child to absorb the vitamins from the intestinal system.

Some improvements in the neurological and visual deficiencies were noted. In the words of the authors, "On changing to oral vitamin E and later with addition of medium chain triglycerides (simple fats) to the diet, a considerable improvement in general well-being, neuromuscular lesions and ophthalmological symptoms was noted." At the time of the report this regime had lasted 67 months and the condition of the girl was regarded as stable.

THROMBOPHLEBITIS

Thrombophlebitis is most simply defined as a thrombus or blood clot in a vein surrounded by an area of inflammation. Although usually occurring in the legs, it is possible for bits of the thrombus to break off and lodge in the arteries of the lung. The resulting pulmonary embolism then becomes a life-threatening situation. Surgery is one of the main stimulants of thrombi; therefore their prevention during any operative procedure becomes of prime importance. Vitamin E has long been advocated as the simplest and most efficient tool in preventing thrombus formation.

One of the main proponents for the prevention of thromboembolic disease by vitamin E is Dr. Alton Ochsner (1968) who stated: "For 15 years I have used alpha tocopherol routinely in the treatment of patients who have been subjected to trauma of any magnitude. None of these patients have had pulmonary embolism." His supplementary regime consisted of giving between 200 and 600 IU of alpha tocopherol daily, either by intramuscular injection or by mouth, beginning no later than the day of surgery (but preferably before) and continuing through the postoperative period. In addition, calcium gluconate was given intravenously (10 ml of a 10 percent solution every 24 or 48 hours). The calcium was an essential part of the treatment.

In a later publication Drs. J. D. and P. B. Kanofsky (1981) reviewed six clinical trials from American and British literature that compared vitamin E–calcium-treated groups with controls in the prevention of thrombi. None used a double-blind design, which meant that there was the possibility of diagnosis of deep vein thrombosis or pulmonary embolism by clinicians who may have been influenced by bias. Nevertheless, the authors concluded that in the control groups, failure to use the vitamin E-calcium treatment doubled the risk of peripheral venous thrombosis; increased the risk of pulmonary embolism sixfold; and increased the chances of fatal pulmonary embolism ninefold. It is believed that vitamin E has this beneficial effect because, as we have seen previously, it appears to inhibit platelet aggregation—an important factor in the formation of a thrombus. Experimental evidence has come from studies on pigs, where inadequate levels of vitamin E were found to induce the formation of vascular thrombosis.

Dr. H. J. Roberts (1978) has refuted the alleged beneficial action of vitamin E in suppressing thrombosis. He has noted that in ten years of patient observation, 46 individuals who were taking high doses (i.e., more than 400 IU daily) of alpha tocopherol had suspected or diagnosed thrombophlebitis. The symptoms of this complaint included discomfort of the lower limbs, with or without edema, and tenderness in the calves and thighs. These complaints disappeared when vitamin E supplementation was stopped and reappeared in two cases when vitamin E was resumed. Pulmonary embolism was confirmed as highly suspect in 57 percent of the patients.

He concludes that vitamin E may encourage thrombosis in patients who already have metabolic cardiovascular or hormonal disorders which predispose to small-vessel disease, platelet aggregation and thrombosis, especially if estrogens (as, for example, in the contraceptive pill) are being taken.

There could be a number of reasons for these opposing claims for the connection between vitamin E and thrombophlebitis. Roberts was merely making observations on patients who claimed to take vitamin E; the trials reported by Kanofsky were controlled studies. The latter trials also used calcium along with the vitamin E, and this mineral could have played an important role.

It may also be expected that in view of the widespread use of high doses of tocopherol in the world, its adverse effects should occur more often than they do.

VITAMIN E AS A THERAPEUTIC AGENT

ANEMIA

One of the few generally recognized uses for vitamin E is in the treatment of hemolytic anemia in premature babies. Hemolytic anemia is characterized by a shortened life of the red blood cell and an increased tendency for it to burst. Once the contents have been released, the hemoglobin is unable to function as an oxygen carrier and the number of red blood cells available is reduced, resulting in the typical symptoms of anemia. A consequence of the shortened survival time of red blood cells in preterm infants is an increase in the blood level of bilirubin. This is a bile pigment which is an excretion product from the disposal of hemoglobin, and in excess it leads to jaundice of the newborn. Bilirubinemia is usually treated in babies by photo-therapy, exposing the child to special sources of light until the level of bilirubin is reduced to normal levels. It is not clear how such phototherapy functions. However, S. J. Gross (1979) studied some forty infants, some of whom were under 1500 grams in weight, and showed that administering vitamin E during the first three days of life enabled the time of phototherapy to be reduced from an average of 107 hours to only 48.

There is a poor transfer of vitamin E from mother to fetus across the placenta so that both premature and full-term newborn babies may have relatively low levels of vitamin E in both tissues and blood. The blood plasma levels of the vitamin in newborn infants average about 15 mg/liter, which is only half that found in normal adults.

The need for supplemental vitamin E in the newborn has been widely recognized, particularly in the premature infant. Human milk is sufficiently rich in vitamin E to satisfy the baby's needs, but cow's milk, frequently used in bottle feeding, contains much smaller amounts. There are numerous studies indicating that vitamin E reduces the hemolysis of the red blood cells of preterm infants (e.g., Graeber, Williams and Oski, 1977). However, recent clinical trials have shown that even in adults certain types of hemolytic anemia respond favorably to vitamin E treatment. This represents a significant step forward in the therapy of an hitherto incurable disease.

Two rare hereditary red blood cell disorders, glutathione synthetase deficiency and chronic hemolytic glucose-6-phosphate dehydrogenase deficiency, are characterized by compromised intracellular reductive capacity and decreased red blood cell survival. The first-named condition is thought to result from inadequate glutathione synthesis during oxidative stress leading to denaturation of hemoglobin and premature removal of affected red blood cells. In the second condition there is lowered production of reduced nicotinamide adenine dinucleotide phosphate (NADPH), leading in turn to decreases in glutathione synthesis, so the end result is similar in both hereditary diseases. Vitamin E in high oral doses (800 IU per day) improved red blood cell survival in both of these disorders. Hence a similar trial was performed with 23 patients suffering from Mediterranean glucose-6-phosphate dehydrogenase deficiency and reported by L. Corash and colleagues (1980) and F. A. Oski (1980).

Three months of vitamin E administration at the dosage of four 200 mg chewable tablets given at one time resulted in decreased chronic hemolysis as evidenced by improved red-cell life span, increased hemoglobin concentration of the blood and decreased reticulocystosis (a measure of red cell production) as compared to baseline values. "Evaluation after one year of vitamin E administration demonstrated sustained improvement in all these indices." Further evidence is required of longer term administration of vitamin E in these disorders, especially the effects at times of hemolytic crises, to determine whether vitamin E has a therapeutic role in this group of blood disorders, but preliminary results are encouraging. Confirmation has now come from European studies.

A related anemia is beta thalassemia or Mediterranean anemia. It is a congenital anemia occurring in populations from countries bordering the Mediterranean and from southeast Asia, and it is characterized by defective hemoglobin synthesis and by ineffective red blood cell formation. Heterozygous beta thalassemia is known as thalassemia minor and is usually asymptomatic, but typical symptoms occur in homozygotes (thalassemia major). In thalassemia major low serum alpha tocopherol levels are usually found. Treatment with the vitamin results in increased blood levels, decreased lipid peroxidation and in some cases prolonged red blood cell survival (Rachilewitz, Shifter and Kahane, 1980).

The treatment of thalassemia minor with vitamin E was reported by R. Miniero and associates (1981) from the University of Turin, Italy at an international symposium. Ten patients were evaluated to determine if vitamin E could reduce oxidative stress and improve anemia. For three months each patient received between 400 and 600 IU vitamin E daily by mouth. In half of them, biochemical parameters showed a reduction of lipid peroxidation and increased red blood cell survival. These encouraging results are being used as a basis for a larger scale study of the benefits of vitamin E in treating beta thalassemia.

There is also preliminary evidence that vitamin E can help in treating sickle-cell anemia. D. Chiv and B. Lubin (1979) found that patients with this disorder have low levels of vitamin E in their blood plasma and red cells. These people appear to have an increased susceptibility of their red blood cells to peroxidation which was corrected in *in vitro* experiments by vitamin E. Confirmation that treating patients with sickle-cell anemia with 450 IU of dl-alpha tocopherol daily reduced the number of irreversibly sickled cells that were circulating comes from studies reported by C. L. Natta (1980). The number of sickle cells in the bloodstream is related to the extent of hemolysis of the blood, so any reduction is beneficial. Prolonged administration of vitamin E is now being investigated to see if it will alleviate other aspects of the clinical condition as a result of a reduction in circulating sickle cells.

THE PREVENTION OF BLINDNESS IN BABIES

Very small premature babies commonly have immature lungs; this leads to respiratory distress, and therefore they have to be kept in an oxygen-rich incubator if they are to survive. Without sufficient oxygen the infants' brain may suffer irreversible damage. With too much oxygen another complication may develop—damage to the blood vessels in the eyes. The condition is called retrolental fibroplasia which, when severe, can lead to permanent blindness. It is the direct result of an oxidative stress.

The connection between excess oxygen and retrolental fibroplasia has been recognized for 50 years. As neonatal medicine has improved, the result has been a higher survival rate among the smallest babies, with a consequent increased risk of developing the condition. Despite a number of research studies it is impossible to recommend a safe level of oxygen for these infants.

Vitamin E, because of its antioxidant properties, would appear to be a natural therapeutic agent for the condition, and it has been tried over the last 50 years with variable results. Twenty-five years separate two of the best controlled studies (W. C. and E. V. Owens, 1949, and L. Johnson, D. Schaffer and T. R. Boggs, 1974). Both sets of investigators concluded that there was a relationship between the prevention of retrolental fibroplasia and the administration of vitamin E as a prophylactic agent. Two more recent studies appear to confirm the effectiveness of vitamin E in this respect.

P. Gunby (1980) reported in the *Journal of the American Medical Association* that high doses of vitamin E appear to result in a reduction in overall incidence of retrolental fibroplasia and a decrease in both the severity and duration of acute stage disease. Healing appears also to be favorably influenced.

The most comprehensive study was reported in the *New England Journal of Medicine* in December 1981 by Dr. Helen Hittner and her collaborators from Baylor College of Medicine and the College of Optometry, University of Houston. They performed a double-blind study (i.e., neither patient nor doctor knows which individuals are being treated) on 101 preterm infants who weighed less than 1,500 grams at birth. These infants had respiratory distress and survived at least four weeks. Two groups were studied. A control group of 51 infants received 5 mg per kilogram body weight of vitamin E per day by mouth. Fifty infants received 100 mg per kilogram body weight of the vitamin also by mouth. The first dose of vitamin E in every case was given within the first 24 hours of life and then daily while in the hospital. Synthetic vitamin E (dl-alpha tocopherol) was used throughout. The state of the retina was evaluated in every child during the third week of life and weekly thereafter. Retrolental fibroplasia was scored on a classification from Grade I (neovascularization of the retina) through Grade IV (retinal detachment), although none were allowed to proceed beyond Grade II without surgical treatment, and none reached Grade IV.

The results of the trial were highly encouraging. There was a significant decrease in the incidence of retrolental fibroplasia in those receiving 100 mg vitamin E per kilogram body weight and none proceeded to Grade III of the disease. When multivariate analysis was applied to both control and treatment groups, the severity of retrolental fibroplasia was found to be significantly reduced in infants given the higher dose of vitamin E.

The researchers conclude that their data indicate that vitamin E does not eliminate the occurrence of mild to moderate grades of retrolental fibroplasia. However, it should be regarded as part of the clinician's armamentarium which can be used to diminish severity of the condition and hence reduce blindness secondary to the disorder. Their advice is not to withhold vitamin E until after oxygen has been given, since early administration of the vitamin allows blood plasma levels to build up and confer protection upon ocular tissue. Sometimes even greater intakes of the vitamin may be justified.

CYSTIC BREAST DISEASE

About 20 percent of American women suffer from noncancerous lumps in the breast tissue known popularly as cysts and clinically as fibrocystic breast disease, mammary dysplasia or fibrous mastopathy. Women with at least some types of fibrocystic breast disease are thought to be at a twofold to eightfold greater risk of developing breast cancer. Even those whose lumps remain benign often experience some discomfort.

As long ago as 1965, reports had come from the Boston University School of Medicine (A. A. Abrams) that moderate to complete relief of premenstrual symptoms in 16 patients with fibrocystic breast disease had been achieved with vitamin E taken orally. Palpable softening of the breasts and a reduction in cyst size were the benefits noted in 13 other patients when given vitamin E. Later studies carried out at Baltimore's Sinai Hospital confirmed these results, claiming that vitamin E relieved breast tenderness, caused cyst regression and on a biochemical note altered adrenal steroid hormone excretion in 20 women (R. S. London, 1978).

A double-blind clinical trial on the use of vitamin E in relieving cystic breast disease was reported by the same Baltimore group headed by R. S. London (1980). Twenty-six patients and eight control subjects were treated with a placebo for four weeks, followed by 600 IU of vitamin E daily for eight weeks. Various blood hormone levels were measured in an attempt to learn whether the vitamin's action is mediated through hormone synthesis or alteration of lipoproteins. All subjects were between 23 and 40 years old (average 34 years), and all were diagnosed as suffering from middle-stage mammary dysplasia.

At the end of the test period ten patients showed a good response, twelve were regarded as fair responders and four gained no benefit. A good response meant that the disease regressed. The lumps went away, and the individuals noticed tremendous clinical improvements. Significant relief in 85 percent of the patients studied is an encouraging clinical response, but hormone changes were also noted.

The vitamin had profound effects in reducing to normal the elevated hormone levels found in most women who have cysts. Since increased amounts of certain hormones have been linked to breast cancer in older women, reducing those levels with vitamin E may possibly prevent cancer from developing. In the women who responded there were other beneficial biochemical changes. Cholesterol carried as HDL increased, and, as we have already seen, this response is thought to give protection from cardiovascular disease.

On the basis of his findings Dr. London recommends that clinicians should try vitamin E as a first-line treatment for benign cystic breast disease. "I think our work highly suggests that vitamin E is effective in these patients," he says. "We found absolutely no side effects in terms of clinical derangements, and it worked in a high percentage of patients. If the clinicians can get symptomatic relief in patients with something as benign as vitamin E, I think it's a reasonable therapy."

Vitamin E may also help as a therapy for breast cancer. Dr. London (1981) has extended his studies on cystic breast disease treatment with vitamin E to postulate that the vitamin's effect on blood steroid hormones may reduce the future risk of breast cancer in the individual. Patients who develop breast cancer have an abnormal pattern of the steroid hormones estradiol, estriol and progesterone in the blood plasma long before the clinical disease manifests itself. In a double-blind study, 88 percent of the 17 patients treated with 600 IU per day of alpha tocopherol showed clinical response to the therapy. There was also a statistically significant rise in the ratio of progesterone to estradiol in those patients with cancer. This ratio is usually abnormally low in this disease. Redressing the balance of hormones with vitamin E could therefore represent a significant step in the prevention and treatment of breast cancer.

RESISTANCE TO DISEASE

It has been reported by Tanaka, Fujiwara and Torisu (1979) that vitamin E enhances resistance to bacterial infection. The evidence by these authors came from studies on mice where the effects of the vitamin on the humoral immune response were studied. Mice were fed a diet supplemented with 0, 20 and 200 mg of vitamin E as alpha tocopheryl acetate per kilogram of food. Using standard immunological tests, it was shown that the antibody response is augmented by dietary supplementation with vitamin E. The study confirmed previous investigations from other research groups in which chickens were given increased protection against E. coli by vitamin E supplementation.

Similar studies on human beings point to an important role for vitamin E in the defense against bacterial infection. The main line of this defense resides in the white blood cells, which have the ability to move toward and engulf microorganisms or foreign bodies that appear in the blood. This process is known as phagocytosis. An important pointer to the role of vitamin E in white blood cells was provided by L. Hatam and H. Kayden (1979), who have reported that normal white blood cells have about 30 times as much vitamin E as red blood cells.

An important collaborative study from several prestigious institutes has shown for the first time that the white blood cells of human beings may be involved in vitamin E physiology (L.A. Boxer and Associates, 1979). In glutathione synthetase deficiency some of the white blood cells become deficient in glutathione, which in one form is needed to dispose of the toxic hydrogen peroxide. A patient with an impaired ability to synthesize glutathione had suffered frequent bouts of ear infection during the first two years of his life. He was treated with 400 IU of vitamin E daily for three months, after which he had no further episodes of bacterial infection for the next 18 months. His brother, who had also inherited glutathione synthetase deficiency, was treated with vitamin E from the fourth day of his life, and he has remained free of infection while on this therapy.

These are preliminary studies, and the relationship of vitamin E to other factors that influence the immune response, for example, vitamin C, has to be worked out, but they do appear to represent yet another function of this versatile vitamin in maintaining good health.

NEW INSIGHT INTO VITAMIN E POTENCY

Vitamin E occurs naturally, and when it does, it is referred to as d-alpha tocopherol. However, d-alpha tocopherol rarely occurs alone, and it is usually accompanied by d-beta tocopherol, d-gamma tocopherol and d-delta tocopherol. All of these differ slightly in chemical structure, but there are gross differences in their biological activity. If d-alpha tocopherol is regarded as 100 percent, the d-beta, d-gamma and d-delta forms are 40 percent, 8 percent and 1 percent, respectively, when measured in the female rat resorption test. Nature is therefore very selective in her production of the E vitamins, but the synthetic chemist is not so fortunate. He is unable to make the d-form exclusively when synthesizing the vitamin in the laboratory; thus the end result is a mixture of the biologically active d-forms and the biologically useless l-forms. Not surprisingly, on a milligram for milligram basis, natural vitamin E as d-alpha tocopherol is more active biologically than the synthesized dl-alpha tocopherol. Hence for many years, based on animal testing, 1 milligram of synthetic dl-alpha tocopheryl acetate was assigned a biological potency of 1 IU, and a milligram of the more active d-alpha tocopheryl acetate was regarded as equivalent to 1.36 IU, that is, some 36 percent more potent. The free-form d-alpha tocopherol, which is rarely used as a supplement because it is less stable than the acetate, was found to be 49 percent more active than synthetic dl-alpha tocopheryl acetate. The difference in spelling—tocopherol or tocopheryl—depends on whether the word is followed by the ester—acetate or succinate—in which case the "yl" form is used.

In recent years the potency of the commercially available dl-alpha tocopheryl acetate has been questioned. When the original international unit standard was established, the tocopheryl acetate was prepared from an entirely synthetic ring (chroman) and a natural (isoprenoid) side chain. One milligram of the acetate of this partially synthetic tocopherol (known as 2-ambo-alpha tocopheryl acetate) was ascribed the biological potency of 1 IU. It was at the time generally called dl-alpha tocopheryl acetate, although this name should really be properly given to the present-day commercially available compound (known as all-rac alpha tocopheryl acetate) which is entirely synthetic both in the side chain and in the chroman ring. Until recently challenged, this latter form has automatically been considered to have the same biological potency as the "2-ambo" semisynthetic form, that is, 1 mg equals 1 IU.

S. A. Ames (1979) has looked at the problems and compared the biological potencies of the two forms of dl-tocopheryl acetates in the rat test. His results show considerable differences between them. If the original standard 2-ambo-alpha tocopheryl acetate is given a value of 1.00, then the natural d-alpha tocopheryl acetate has a relative potency in the long-accepted rat fetal resorption assay of 1.66. This is considerably higher than the currently accepted value of 1.36. Preparations of the modern material all-rac alpha tocopheryl acetate similarly compared had a relative potency of 0.81. When this was standardized against the natural d-alpha tocopheryl acetate, it had a relative potency of only 0.52. What it all means is that in this test at least, all synthetic vitamin E acetate is only half as active as the natural material.

These results led M. K. Horwitt (1980) to study how active the various preparations of vitamin E were in human beings. Vitamin E-depleted subjects (all males) were given supplements of the various tocopheryl acetates for 138 days and the blood levels were measured. Daily doses of 7.5 mg, 15 mg, 60 mg and 240 mg of natural d-alpha tocopheryl acetate were compared with 10 mg, 20 mg, 80 mg and 320 mg of the synthetic variety of the vitamins. When evaluated, he found that all-rac alpha tocopheryl acetate (modern synthetic material) may have no more than half the biological potency of the natural d-alpha tocopheryl acetate when used as a supplement in E-depleted subjects. On the basis of these studies, which confirm those of Ames, Horwitt suggests that present-day synthetic vitamin E should be allotted only half the biological potency of the natural form of the vitamin (d-alpha tocopheryl acetate) when calculating human requirements. The previously accepted figure was 74 percent.

These conclusions by Horwitt stimulated other studies on the relative potencies of semisynthetic vitamin E acetate and all-synthetic vitamin E acetate, and two papers provide contrary evidence. The first was from L. Machlin and M. Brin (1981) of Hoffman-la Roche, New Jersey, and their results were based on the curative effects of vitamin E on muscle dystrophy in E-deprived rats. They found that the 2-ambo-alpha tocopheryl acetate partially synthetic form displays only 92 percent of the activity of the all-rac alpha tocopheryl acetate completely synthetic form. They concluded that both were substantially the same, so that modern synthetic vitamin E acetate may be regarded as having 74 percent of the potency of the natural material.

H. Weiser and M. Vecchi (1981) report somewhat different results from Hoffman-la Roche in Basel, Switzerland. They used the rat resorption test and found that the all-rac alpha tocopheryl acetate (all-synthetic) was 9 percent less active than the 2-ambo-alpha tocopheryl Jersey group. They also concluded that there was no statistically significant difference in the two synthetic forms.

These groups differ from Horwitt's conclusions in another way. Horwitt claimed that natural vitamin E is lost from the blood at a slower rate than the synthetic vitamin is. The Hoffman-la Roche teams claimed to demonstrate an equivalent loss of both forms, using the same data. There is of course no guarantee that the relative activities of various tocopherols established by animal experiments are the same as those in humans. Additional evaluation in humans is therefore considered desirable.

In view of this conflicting evidence, there is little doubt that the safest course in supplementation is to use natural vitamin E, that is, d-alpha tocopheryl acetate, whenever possible. On a well-established and generally agreed basis of one milligram of the natural acetate being equivalent to 1.36 IU, a daily dose measured either by weight or by biological potency is simple to calculate.

REFERENCES

Abrams, A. A. 1965. *New Engl. J. Med.* 272:1080.

Ames, S. A. 1979. *J. Nutr.* 109:2198.

Azizi, E., Zaidman, J. L., Eshchar, J. and Szeinberg, A. 1978. *Acton Paediat. Scand.* 67:797.

Barboriak, J. J. 1982. *Amer. J. Clin. Path.* 77:371.

Barrett, M. and O'Regan, S. 1980. *Prostaglandins and Medicine* 5:337.

Binder, H. J. and Shapiro, H. M. 1967. *Amer. J. Clin. Nutr.* 20:594.

Boxer, L. A., Oliver, J. M., Spielberg, S. P., Allen, J. M. and Schulman, H. D. 1979. *New Engl. J. Med.* 301:901.

Chiv, D. and Lubin, B. 1979. *J. Lab. Clin. Med.* 94:542.

Corash, K., Spielberg, S. P., Bartsocas, C., Boxer, L. A., Steinherz, R., Sheetz, M., Egan, M., Schlessleman, J. and Schulman, J. D. 1980. *New Engl. J. Med.* 303:416.

Cornwell, D. 1979. *Lipids* 14:194.

Farrell, P. M., Bieri, J. G., Fratantoni, J. F., Wood, R. E. and Di Sant'Agnese, P. A. 1977. *J. Clin. Invest.* 60:233.

Forster, W. 1980. *Acta Med. Scand.* (Suppl.) 642:47, 35.

Graeber, J. E., Williams, M. L. and Oski, F. A. 1977. *J. Pediat.* 90:282.

Gross, S. J. 1979. *Pediatrics* 64:321.

Gunby, P. 1980. *J. Amer. Med. Assoc.* 243:1021, 1025.

Gwebu, E. T. 1980. *Res. Comm. in Chemical Pathology and Pharmacology* 28:361.

Haeger, K. 1974. *Amer. J. Clin. Nutr.* 27:1179.

Hatam, L. and Kayden, H. 1979. *J. Lipid Res.* 20:639.

Hatam, L. and Kayden, H. 1981. *Amer. J. Clin. Path.* 76:122.

Hermann, W. J., Ward, K. and Faucett, J. 1979. *Amer. J. Clin. Path.* 72:848.

Hittner, H. M., Godio, L. B., Rudolph, A. J., Adams, J. M., Garcia-Prats, J. A., Friedman, Z., Kautz, J. A. and Monaco, W. A. 1981. *New Engl. J. Med.* 305:1365.

Horwitt, M. K. 1980. *Amer. J. Clin. Nutr.* 33:1856.

Howard, D. R. 1982. *Amer. J. Clin. Path.* 77:86.

Johnson, L., Schaffer, D. and Boggs, T. R. 1974. *Amer. J. Clin. Nutr.* 27:1158.

Kanofsky, J. D. and Kanofsky, P. B. 1981. *New Engl. J. Med.* July 16, 1973.

London, R. S. 1978. *Breast* 4:19.

London, R. S. 1981. *Cancer Research* 41:3811.

London, R. S., Sundaram, G. S., Schultz, M., Naier, P. P. and Goldstein, P. 1980. *J. Amer. Med. Assoc.* 244:1077.

Machlin, L. and Brin, M. 1981. *Amer. J. Clin. Nutr.* 34:1633.

Miniero, R., Canducci, E., Ghigo, D., Saracco, P. and Vullo, C. 1981. 1st Europ. Symp. on Vitamins. New Aspects in Prevention and Therapy.

Natta, C. L. 1980. *Amer. J. Clin. Nutr.* 33:968.

Ochsner, A. 1968. *Postgrad. Med.* 44:91.

Oski, F. A. 1980. *New Engl. J. Med.* 303:454.

Owens, W. C. and Owens, E. V. 1949. *Amer. J. Ophthalmol.* 32:1631.

Passeri, M. and Butturini, U. 1981. 1st Europ. Symp. on Vitamins. New Aspects in Prevention and Therapy.

Rachilewitz, E. A., Shifter, A. and Kahane, I. 1980. Haematology Service, Hadassah Univ. Hosp. and Biomembrane Res. Lab. Hebrew Univ., Hadassah Med. School, Jerusalem.

Roberts, H. J. 1978. *Lancet*, January 7, 49.

Roberts H. J. 1981. *J. Amer. Med. Assoc.* 246:129.

Szczeklik, A., Skawinski, S., Gluszko, P., Nizankowski, R., Szczeklik, J. and Gryglewski, R. J. 1979. *Lancet*, May 26.

Tanaka, J., Fujiwara, H. and Torisu, M. 1979. *Immunology* 38:727.

Weiser, H. and Vecchi, M. 1981. *Int. J. Vit. and Nutr. Res.* 51:100.

Wilson, R. B., Middleton, C. C. and Sun, G. Y. 1978. *J. Nutr.* 108:67.

Yokata, F. 1981. *Atherosclerosis* 38:249.

Vitamin E Pioneers Were Right:
E Fights Heart Disease and More

Evan and Wilfrid Shute knew they were on to something when they discovered vitamin E in 1933, but even they may not have realized the tremendous impact that alpha tocopherol [vitamin E] would eventually have on medicine today.

Susan Carlson, R.Ph. and the vice-president of J.R. Carlson Laboratories in Arlington Heights, Illinois, vividly remembers how the Shutes' discovery touched her own life:

"In his mid-50s," she told *Health News & Review*, "my father began experiencing angina [heart] pain. He didn't feel well enough to work. His doctors prescribed nitroglycerine and other medications, but they did not remove the pain. He was a pharmacist who had been active both in manufacturing and retailing.

"In 1964 we heard of Wilfrid and Evan Shute's work with vitamin E. We were very skeptical, but after visiting the Shute Institute Medical Clinic in Canada and beginning a specific vitamin E program, Dad's pains were gone and he returned to the work he loved," Carlson continued.

Interestingly, her father's angina returned when he tried another type of the vitamin. That's when the Carlsons realized the importance of a good vitamin E preparation, Susan Carlson added.

"Dad was just one of the many thousand patients of Dr. Shute. His results were spectacular, and since vitamin E first touched home with Dad's early experiences, I have been actively involved with many aspects of vitamin E."

The Shute brothers were brilliant and considered geniuses by some. Their father was a physician and their mother was a strong influence in their early years. Their home lives and educations were focused on medicine.

Evan, the eldest brother, set two records in his native Canada when he passed the high school entrance examination when he was only 9, and then entered the University of Toronto at age 14.

STRONG COMMITMENT

Susan Carlson recalled, "Wilfrid once explained to me that his mother was somewhat disappointed with him, for he did not enter the University until he was 15! A third brother, Wallace, who also became a physician, entered the University at age 16."

The brothers would need that strong family background and commitment to ideals. As is the case with many pioneers in medicine, the brothers' work was rejected for a long time by their peers, the medical establishment and even their own community.

Still they persevered, convinced that the vitamin would revolutionize the treatment of many types of diseases and prove especially valuable in treating and preventing heart and circulatory conditions.

Because prominent medical journals would not print their revolutionary articles, the Shute Institute published its own journal, *The Summary*, and sent it to medical libraries around the world free of charge. Wilfrid and Evan each authored books on vitamin E, and Wilfrid's *Vitamin E for Ailing and Healthy Hearts* became a number-one best seller in the U.S.

"Today, of course, research is not only substantiating what the Shute brothers documented and reported, but discovering the biochemical principles behind it, helping us to understand why E can be useful for a broad spectrum of health conditions," Carlson said.

And the medical community is finally beginning to accept vitamin E as a powerful ally in the battle for health, the pharmacist added.

"Wilfrid and Evan Shute lived, ate and breathed vitamin E for nearly 40 years, supported by loving families and the knowledge that vitamin E could help so many. I remember them as warm, caring, brilliant men, whom I was very proud to know and deeply respected," she concluded.

WHY WE NEED E SUPPLEMENTS

Is it necessary to take supplements of E? Surely we could get enough from a healthful diet? Yes, in centuries past, but not today. Alpha tocopherol is found in wheat germ, seeds, nuts, and the oils of these products, but, unfortunately, modern food processing methods strip most supermarket oils of this beneficial vitamin.

Refining, processing and storage stages of food handling destroy some vitamin E in virtually all foods containing this essential nutrient. E in foods is destroyed by oxygen, and this oxidative process is accelerated by heat, light, and freezing.

The newest research suggests that the amounts of E consumed in typical diets is not enough to counteract the free-radical cell damage that can compromise health and hasten aging. Furthermore, the Recommended Dietary Allowance of 15 IU of E is barely adequate to prevent deficiency disease in most people. Many people need at least 10 times that, the Shutes found, and even more for therapeutic use.

Many diets are "marginally deficient" in E. According to a food consumption survey done by the U.S. Department of Agriculture in 1985, 70% of women were getting less than the RDA of vitamin E from their diets, while 41% were getting less than 70% of the RDA.

Furthermore, in two recent studies which appeared in the *American Journal of Clinical Nutrition and Clinical Nutrition,* researchers examined normal, healthy, people who consumed "adequate diets." Despite their apparent good health, after supplementation with vitamin E, all showed "a significant decrease in a marker of cell damage."

In fact, according to the late Evan Shute, "No substance known to medicine has such a variety of healing properties as alpha tocopherol."

Vitamin E has the power to:

- Reduce the oxygen requirement of tissues, providing immediate help in cases of diminished oxygen and/or blood supply
- Decrease the insulin requirement in some diabetics
- Melt fresh clots (thrombosis), preventing death of the vein or artery
- Increase circulation in surrounding smaller blood vessels
- Dilate capillaries, bringing more blood and oxygen to burned areas, for example, for faster healing
- Regulate fat and protein metabolism
- Prevent the overproduction of scar tissue and sometimes even remove excess scar tissue
- Mobilize and increase platelets, affecting the blood clotting process.

All of these actions make vitamin E appropriate in treating a very wide range of problems, including: heart disease, arteriosclerosis, angina pectoris, congestive heart failure, diabetes, burns and scarring, miscarriage and sterility, as well as certain birth defects.

As a powerful antioxidant, this vitamin may also help prevent cancer, many of today's "E" experts believe. The Shute brothers' contribution to medicine, although belatedly recognized, will be remembered as one of the greatest in current history. Their work continues at the Shute Medical Clinic of London, Ontario, Canada.

MARY ELLEN HETTINGER

Research Shows Roles for Vitamin E
in Ills from Cataracts to Cancer

Vitamin E, discovered in the early part of this century, has had a colorful and a controversial history rife with fantastic claims of skin rejuvenation and even penile growth. Alas, the truth is less spectacular as it relates to human vanity. But vitamin E's implications for our overall health and well-being have proven true well beyond our expectations.

Although a myriad of uses for this antioxidant are being uncovered, some of the most intriguing include E's multifaceted action as an immune system booster. Because of its antioxidant nature, it defends the body against free radicals (molecular byproducts considered to be responsible for side effects of aging, and also implicated in some cancers). It also appears to bolster cell membranes, strengthening their defenses against pathogenic bacteria and viruses.

PIONEERS LINK E AND HEART DISEASE

Two Canadian physicians, Drs. Evan and Wilfrid Shute, were the visionaries behind vitamin E's role in treating and preventing heart disease in the 1940s. Dr. Wilfrid Shute was the first to note that the tremendous rise in cases of heart failure occurred at the same time wheat germ was eliminated from flour through modern milling practices. Wheat germ is naturally rich in vitamin E. The Shute brothers were the first to question the role of atherosclerosis and fat in the development of heart disease because of this.

The brothers' theory that E helped prevent heart attacks has since been proven in a number of cell and animal studies which demonstrated that E inhibits blood platelets from clumping. Other studies showing E's effectiveness against free radicals have testified to its role in preventing damage that often accompanies circulatory problems.

In fact, in 1991, researchers at the University of Toronto reported that a study showed that large doses of pure vitamin E administered daily from two weeks before patients had coronary bypass surgery reduced the "metabolic dysfunction" in the heart muscle that typically follows this surgery.

Terrence Yau, M.D., reported at the 63rd Scientific Sessions of the American Heart Association that vitamin E "is the only antioxidant to penetrate the lipid membrane around the heart muscle cell, to reach the sites where free radicals do their damage."

Since the Shute brothers' forays into vitamin E therapy, many more uses for it have been found—especially since current research shows most Americans are likely to be deficient.

Patrick Quillen, Ph.D., told *Let's Live* magazine that "long-term subclinical deficiencies of vitamin E among Americans probably surface as common diseases (such as heart disease, cancer, senility, allergies, cataracts and premature aging) rather than a neat and concise vitamin deficiency disease."

WHO NEEDS VITAMIN E?

Among the many people who can benefit from this fat-soluble antioxidant are the elderly, since accumulated oxidative damage is considered to be a prime cause of cataracts in the elderly. In *Nutrition Today*, November/December 1988, Drs. Edwin Bunce and John Hess of Virginia Polytechnic Institute wrote, "The presence of liberal quantities of vitamin E can diminish oxidative damage in the lens." Since cataracts take years to advance, up to 400 IU of E each day may retard their development—especially if taken earlier in life.

Another benefit for the elderly provided by this nutrient is improved immune response. This was found after a group of healthy senior citizens took 400 IU a day for one month. Reporting on this study at the Vitamin E Symposium, S.N. Meydani, Ph.D., called E "a single nutrient supplement (that) can enhance immune responsiveness in the elderly."

But they are by no means the only group of people helped by regular dietary supplementation of this vitamin. Athletes and weekend exercisers alike should include E as part of their fitness regime, because recent studies show that a vigorous workout can damage cells that don't have adequate protection from vitamin E. According to Dr. Lester Packer, who has pioneered the study of oxidative damage during exercise, exercise causes the body to use from 10 to 20 times the normal amount of oxygen. This creates more free radicals and boosts the risk of long-term cell damage. E's antioxidant action can help prevent this damage.

For women, vitamin E is beneficial both by itself and in conjunction with other nutrients. In a study of 40 women with premenstrual syndrome (PMS), 22 women were given vitamin E while 19 took a placebo daily. After three months, the group that received vitamin E reported they felt less fatigued, had fewer headaches and noticed less of a craving for sweets. One third of those treated with E said their physical and emotional symptoms were relieved, while only 14 percent of the control group felt their symptoms had lessened.

Vitamin E is also proving helpful for women during menopause. Dr. Schuyler Lininger, Jr., recommends 800 IU a day for hot flashes, and also to treat menstrual cramps. The dosage should be lowered to a maintenance dose after symptoms are alleviated.

According to the *International Journal of Cancer* in 1989, vitamin E intake was associated with a significantly lower risk of cervical cancer. Use of vitamin E and A supplements was also related to a decrease in the risk of invasive cervical cancer.

The Institute for Breast Disease of the New York Medical College has been conducting research on the effects of vitamins A and E on breast cancer patients. The study shows that from 50 to 60 percent of the patients who were experiencing impaired immunity against their own tumors had improved immune response after taking either vitamin. Furthermore, when both vitamins were taken together, 80 percent of the patients improved.

Vitamin E may be linked in lung cancer cases as well. A case-control study of serum vitamin A, E and C in lung cancer patients written up in *Nutrition and Cancer* in 1990 showed that lung cancer patients had "significantly lower mean serum levels of carotenoids, vitamin E and total cholesterol than controls. . . . Vitamin E was lower in hospitalized persons with lung cancer than in other hospitalized persons, even after adjusting for total cholesterol levels."

Still others may benefit from vitamin E supplementation, among them rheumatoid arthritis sufferers, patients with Parkinson's disease and diabetics. Children with sickle cell anemia are particularly low in this vitamin, as are children with juvenile chronic arthritis, and long-term deficiencies of E have been associated with neurological abnormalities. In short, virtually everyone could benefit.

HOW MUCH E?

The RDA for vitamin E is 15 IU, but most American diets don't even come close to this minimum amount. Although people taking anti-clotting drugs or with liver disease should not take vitamin E without their physician's supervision, most of us can benefit from E supplements. Vitamin E's toxicity is low, animal studies have shown no mutagenic, carcinogenic or teratogenic effects, and doses as high as 3.2 grams a day have resulted in few if any undesirable side effects. For most of us, 200 IU a day is probably sufficient to reap its many benefits.

MARY ELLEN HETTINGER

Vitamin E Is for Elephants

The benefits of vitamin E for humans—in preventing and treating athero-sclerosis, lowering blood pressure, preventing blood clots and bacterial infections and as a general aid to longevity due to its antioxidant action—have been proven. But now animal nutritionists are discovering that E is just as effective on elephants, and may even help save them, the black rhino and other endangered species.

Dr. Ellen S. Dierenfeld of the New York Zoological Society says meeting the nutritional needs of animals in captivity is imperative for the survival of the species.

"Black rhinos, elephants and many other species are rapidly vanishing from the earth. One hope for preserving these magnificent creatures for future generations lies in a better understanding of their nutritional needs," the zoo staff nutritionist reported at a 1990 Federation of American Societies for Experimental Biology meeting.

She also presented the preliminary findings of vitamin E levels in plants eaten by black rhinos in Kenya and Zimbabwe. These studies showed that many natural foods contain higher vitamin E levels than those found in typical zoo diets.

Vitamin E deficiency affects a large cross-section of zoo animals. Over the past four years, Dr. Dierenfeld studied hundreds of animals from croco-diles, eagles, rhinos and antelopes to gorillas and giraffes, and collected data to examine the scope and causes of vitamin E deficiency-related problems so preventive measures could be implemented. Deficiencies in this essential nutrient affect different muscle systems in animals, the expert explains:

"In elephants and gorillas, the deficiency often results in heart disease. In antelopes and other hoofed animals, thigh muscles are a frequent site of vitamin E deficiency-induced disease. Giraffes are likely to develop disease in the tongue muscle. When that happens, giraffes cannot feed properly and death by starvation may result."

One reason vitamin E shortages may become a problem in zoo animals is that these creatures tend to live longer than they do in the wild. Just as it does in humans, longevity may increase the need for vitamin E.

But supplementing a wild animal's diet with anything is not as simple as it sounds. You can't tell a peaked pachyderm to pop a pill.

To coax elephants, which, like humans, have a life-span of 50-70 years, into taking their regular dose of vitamin E, the keepers at New York's Bronx and Central Park Zoos hollow out a loaf of French bread and stuff it with a powdered form of the nutrient. The elephants eagerly chow down.

"With so many animals at risk in the wild, our captive populations may be the gene pools for the survival of many exotic species," Dr. Dierenfeld warns. So increasing survival and reproduction rates of zoo animals is top priority around the world.

"Supplementation of animal diets with vitamin E appears to be making a significant contribution to the success of these programs," she concludes.

SELENIUM

How It Protects Against Cancer, Heart Disease, Arthritis and Aging

RICHARD A. PASSWATER, PH.D.

SELENIUM AROUND THE WORLD

Large-scale studies in China and Finland, involving thousands—sometimes tens of thousands—of subjects, have demonstrated conclusively the protective role of the trace mineral selenium in both cancer and heart disease, and each new research effort in the United States and other countries adds to the evidence. Dr. Passwater, a pioneer selenium proponent, presents important information on the lifesaving properties of this little-known nutrient.

Selenium is a trace element (mineral) that is vital to your health. Just like the minerals iron and calcium, it is needed in your diet or you will die of malnutrition. If you do get some—but not enough—selenium in your diet, you won't develop outright malnutrition, but will instead have greater chances of getting cancer, heart disease, and arthritis and of experiencing accelerated aging. Now there is exciting and strong evidence that the optimal selenium intake will prevent or reduce the incidence of many deadly diseases. This chapter tells the dramatic selenium story and explains how proper selenium nutrition can safely improve and lengthen your life.

BACKGROUND

It is gratifying to see that the research that I performed in the early 1960s showing that selenium increases the life span and prevents cancer has now been accepted by most scientists and physicians involved in those areas of research. Also, it has been exciting to see that researchers have expanded animal studies to show that selenium is protective against heart disease, as well as protective and sometimes curative in arthritis and other diseases. Selenium is not a wonder drug. These diseases are all dependent on a common factor called a "free radical," and selenium is a nutrient that stimulates the body's defense against free radicals.

While "free radical" is not quite yet a household word, the term is in common use among the most knowledgeable of those interested in improving their lives with optimal nutrition. Our interest in free radicals is due to their high reactivity with vital body components. It is not necessary that we understand what free radicals are or how they do their damage, but it does help if we have a "word picture" conceptual use of the term. A simplified definition of free radicals is given in Box 1. (See Appendix A for more about free radicals.)

BOX 1

FREE RADICALS

Chemical compounds consist of two or more elements that are held together as molecules by the force of chemical bonding. The bonding involves electrons, which are negative parts of the atoms of the elements. The arrangement of the electrons determines the stability of the compound. A stable compound has electrons that are in pairs—think of it as a molecular buddy system. If an electron does not have a partner, it can become very reactive and unstable. It will seek out another electron to pair up with—even if it has to capture or steal the electron from another molecule and disrupt or destroy that molecule. A molecule or atom with an unpaired electron is called a free radical.

Please note that electron pairing is different from electron balance and total electron charge or ionization state. A free radical may be a neutral or a charged molecule or atom.

The pace of research on selenium and health is very brisk right now, and many scientists and research physicians are entering the field because of the strength of the research results and the promise of even more health benefits to come. Now scientists often start their investigations without thoroughly reviewing the works of the pioneers that preceded them, including Coombs, Schrauzer, Scott, Schwarz, Shamberger, Spallholtz, Tappel and myself. Of these selenium pioneers, only Schrauzer, Shamberger and I experimented with selenium as an anti-cancer nutrient. If the newcomers, with their broad array of talent and sophisticated skills, would dig out the published studies of the 1960s and early 1970s, they would find that much of what they are publishing as new discoveries has already been published—admittedly, however, based on the less sophisticated experimental techniques of those times.

As newcomers enter the field, they find that there are hundreds of studies over three decades involving thousands of people and laboratory animals. My first scientific presentation of my 1960s research showing that selenium in synergistic combination with other nutrient antioxidants (anti-free-radical compounds) slowed the aging process in laboratory animals was at the twenty-third Gerontological Society Meeting in Toronto in October 1970. A confirmation of the anti-free-radical power of my synergistic formulation was reported in *Pathological Aspects of Cell Membranes* (Academic Press, 1971) by Dr. A. L. Tappel of the University of California at Davis. My first scientific presentation of how selenium and other nutrient antioxidants in synergistic combination prevented cancer appeared in the magazine *American Laboratory* in May 1973. Earlier presentations of my research were in patent applications and news articles. (See Box 2 for a bibliography of reports on my early research on this topic.)

These studies were small-scale experiments involving small laboratory animals. Few scientists thought that the results would apply to humans in the real world. Few scientists wanted to risk their reputations and future funding by conducting the needed clinical trials with only laboratory animal studies and a strange new theory about "free-radical pathology" as the supporting evidence.

The good news is that we pioneers kept hammering away, ex-

BOX 2

BIBLIOGRAPHY OF THE AUTHOR'S EARLY PUBLICATIONS
ON THE ANTI-CANCER ACTIVITY OF SELENIUM

In the scientific press:

1. *The Gerontologist*, 10(3):28, Oct. 1970
2. *Chem. & Eng. News* 48:17 (Oct. 26, 1970). Followup: May 10, 1971
3. *Geriatric Focus*, March–April 1971
4. *American Lab* 3(4):36–40, April 1971
5. *American Lab* 3(5):21–25, May 1971
6. *American Lab* 5(6):10–22, May 1973
7. *American Lab* 8(4) 32–47, Aug. 1976

U.S. Patent Numbers 39140 and 97011, and patents in various other countries.

In the general interest press:

1. *Washington Daily News* p. 5, Sept. 15, 1970
2. *Prevention* 23(12) 104–110, Dec. 1971
3. Reuters News Agency report, Oct. 23, 1970
4. *Ladies' Home Journal* 70, 129–131, July 1971
5. Kugler, H., *Slowing the Aging Process*, Pyramid, NY, 1973
6. Rosenfeld, A., *Prolongevity*, Knopf, NY, 1976

panding our experiments, lecturing our colleagues and daring somebody to prove us wrong. Unfortunately, some of us were often chastised or labeled "quacks" by those not able to understand free-radical pathology. Therefore, we had to become "activists" to bring this important research before as many scientists as we could. The great news is that the new scientists who entered the field brought with them new skills and capabilities that produced different kinds of evidence that selenium did prevent cancer, heart disease and arthritis and did slow the aging process. Here is a look at the exciting new evidence involving clinical trials, epidemiological studies and laboratory studies. You don't have to be a biochemist to understand how strong the evidence is.

A brief explanation as to how selenium prevents cancer is given in the diagram below.

CANCER

Selenium prevents cancer. There is even evidence that selenium may help cure cancer. Selenium by itself can't protect all people from all types of cancer, but it definitely reduces the incidences of all types of cancer studied so far in large populations. Some individuals may have genetic weaknesses, or be so undernourished that their immune system can't function, or be so overwhelmed with chemicals that cause cancer, that they don't have a chance. However, most people are not so unfortunate, and selenium will reduce their risk of getting

Properties and functions of selenium that may be related to its anticarcinogenic action

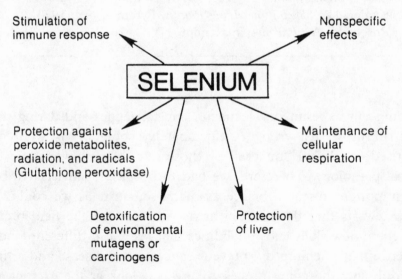

Source: Schrauzer, G. 1978. *Inorganic and Nutritional Aspects of Cancer.* New York: Plenum Press, p. 330.

cancer by strengthening their immune system and protecting their vital cell components against free-radical attack.

Through hundreds of laboratory studies, case-controlled clinical studies and epidemiological studies, it has been consistently demonstrated that the better the selenium nutriture of a person, the less chance of cancer. The evidence for a prophylactic role for selenium is without a doubt stronger than for any other factor, including the nutrient beta-carotene, dietary fiber, crucifers or any other food factor recommended as potential cancer-preventive agents by the American Cancer Society, National Cancer Institute, and other official bodies.

The evidence includes the following types of study:

Clinical: prospective, retrospective
Epidemiological: blood levels, food intake, soils
Animal: life span, spontaneous cancer; carcinogen-induced (dietary, contact); virus-induced (not inoculated, inoculated); transplanted cancer tissue; inoculated cancer cells
Therapeutic

The protective action of selenium against every type of cancer studied has been demonstrated regardless of whether the cancer-causing agents have been introduced in the laboratory or naturally, chemically or virally induced, inoculated or transplanted.

The clinical confirmation that cancer probability correlates inversely with a person's blood selenium content (the higher the selenium, the less chance of cancer) was shown epidemiologically in the 1970s by Dr. Raymond Shamberger and clinically in the *New England Journal of Medicine* by Harvard's Dr. W. C. Willet, and colleagues in 1983.

There is no need to review the hundreds of tests. Let's just start with six studies that should catch your attention. Here is a brief summary of the major points they make (the studies are discussed in greater detail in the next section, and identified here by the name of the principal author in parenthesis):

1. Considering selenium blood levels alone, those persons in the *lowest* fifth of all blood selenium levels *have twice the incidence of cancer* as those in the highest fifth (Willett, 1983).

2. Total cancer mortality is *three times higher* in persons having *blood selenium values below a certain value* than the incidence of cancer in those above this value (Yu, 1985).

3. Considering selenium blood levels alone, those persons in the *lowest* tenth of all blood selenium levels *have six times the incidence of* cancer as those in the highest tenth (Clark, 1984).

4. Both selenium and vitamin E are needed together to prevent cancer (Horvath, 1983).

5. When considering both selenium and vitamin E blood levels, those persons in the lowest third of blood vitamin E level and also having a low blood selenium level had *more than eleven times the incidence of* cancer as those in the upper two-thirds of blood vitamin E and selenium levels (Salonen, 1985).

6. Still another researcher concludes that "selenium should be considered not only as a preventive, but also as a therapeutic agent in cancer treatment and may act additively or synergistically with drug and X-ray treatments" (Milner, 1984).

I hope those studies have your attention. The next section describes them in detail. The section also includes graphic illustration of several other studies indicating the inverse relationship between cancer incidence and selenium intake. Figures 1 through 3 deal with the occurrence of cancer in the United States; Figure 4 relates selenium intake and breast cancer in several countries; Figure 5 shows the results of experiments with laboratory animals in which cancers were induced.

The epidemiological studies by themselves do not prove anything, but combining them with the clinical studies and laboratory experiments allows a valid conclusion to be inferred.

SIX STUDIES OF IMPORTANCE

The Willett Study. This study is of major importance not only for its research but for its influence. The Willett study was conducted by a well-respected group of researchers, and the work was done at

FIGURE 1. ZERO CANCER EXTRAPOLATIONS

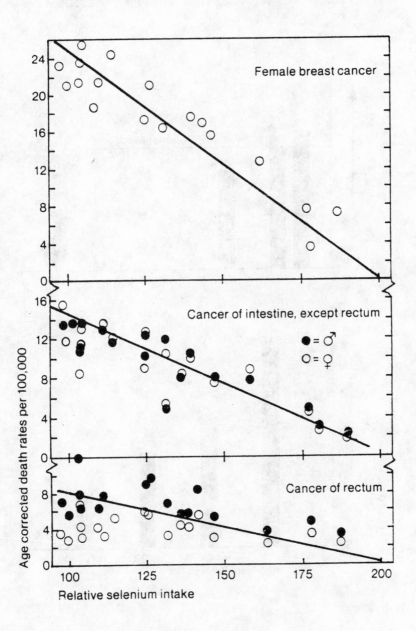

Source: Schrauzer, White, and Schneider, 1977. *Bioinorganic Chem.* 7:37.

FIGURES 2 AND 3. CANCER DEATH RATE VERSUS SELENIUM LEVEL

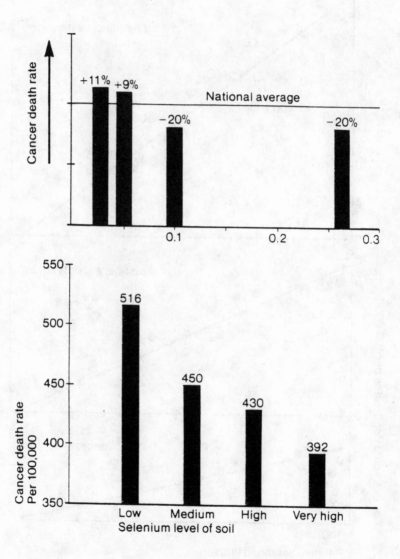

Sources: Passwater drawings based on data from Shamberger, R. and Frost, D. 1969. *Canadian Medical Association Journal* 100:682.

FIGURE 4. RELATIONSHIP OF SELENIUM INTAKE AND
BREAST CANCER MORTALITIES

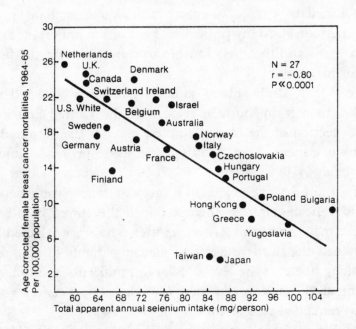

Source: Schrauzer, G., White, D. and Schneider, C. 1977. *Bioinorganic Chemistry*, vol. 7. p. 36.

FIGURE 5. PROTECTIVE EFFECT OF SELENIUM AGAINST
CARCINOGEN-PRODUCED CANCER IN ANIMALS

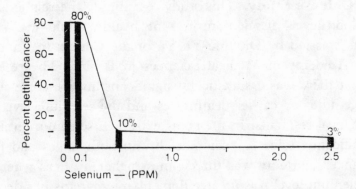

Source: Passwater drawing based on data from Harr, J., Exon, J., Whanger, P. and Weswig, P. 1972. *Clinical Toxicology* 5(2):187–94.

major centers of learning: Harvard, Johns Hopkins, Duke, the University of Texas and other respected colleges and universities. The results were published in a major medical journal, rather than an obscure scientific periodical. Many physicians read of the importance of blood selenium levels and their relationship to cancer risk for the first time, thanks to this study.

In the Willett study, blood samples had been collected in 1973 from 4480 men from fourteen regions of the United States. At the time of collection of the blood samples, none of the men had detectable signs of cancer. The blood samples were preserved and stored for later analysis.

During the next five years, 111 cases of cancer were detected in the group. The researchers then retrieved the stored blood samples from these men, and from 210 other men who were selected because they matched the newly developed cancer patients in age, sex, race and smoking history. The levels of several nutrients and other factors were compared between the men who developed cancer and those men who remained free of cancer.

One difference stood out as being highly significant. The risk of cancer for subjects in the lowest quintile (fifth) of blood selenium was twice that of subjects in the highest. (W. C. Willett et al., "Prediagnostic Serum Selenium and Risk of Cancer." *Lancet* 11:130-4, July 16, 1983)

The Chinese Study. This study, examining the relationship between blood levels of selenium in 1458 healthy adults in 24 regions of China, was led by Dr. Shu-Yu Yu of the Cancer Institute of the Chinese Academy of Medical Sciences in Beijing. The researchers found that there was a statistically significant inverse correlation between age-adjusted cancer death rates and the selenium levels in the blood of local residents. In the areas with high selenium levels, there was significantly lower cancer mortality in both males and females. Total cancer mortality was three times higher in areas where mean blood selenium level was greater than 11 micrograms per deciliter of blood than where it was 8 micrograms per deciliter. (Shu-Yu Yu et al., "Regional Variation of Cancer Mortality Incidence and Its Relation to Selenium Levels in China." *Biological Trace Element Research* 7:21-9, January-February 1985)

The Clark Study. Dr. Larry C. Clark and colleagues at Cornell determined the blood selenium levels in 240 skin cancer patients and compared the results to those from 103 apparently healthy persons living in low-selenium areas. The mean blood selenium level for the skin cancer patients was significantly lower than that of the apparently healthy individuals. After adjusting for age, sun damage to the skin, blood beta-carotene and vitamin A levels, and other factors, the incidence of skin cancer in those persons in the lowest decile (tenth) of blood selenium was 5.8 times as great as those in the highest decile. (L. C. Clark et al., "Plasma Selenium and Skin Neoplasms: A Case Controlled Study." *Nutrition and Cancer* (6:13-21, January-March 1984)

The Horvath Study. The preceding three studies have dealt with real people, but let's look at an important laboratory animal study for a moment. Most scientific experiments examine one variable at a time to study the effect of just that one variable. This reduces confusion from confounding factors. Yet the body is not a simple laboratory; it is a biologically complex mechanism that functions independently of science's effort to study it. While this chapter is written primarily about selenium, I want to stress that total nutrition is important. If you are grossly deficient in vitamin A or vitamin E, the correct amount of selenium will not make up for all the deficiencies.

However, there is more to the relationship than balanced total nutrition. There is a special synergistic relationship among all the antioxidant nutrients, but especially vitamin E and selenium. This has been the essence of my research and the basis for my patents and publications. In 1983, a sophisticated study published by Drs. Paula Horvath and Clement Ip clarified this synergistic relationship of vitamin E and selenium.

They found that vitamin E and selenium must both be present to prevent the proliferating phase of cancer. Their evidence indicates that it is not the amount of selenium-containing glutathione peroxidase that is critical but the amount of microsomal peroxidase activity, which is stimulated only by the presence of both vitamin E and selenium. (P. M. Horvath and C. Ip, "Synergistic Effect of Vitamin E and Selenium in the Chemoprevention of Mammary Carcinogenesis in Rats." *Cancer Research* 43:5335–41, November 1983)

The message here is that scientists should not be studying the correlation between blood selenium levels alone and cancer but studying the blood levels of vitamin E and selenium together. Studying selenium alone, we do in fact find that there is a substantial reduction in cancer risk with the higher blood levels of selenium. But we find the same relationship with vitamin E and some types of cancer—the more vitamin E in the blood, the lower the incidence of cancer. As an example, consider the report in the *British Journal of Cancer* (49:321–324, 1984) by Dr. N. J. Wald that showed that women in the lowest quintile of vitamin E levels had 5.2 times the risk of cancer as women in the highest. However, when a person's blood is rich in both vitamin E and selenium, the protection given that person is far more than that of adding the vitamin E protection and the selenium protection together.

If a person has a normal blood level of selenium, but is very deficient in vitamin E, that person will not have a good defense against cancer. Conversely, if a person is a little low in selenium— but well fortified with vitamin E—then that person may be more resistant to cancer.

Since the vitamin E blood level can affect the usefulness of selenium, researchers should be looking at the combined levels, not just a simple selenium level. Once researchers catch on to this relationship, we will see even more dramatic results. This becomes apparent in the next study.

The Finnish Study. Dr. Jukka Salonen and his colleagues at the University of Kuopio (Finland) have been studying over 12,000 Finns for several years. The study is known as the North Karelia Project. Four years after drawing blood samples from these 12,155 persons, 51 had died of cancer. They were matched by age, sex and smoking habits with others, and their blood samples were compared.

In this study many factors were examined, but most important, both vitamin E and selenium levels of the blood were examined in combination. The relative risk of cancer mortality for the third of people with blood selenium levels below 47 micrograms per liter of blood compared to those with higher levels was 5.8 to 1. But of more importance is the finding that, for people with low selenium levels who also had vitamin E levels in the lowest of values, risk of death from *cancer compared to persons with both selenium and vitamin E levels in the upper two-thirds of values was* 11.4 to 1. (J. T. Salonen et al., "Risk of Cancer in Relation to Serum Concentrations of Selenium and Vitamins A and E." *British Medical Journal* 290: 417-20, February 9, 1985)

The Milner Review. Dr. John A. Milner of the University of Illinois has been studying selenium and cancer prevention for more than a decade. Most of Dr. Milner's studies involve transplanting or inoculating cancer cells into mice receiving different levels of selenium. He has found that selenium inhibits the development of such cancer.

Dr. Milner's conclusion is that selenium should be considered not only as a preventive but also as a therapeutic agent in cancer treatment. There is evidence, which will be presented here later, that selenium may act additively or synergistically with drug and x-ray treatments. (J. A. Milner, "Selenium and the Transplantable Tumor." *Journal of Agricultural and Food Chemistry* 32:436–42, May–June 1984)

Nutrition Reviews Brings the News to the Nutritionists. These six studies will eventually have a major impact on cancer research. However, the subject is still new to most researchers and especially so to those who hold fast to the notion that diet and cancer are not related. To begin to educate such "old-line" nutritionists, the conservative nutrition journal *Nutrition Reviews* published an issue devoted to the topic.

Drs. Gerald Combs and Larry Clark of Cornell present an excellent review of selenium's protective roles against cancer in the November 1985 issue of *Nutrition Reviews*. Their review article is entitled "Can Dietary Selenium Modify Cancer Risk?" and the evidence that they present is quite convincing (43:325–31). They provide 97 references for the serious scholar to pursue. Most scientists who bother to read those 97 reference articles will become selenium fans, but there are five times that many in the literature, and they should be read to really understand the depth of the research that supports the hypothesis.

Since *Nutrition Reviews* is widely read by nutritional scientists—and keep in mind that nutritionists usually are not regular readers of the journals on cancer research—the importance of selenium may finally be appreciated by nutritionists.

Blood Level of Selenium Is Critical. One important aspect of selenium research is that blood or hair levels of selenium are of major importance. It is not just simply a matter of what foods one eats, or how much selenium is present in those foods. Foods vary greatly in their selenium content, and just as important, food selenium varies greatly in its availability to the body. Sometimes the food selenium is present in a form more readily assimilated than other forms, and sometimes the selenium is "tied up" with other compounds such as mercury and is unavailable to the body. This is why selenium supplements are important, as they are bioavailable and in measured doses. The importance of blood levels will become clearer in the following section concerning the use of selenium in cancer therapy.

CANCER THERAPY

In the early 1970s, when it was clear that optimal intake of selenium was protective against cancer in laboratory animals, Dr. Gerhard Schrauzer of the University of California at San Diego and I called for clinical trials to test for this capability in humans. Dr. Schrauzer had completed a series of experiments that showed that optimal selenium intake could reduce the natural occurrence of breast cancer in mice by nearly 90 percent to only 12 percent of the normal cancer rate. (G. Schrauzer and D. Ishmael, *Annals of Clinical Laboratory Science* 4:441–7, 1974). He told the National Cancer Institute in 1978 that the key to cancer prevention lies in assuring adequate selenium intake.

Dr. Schrauzer stated in a 1978 article in *Family Circle* that if every woman in America started taking selenium (supplements) today or had a high-selenium diet, within a few years the breast cancer rate would decline drastically. He also remarked that if a breast cancer patient has low selenium levels in her blood, her tendency to develop metastases (other tumors) is increased, her possibility for survival is diminished and her prognosis in general is poorer than if she had normal levels.

These observations were based on the experience of a group led by Dr. K. McConnell and may have been what set several surgeons looking to see if better selenium and other nutrient antioxidant nourishment would improve patients' chances of recovery. And guess what—they do.

Recent results in treating cancer patients with selenium have been astonishing! However, there are successful reports in the medical literature going back to the 1950s that were missed even by the selenium pioneers working with laboratory animals. In 1956 four leukemia patients were given an organic compound that contains selenium called slenocystine. In all four cases, a rapid decrease of the total leukocyte count was observed, as well as a reduction in spleen size. The most striking results were obtained in the cases of acute leukemia. (A. Weisberger and L. Suhrland, *Blood* 11:19, 1956)

In 1975, as referred to above, Dr. McConnell noticed a link between the survival times of 110 cancer patients and their blood selenium levels. Dr. McConnell and his colleagues concluded that those patients with the lowest blood selenium levels were more likely to have far-spreading cancer, multiple tumors located in different organ systems and multiple recurrences. (K. McConnell, W. Broghamer, A. Blotcky and O. Hurt, *Journal of Nutrition* 105:1026–31, 1975; W. Broghamer, K. McConnell and A. Blotcky, *Cancer* 37:1384, 1976)

Conversely, those patients whose cancers were confined and who rarely suffered recurrences all had higher (but still subnormal) selenium levels. These same researchers determined in 1978 that the blood selenium levels of breast cancer patients were lower than in women in the same age brackets without breast cancer. (K. McConnell, *Advances in Nutrition Research*, vol. 2, ed. by H. Draper. New York: Plenum Press, 1979, p. 225)

Several surgeons and oncologists are now using selenium and other antioxidant nutrients to successfully treat cancer. However, since such adjunct nutritional therapy may be considered "experimental" in the legal sense in the case of malpractice suits, these doctors do not wish to be publicized. Also, there is that ever-present concern among doctors not to appear to be food faddists or quacks by using food supplements in new ways. But physicians should now recognize that the wealth of data and truth is on the side that selenium helps the body overcome cancer and it is criminal *not* to use selenium supplements as adjunct therapy. For the good of humankind it is now time for all of these researchers to put their fears behind them and speak up— and let their results do the talking.

In 1983 I reported in my book *Cancer and Its Nutritional Therapies: Updated Edition* (Keats Publishing) that Dr. R. Donaldson of the St. Louis Veterans Administration Hospital orally reported his results to the National Cancer Institute (May 9, 1982) and the Annual Meeting of VA Surgeons (1980). These reports showed remarkable results for the use of selenium in treating terminally ill cancer patients and emphasize the need for further large-scale investigation of such use. Dr. Donaldson's studies and their results have not yet been published in professional literature, perhaps because they are considered preliminary, but the bare facts of this work are important enough to merit mention here.

At the time of Dr. Donaldson's presentation to the National Cancer Institute, he had 140 patients enrolled in his study. According to the data that I have, all the patients who entered his study were certified as being terminally ill by two physicians after receiving the appropriate conventional therapy for their particular cancer. Some of the patients who entered the program with only weeks to live were alive and well after four years, and with no signs or symptoms of cancer. Not all patients were cured, but all had reduction in tumor size and pain. It is unfortunate that they did not receive the selenium until they were pronounced incurable. This research may well change cancer therapy in the future.

It is important to realize that the dramatic improvements did not occur until sufficient selenium was ingested to bring the patient's blood selenium level up to normal. Sometimes this could be achieved in a few weeks with 200–600 micrograms of selenium per day, while for other individuals as much as 2000 micrograms per day were required to normalize the blood selenium levels.

No signs of toxicity were observed in any patient—even in the autopsies of the 37 patients who were helped, but not cured by the therapy. It should also be pointed out that other antioxidant nutrients, vitamins A, C and E, were also used in the program.

It's time to cease debating the possibility that selenium helps cure cancer and move into large controlled clinical trials.

HEART DISEASE

It is not surprising that selenium is protective against heart disease. The main reason that early researchers were studying selenium was that selenium deficiency in livestock caused heart and muscle disease. In cattle and sheep, selenium deficiency caused white muscle disease, which produced chalky striations of calcium in the muscles. In swine, selenium deficiency produced mulberry heart disease, which is named after the mulberry color of the heart tissue due to the blood infiltration. Another characteristic of mulberry heart disease is that when you lay a surgically removed mulberry-diseased heart on a table, it collapses. A healthy heart maintains a firm structure; selenium deficiency tends to weaken all muscle structure.

Livestock graze in a limited area and have a limited diet. It has always been thought that since people have a more diverse diet with foods coming from widely varied regions, humans would never experience such gross selenium deficiency as seen in cattle and swine. Wrong. In 1981, the *New England Journal of Medicine* (304(21): 1304–1305) reported a case of cardiomyopathy in a young girl eating a diet essentially of hot dogs and cereal. After selenium supplementation, she improved dramatically and the disease was corrected.

But selenium's role in protection against heart disease is not limited to the health of the tissue or affected only by gross selenium deficiency; subclinical deficiency plays several roles in heart-related problems. In 1965, Dr. K. O. Godwin found that animals fed low-selenium diets developed abnormal electrocardiograms and blood pressure disturbances.

In *Supernutrition* (Dial Press, 1975; Pocket Books, 1977) I reported that a veterinary drug called Seletoc, a combination of selenium and vitamin E, had been in use since 1962 to successfully treat degenerative heart disease. In 1972, a variation of the formula, called Telsem, was reported to be 92 percent effective against recurring angina pectoris in dogs and was undergoing clinical trials in Mexico. The wide availability of selenium as a food supplement may have discouraged the completion of those trials. A drug has to produce a high profit margin to pay for the clinical trials, and the wide availability of inexpensive supplements removed the profit incentive.

However, research on the role of selenium in protection against heart disease continued. In 1976, Drs. Ray Shamberger and Charles Willis of the Cleveland Clinic reported that persons living in low-selenium areas had three times more heart disease than those in selenium-rich areas. Tables 4 and 5 show this relationship in greater detail. Dr. Johan Bjorksten found that in Finnish counties having 0.1 part per million (ppm) or more of selenium in the drinking water, the heart disease death rate in persons 15-64 was only one per 1730 persons. This compares to one heart disease death per 224 persons of the same age in counties where the drinking water contains 0.05 ppm or less of selenium. The relationship between low soil selenium and increased rates of heart disease still holds.

In the mid-1970s, the relationship between selenium deficiency and high blood pressure was being pursued. One link between selenium deficiency and high blood pressure was a reduction in prostaglandin levels. Another link was that selenium detoxifies cadmium, which is known to elevate blood pressure.

A DISCOVERY IN CHINA—KESHAN DISEASE

China has a huge low-selenium belt running diagonally from the northeast to the southwest. A form of heart disease called Keshan disease is prevalent in this low-selenium area. Keshan disease resembles the mulberry heart disease described earlier. The people most

TABLE 4

WORLD HEART DISEASE RATES VERSUS SELENIUM INTAKE

Country	Selenium Intake micrograms/day	Coronary Heart Disease Rate
Finland	25	1009
USA	61	870
Canada	62	722
Ireland	75	722
Australia	76	867
Norway	82	602
Greece	92	236
Poland	94	301
Yugoslavia	99	232
Bulgaria	108	331

Selenium intake and coronary heart disease deaths per 100,000 in 55- to 64-year-old males in ten countries

Source: Data with exception of Finland from Shamberger, R., Gunsch, M., Willis, C. and McCormack, L. 1975 *Trace Substances in Environmental Health* ix ed. D. Hemphill. Columbia: University of Mississippi Press, pp. 15–22. Author has corrected the Finnish figures to those used by Dr. Johan Bjorksten and Dr. Pekko Koivistoinen, head, Dept. of Food Chemistry and Technology, University of Helsinki.

susceptible to this disease are children and women of child-bearing age.

A study of the effects of selenium supplements of Keshan disease was initiated in 1974. In Nianning County, selenium supplements were given to 4510 children selected at random, while 3985 others made up the control group receiving the placebo. The following year these two groups were increased to 6709 and 5445, respectively. The results were so dramatic that the control group was abolished in 1976 and all children were given selenium supplements. Thus, 99 percent of the children aged one to nine in four communes in the county participated in the clinical trial.

As reported in the *Chinese Medical Journal* and *Lancet*: "In 1974, of the 3,985 children in the control group, there were fifty-four cases of Keshan disease (1.35 percent), while only ten of the 4,510

TABLE 5

U.S.A. HEART DISEASE DEATH RATES AND SELENIUM

Disease	Selenium levels			
	Very high	High	Medium	Low
Coronary	774	818	893	962
Hypertensive	34	53	64	71
Cardiovascular Renal	1045	1149	1252	1308
Cerebrovascular	108	138	159	139
Coronary	220	225	249	306
Hypertensive	27	39	47	53
Cardiovascular Renal	413	428	474	539
Cerebrovascular	89	94	109	104

Age-specific death rates per 100,000 for white males or females, age 55–65, 1959–1961. Selenium level classification, above 0.26 is very high, 0.10 to 0.25 is high. 0.06 to 0.09 is medium, and 0.01 to 0.05 is low.

Source: Shamberger, R. May 11–13, 1976. *Proceedings of the Symposium on Selenium-Tellurium in the Environment.* University of Notre Dame, p. 265.

selenium-supplemented children fell ill to the disease (0.22 percent). The difference in the morbidity rate between the two groups was highly significant.

"Again a significant difference was shown in the 1975 figures with fifty-two of 5445 children in the control group (0.95 percent) and only seven of the 6767 in the treated group (0.1 percent).

"As a result of this data that showed that oral administration of selenium had positive effects in the prevention of Keshan disease, all the children were given selenium supplements from 1976 on. In consequence, only four cases occurred out of the 12,579 children in 1976, further lowering the rate of 0.03 percent. *In 1977, there were no fresh cases among the 12,747 treated children.*" (*Chinese Medical Journal* 92 (7): 471–476, 1979; *Lancet,* October 28, 1979, p. 890.)

ATHEROSCLEROSIS AND COMMON FORMS
OF HEART DISEASE

Persons with low selenium blood levels develop significantly more heart disease than those with higher levels of selenium blood levels. In 1982, Dr. J. T. Salonen and his Finnish colleagues published an interesting prospective clinical study (*Lancet* 2:175). Blood samples were collected from approximately 11,000 Finns who were free of heart disease in 1972, and stored for analysis at a later date. During the next seven years 367 of these volunteers suffered a heart attack or died of heart disease. These subjects were matched with 367 volunteers of the same sex, age, lifestyle, etc., who remained free of heart disease, and the stored blood samples from these 724 individuals were retrieved and analyzed for selenium concentration.

The average selenium level in the blood from those who became stricken with heart disease during the seven-year period was significantly lower than the average blood selenium level from those who remained free of heart disease. A blood selenium level of less than 45 micrograms per liter was associated with a two- to threefold greater risk of heart disease as compared to subjects with higher blood selenium levels.

Another study demonstrated that there were actually fewer cholesterol deposits in the arteries of persons with higher levels of selenium in their blood. Drs. Julie Ann Moore, Robert Noiva and Ibert C. Wells of the Creighton University School of Medicine followed up the study led by Dr. Salonen by measuring the amount of selenium in the blood of patients about to have their arteries examined by arteriography (angiogram). In the 106 patients the extent of observed cholesterol deposits was inversely correlated with selenium level—the lower the selenium level, the more likely the presence of cholesterol deposits and the greater the extent.

The highest average selenium value (136 micrograms per liter) was found in those persons free of coronary blockage. Patients with the lowest average blood selenium level were found to have blockage of three coronary arteries. Patients with one or two blocked coronary arteries had intermediate blood selenium levels.

It is significant to know that selenium reduces heart disease incidence and death rate, yet scientists always want to know how and why. Part of the answer is that selenium is protective against heart disease by keeping arteries free of cholesterol deposits. But selenium also helps keep the blood "slippery." Since a heart attack is usually caused by a clot forming in a coronary artery which prevents oxygen from reaching the heart tissue serviced by that artery, having fewer cholesterol deposits on which clots can form, and "slippery" free-flowing blood, certainly diminishes the possibility of a clot forming.

Arteries produce a substance called prostacyclin which prevents blood clots. However, if oxidized fats are present in the blood, prostacyclin production is reduced, and the blood tends to clot. Selenium reduces the oxidation of fats in the blood and tissue, thereby helping to keep the prostacyclin level normal. Thus, the blood retains its normal—and appropriate—"slipperiness." This is different from anticoagulant drugs that can cause the blood to become so "slippery" that bleeding cannot be controlled or that spontaneous bleeding occurs.

Two studies published in 1984 examine this role of selenium. One is by Dr. N. W. Stead and colleagues as published in the *American Journal of Clinical Nutrition* (39:677) and the other is by Dr. R. Schiavon et al., in *Thrombosis Research* (34:389). The net effect was demonstrated in laboratory animals that had their coronary arteries tied off so as to produce the same effect as a blockage due to a clot in the coronary artery. Two teams of researchers found that selenium greatly reduced the damage to the heart caused by the stoppage of blood. (Koeler et al., *Kardiologiya* 25:9, 72–6, 1985 and Litvitskii et al., *Kardiologiya* 22:7, 94-8, 1982)

Selenium has thus been shown to be protective against heart disease by livestock animal studies, laboratory animal studies, epidemiological studies and human clinical studies. In addition, several mechanisms have been delineated through which selenium provides this protective action. These mechanisms include maintaining the integrity of heart and artery tissue, regulation of blood pressure, regulation of blood clotting and "slipperiness" and the reduction of plaque or cholesterol deposits in arteries.

A gallery of some of the most important figures
in the development of antioxidants and of
some of the authors represented in this book

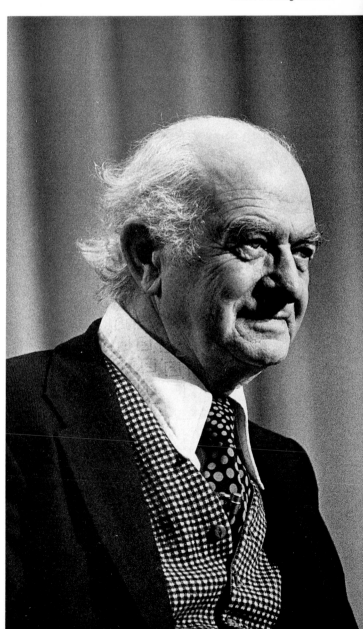

Linus Pauling Institute

*Two-time Nobel Prize laureate LINUS
PAULING, Ph.D. did more than anyone
to popularize the most widely used of the
antioxidants, vitamin C—by tying it to the
treatment and prevention of one of the most
prevalent, annoying and intractable
ailments, the common cold. His book* The
Nature of the Chemical Bond
revolutionized chemistry and biochemistry

In Hungary in 1932 ALBERT SZENT-GYÖRGYI, M.D., Ph.D. discovered and synthesized vitamin C, which brought him a Nobel Prize five years later. At the same time he discovered "vitamin P"—bioflavonoids—first hailed as of major nutrient Importance, then derided as valueless, now seen once again as essential to good health. He was for many years Scientific Director of the National Foundation for Cancer Research at Woods Hole, Massachusetts.

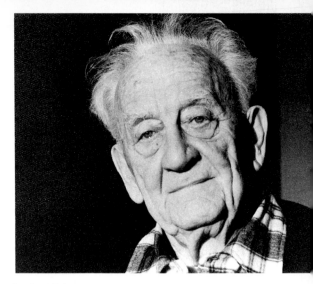

Marine Biological Laboratory

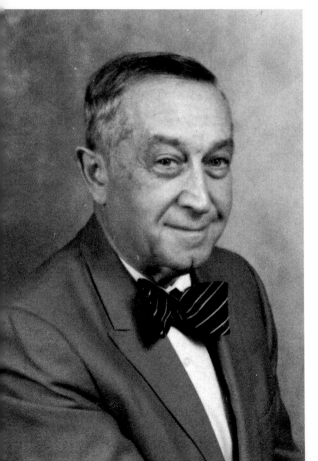

Biochemist IRWIN STONE, D.Sc. was investigating the curative properties of vitamin C within a few years of its discovery by Szent-Györgyi and spreading the word of its effectiveness even before Dr. Pauling. In 1934 he received the first patents on the use of the vitmain.

WILFRID E. SHUTE, M.D. and physician brother Evan discov vitamin E in 1933, pioneered its use for h health, and explored its use in burns other conditions, treating more than 30, patients at their famous institut London, Ontario. Wilfrid wrote the pop Vitamin E for Ailing and Heal Hearts and Evan wrote The Heart Vitamin

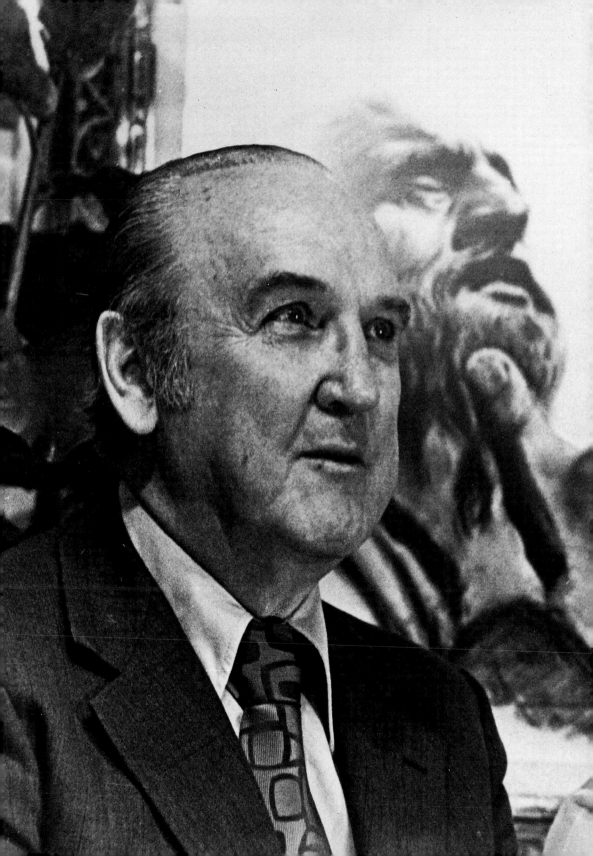

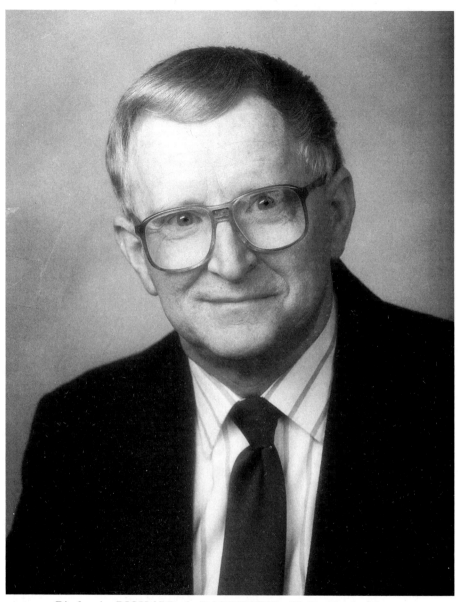

Biochemist RICHARD A. PASSWATER, Ph.D. (Antioxidants,
Beta-Carotene, Selenium, Pycnogenol) *has shared the fruits
of his laboratory work in many books, including several on antioxidant
nutrients; two of his books popularized the term
"supernutrition."*

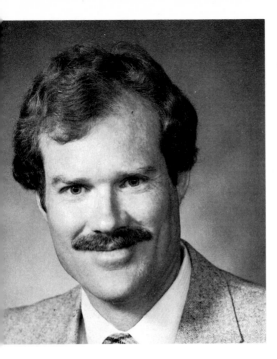

His consuming interest in nutrition has made
JEFFREY BLAND, Ph.D.
(Bioflavonoids) *a nationally known figure in
the field, with books, lectures, articles
and seminars, and, indeed, his own health
communication firm.*

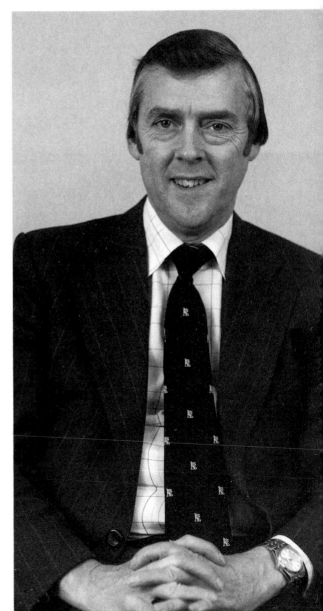

*Chemist and teacher LEN MERVYN, Ph.D.
(Vitamin E) earned awards in Europe
and America for his work with vitamin B12.*

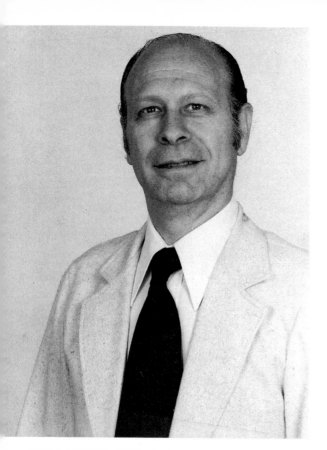

WILLIAM H. LEE, R.Ph., Ph.D.
(Coenzyme Q-10) *used his academic
and practical background in pharmacology
and herbal studies to produce a number
of books and pamphlets on nutrition and its
relationship to health.*

JACK CHALLEM (Vitamin C) *is wide
known for his many books and articl
and is a frequent contributor to health-orient
periodicals, for which he intervieu
Linus Pauling and Wilfrid Shute, amo
many othe*

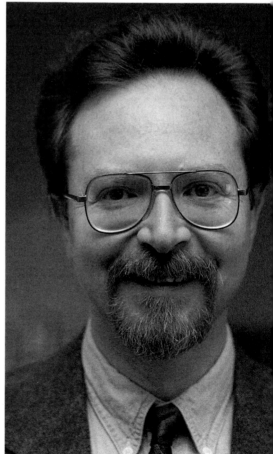

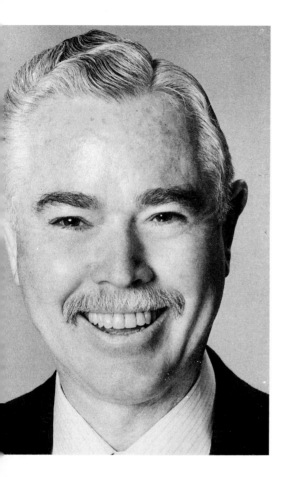

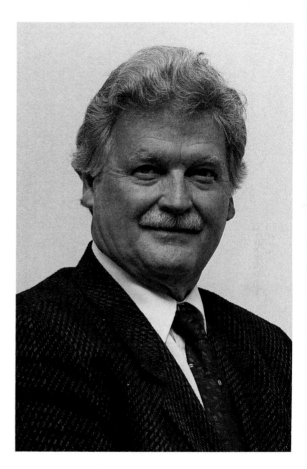

FRANK MURRAY (Ginkgo Biloba) *has written or coauthored nearly 30 books on health and nutrition, and is editor of* Better Nutrition, *a magazine reaching 470,000 readers.*

J. AUGUSTE MOCKLE (Phytomedicines) *has researched the properties of medicinal plants both in France and in Canada and continues to consult in that field.*

DAVID J. LIN (Free Radicals) *has covered the complex area of free radical biochemistry in a popular book and several articles.*

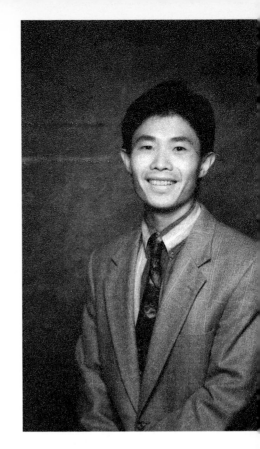

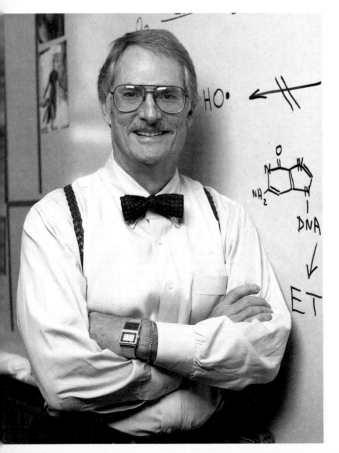

WILLIAM A. PRYOR, Ph.D. (Foreword), *Director of the Biodynamics Institute at Louisiana State University, has investigated for many years the action of antioxidants against free radicals.*

ARTHRITIS

Arthritis is a multifactorial disease for which there is no agreed-upon cause or cure. Although the cause is not agreed upon, there is evidence that selenium relieves the symptoms. There is also evidence that selenium deficiency—or a general deficiency of the other antioxidant nutrients (vitamins A, C and E) plus selenium—contributes to the development of arthritis. The deficiency of the antioxidants allows the formation of excess free radicals which produce the pain and swelling of arthritis.

Superoxide dismutase (SOD), an enzyme that serves as an antioxidant, is also deficient in persons with arthritis. When additional SOD is injected into arthritic joints, significant reduction of swelling and pain is observed. There is evidence that the antioxidant enzyme glutathione peroxidase, which contains four atoms of selenium in every molecule, also reduces swelling and pain in arthritic joints.

Veterinarians have used a formulation containing 1000 micrograms of selenium and 68 IU of vitamin E successfully for years in treating arthritic horses. The injections of SOD provide quicker results, but the selenium and vitamin E does work well. Now the same relief is being reported in people.

At the May 1980 meeting of selenium researchers, Norwegian scientists reported the beneficial results of selenium against arthritis: "In rheumatoid arthritis, it has been suggested that superoxide (free) radicals and lipoperoxides (also free radicals) can be generated in the tissues and accelerate the progression of the disease. Since selenium is a component of the protective enzyme glutathione peroxidase, we determined the blood levels of selenium in a group of twenty-three rheumatoid arthritis patients." (J. Aaseth et al., *Second International Symposium on Selenium in Biology and Medicine*, Texas Technical University, Lubbock, Texas, May 1980) The researchers found that the arthritis group did have depressed selenium levels compared to the reference group. At the same conference, Dr. E. Crary of Smyrna, Georgia, had already treated patients having traumatic arthritis with selenium plus the antioxidant nutrient vitamins A, C and E, success-fully relieving the pain in their traumatized joints.

In 1982, the British Arthritic Association conducted a three-month trial of a formulation containing selenium plus vitamins A, C and E. The trial included some of the worst cases, and yet 64 percent re-ported considerable reduction in pain within the three months. Many continued the supplement and found continuing reduction in pain.

Among the patients was Mr. Charles Ware, 74, the British Ar-thritic Association's president, who developed arthritis of the hip after a fall during World War II. He told newspaper reporters, "I thought that I would never get rid of the pain. But now I have full movement of my hip and no pain whatever." The British Arthritic Association is now recommending selenium plus the antioxidant vitamins A, C, and E to all its members.

Following newspaper accounts of this successful trial, the British magazine *Here's Health* distributed this same formulation of selenium plus the vitamins A, C, and E to 1000 volunteers. Replies to a fol-lowup questionnaire were received from 418 of the volunteers. Im-provement was noted by 315 (75 percent).

A Danish study was published in 1985 that confirmed the 1980 Norwegian study. Blood selenium concentrations were measured in 87 patients with rheumatoid arthritis. The researchers headed by Dr. U. Tarp found significant differences in patients of the three distinct courses of the disease. The group having an active, disabling disease of long duration had a very reduced selenium level (65 mcg). The group with protracted but mild disease had a slightly reduced level (74 mcg). The group with mild disease of short duration had a slightly (but not statistically significant) reduced blood selenium level (76 mcg). The researchers concluded, "A low selenium level may thus be a further factor in the pathogenesis of rheumatoid arthritis." (*Scandinavian Journal of Rheumatology* 14:97–101, 1985)

Japanese researcher Dr. Masaru Kondo has found that treating persons with arthritis with 350 micrograms of selenium and 400 IU of vitamin E daily, plus injecting white blood cells from healthy people is very effective. All seven of his first patients improved dramatically, and five of the seven were essentially free of the disease by the time he wrote his report. (*Biological Trace Element Research* 7:195–198, May–June 1985)

When the white blood cell injections were given without the antioxidant supplements, only one of thirty rheumatoid arthritis patients obtained a complete remission. All patients had severe joint pains for over four years prior to the treatment, and their rheumatoid factor titer (RFT) was initially high (average 379). The five patients experiencing complete remission also had their RFT return to a normal of less than four. The remaining two patients had diminished joint pain and increased joint mobility.

This chapter has presented a sampling of the research that shows that selenium is protective against cancer, heart disease and arthritis. More details on this research plus the role of selenium in the protection against other diseases is found in my book *Selenium as Food and Medicine* (Keats Publishing).

Why Selenium May Be the Secret of Your Longer Life

A little-known mineral may well be the secret of adding extra years to your heart—and so to your life—if the initial results from current research prove to be widely applicable. The mineral is selenium, whose use as a protector against cancer has long been known. Recently, doctors have decided to investigate the relationship of selenium to the health of the heart, and have come up with indications that selenium therapy could well reverse the trend of the nation's leading killer.

Kaarlo Jaakkola, M.D., of the University of Jyvaskyla in Finland, astounded medical colleagues when, as the head of a research team, he announced that selenium together with vitamin E could reduce chest pains.

Dr. Jaakkola found that by giving selenium to a group of thirty patients with ischemic heart disease (a condition characterized by narrowed coronary arteries), he could produce remarkable improvements in their condition. All the patients were troubled with moderate to severe chest pain. At the beginning of the experimental treatment, they were taking large supplies of prescribed nitroglycerin as well as other medication to relieve their symptoms.

Dr. Jaakkola prescribed a daily supply of selenium together with vitamin E and told the heart-troubled patients to continue taking their medications. He reports, "We saw improvements within two weeks. Then we saw maximum benefits after four to eight weeks."

This combination was reported as most beneficial for those troubled with ischemic heart disease. The nutrients played an important role in the intracellular antioxidant defense mechanism, protecting cells from damaging lipid peroxides, thus preventing the rancidity of important cells and guarding against invasion of free radicals or waste products that could be damaging to the heart. Selenium also protects against platelet hyperaggregation, or sticky platelets that could cause a fatal stroke.

SELENIUM WASHES OUT FREE RADICALS

A noted internist and cardiologist, Arnold Fox, M.D., former assistant professor of medicine at the University of California at Irvine Medical School, has found that selenium has a unique heart-saving effect, that of unblocking, controlling and washing out free radicals.

"Rusting is a form of oxidation. As oxygen is used in the course of normal reactions within the body, free radicals can be formed. These are unstable compounds with a propensity toward reacting with other compounds in a hasty, and quite often dangerous, fashion."

Dr. Fox has found that selenium, along with other nutrients, can control free radical formation. Why is this so? Because selenium is an antioxidant. "Antioxidants help control, that is, suppress, the rate of oxidation, and hence a free radical formation." He cautions that "free radicals can be involved in a circular series of reactions which increase the risk of heart attack with every step."

A pioneer researcher in the use of this heart-saving mineral, Dr. Raymond Shamberger of the (Ohio) Clinic, joined with other researchers to extol the importance of selenium. Speaking before the 1976 annual meeting of the Federation of American Societies for Experimental Biology, he announced that if you live in a selenium-reduced area, you are three times as much at risk of dying of heart disease as is someone in a selenium-rich area.

He identified these deficient areas: Connecticut, Illinois, Ohio, Oregon, Massachusetts, Rhode Island, New York, Pennsylvania, Indiana, Delaware and the District of Columbia.

Other areas may not be as severely deficient in selenium, but shortages can create problems, even at a small level. This suggests strongly that supplemental intake of selenium may be desirable, even outside selenium-poor regions. "If selenium has an effect on heart disease—and the evidence points to it—then Americans are probably 100 to 150 micrograms short in their selenium intakes. A supplementation of the American diet could bring about the desired increase of the total intakes to about 250 to 350 micrograms per day."

A GIFT PACKAGE OF HEALTH BENEFITS

When you take your doctor-approved selenium, you will nourish your heart muscle, shield yourself against reactions should you sustain heart problems, help to give yourself a better-balanced blood pressure and protect against deposit formation along your arteries. In short, you may be taking out the best heart insurance policy available!

Garlic ... Ancients' Answer to Poison Now Modern Remedy for Blood Clotting and Variety of Human Ills

Progress, or what is called progress, brings with it a collection of poisons, but polluted air, polluted water, stress and the other ills we are now heir to may be relieved by an herbal remedy cherished by the ancients as an answer to their poisons.

That remedy is garlic.

For centuries, people have extolled the extraordinary powers of garlic. In 3,000 B.C. the Babylonians used it against disease. The ancient Egyptians gave garlic to slaves to increase their ability to work harder and longer and to soldiers to instil courage in battle. It was the one herb the Hebrews missed during their exodus from Egypt as Moses searched for the Promised Land. Dioscorides, a physician of ancient Greece, wrote, "It clears the arteries," while an ancient Roman commented, "It cures coughs also, and suppurations of the chest, however violent they may be."

Aristophanes believed that garlic juice could restore a man's flagging virility; the Persians thought it had the power to prevent "stagnation of the blood"; it was used as a laxative, sudorific, diuretic and as an antidote to poison. During the Middle Ages it was said to ward off the plague and American doctors used it until early in this century against asthma, whooping cough, typhus and cholera.

This aromatic herb has come into its own in modern times as research in nutrition and wholistic medicine indicates that the healthful and curative power revered by the ancients can serve us just as well.

What is it in garlic that makes it work?

According to the U.S. Department of Agriculture, garlic contains the following:

protein	**carotene**
vitamin A	**selenium**
vitamin C	germanium
vitamin B complex	calcium

phosphorus   iron
potassium   allicin

Germanium and selenium are considered to be the most important minerals supplied by garlic, with selenium recently recognized by the govern-
ment as being essential to life. It is a strong antioxidant and necessary for
the health of the heart muscle. It can improve the function of the mitochondria (the energy-producing units of cells) by protecting them from lack of
oxygen. Selenium is also required for the production of a hormone-like
substance called prostaglandin which helps to regulate blood pressure. It is
also a component of an enzyme, glutathione peroxidase, which protects cells
against oxidative damage. Selenium is required to maintain resistance to
many diseases, yet selenium-deficient soil, modern fertilization practices and
the spread of acid rain have reduced the amount of this trace mineral in
our foods.

Germanium has been the subject of research abroad, although little has
been done in this country, and is reputed to be effective in the treatment
of cancer.

Most of the laboratory and clinical research on garlic has been done on
allicin. Technically, allicin is known as allyl allylthiosulfinate and is created
in garlic through the combination of an enzyme and an animo acid. Allicin
is believed to be responsible for garlic's antibacterial action; it destroys the
bacteria that cause strep throat, staph infections, typhoid and dysentery.
But garlic must be crushed to initiate this bactericidal action; crushing the
cloves causes the enzyme aliinase to interact with the amino acid alliin,
forming allicin—and also, unfortunately, releasing the powerful odor and
sometimes creating "garlic breath." The power is directly related to the
odor and is easily destroyed if it is heated. Commercial packagers have
found a way to extract the volatile oil from garlic cloves and put it into
capsules. Two capsules three times a day with meals is adequate and most
people do not experience the odor or taste. It's a small price to pay for
the benefits.

Recent studies suggest that garlic does indeed have the power to "clear
the arteries." It may be more accurate to say it can keep them clear of the
fatty deposits that herald atherosclerosis and the risk of heart disease. It also
gradually reduces the cholesterol level. What's more important, it reduces
the low-density-lipoprotein (LDL) cholesterol that raises heart disease risk.

Garlic also serves as an added protection against internal clotting. The
clotting procedure is a protective measure and without it we would bleed
to death from any tiny wound. However, if clotting should occur within

one of the blood vessels, it could lead to a serious condition and possibly death. Garlic helps protect the body against spontaneous clotting by making blood platelets less "sticky" so they won't clump together too easily. If they can flow past each other, they are less likely to block a small vessel and become a clot. Garlic also promotes the natural action of certain blood chemicals that dissolve clots that have begun to form.

Vegetarians learned that complete protein (protein that supplied the body with all the essential amino acids) could be obtained by eating rice and beans or corn and beans in the same meal. Our neighbors living on a so-called "primitive diet" have known that for centuries. Now we can take another lesson from the countries of the Mediterranean and Latin America. Garlic is a mainstay in their cooking, and it's no coincidence that those countries have much lower heart disease rates than our own.

There are odorless garlic products available. Kyolic, an aged and purified garlic extract, was developed in the 1960s in Japan and is available in the U.S. in health food stores.

American medicine is just beginning to catch up with the folk remedies. They offer a great advantage over the powerful drugs prescribed so casually, which have side effects ranging from minor to serious to severely dangerous to the individual taking them. Science should pay greater attention to the herbal remedies that cure more slowly but more thoroughly.

Folklore, Old Wives Were Right

*Garlic Stimulates the Immune System, Fights Free
Radicals, Inhibits Tumors*

Although garlic and other members of the allium family have been mainstays
of folk medicine and international cuisines for thousands of years, it has
only been rather recently that scientific research has proven the many health
benefits of garlic and onions. Ongoing research has shown that garlic, *Allium
sativum*, is useful in the treatment of various forms of cancer, for lowering
high blood pressure, as a stimulant for the immune system, for reducing
cholesterol and triglyceride levels in the blood, and for offsetting free-radical
damage and heavy-metal intoxication among other things.

REDUCED CHOLESTEROL

At a seminar entitled "Garlic: An International Dialogue on Cardiovascular Benefits," held in April 1991 in New York, results of a German study
involving 261 patients revealed that garlic tablets helped to reduce cholesterol levels by an average of 12 percent while lowering triglyceride averages
by 17 percent. Both of these substances have been implicated in the development of cardiovascular disease.

"These findings suggest that using a concentrated form of garlic powder
is safe and, if additional studies confirm the preliminary data, may prove
effective as a diet supplement for lowering cholesterol or as a substitute for
some cholesterol-lowering drugs," said Marvin Moser, M.D., clinical professor of medicine at Yale University School of Medicine.

In the study, conducted by the German Association of General Practitioners, volunteers were given 800 mg of garlic powder or a placebo daily
for four months. All participants had a cholesterol reading of 200 mg/dl,
the ideal count, or higher.

For the patients who had cholesterol levels over 300 mg/dl, which is very
high, garlic decreased the blood levels of the fat-like substance by 16 percent. In the placebo group, the drop was 7 percent. For the participants
who had cholesterol readings of between 250 and 300 mg/dl, garlic brought

the level down 14 percent. In the placebo group, the reduction was only 1 percent.

Garlic reduced cholesterol levels by 7 percent in the volunteers who had readings of between 200 and 250 mg/dl. And in the placebo group, the readings went down 3 percent.

GARLIC THERAPY

In Germany, where garlic has been studied extensively, numerous trials have demonstrated the efficacy of using garlic as a therapeutic agent. As an example 12 studies, which involved some 700 patients, showed that garlic lowered total cholesterol an average of 11 percent.

Eleven studies, with over 650 people participating, have found a reduction in blood pressure in those who continued with the therapy for the duration of the study. For patients with mild to moderate hypertension (90 to 106), decreases in diastolic blood pressure were in the 5 to 16 percent range, depending on the dosage and blood pressure measurements at the beginning of the study.

In 10 of 11 clinical trials, garlic lowered triglycerides from 5 to 35 percent. These studies involved over 640 patients.

At the First World Congress on the Health Significance of Garlic and Garlic Constituents, held Aug. 28–30, 1990 in Washington, D.C., more than 50 prominent garlic researchers from 15 countries discussed the lipid-lowering, cancer-preventing and anticoagulatory properties of garlic.

Dr. Asaf A. Quereshi, Dr. Robert I. Lin, Dr. Niloer Quereshi and Dr. Naji Abuirmeileh discussed their study, which showed substantial protective effects of aged garlic extract in reducing cholesterol levels. Using chickens for their model, they found that garlic reduced total cholesterol by up to 30 percent; low-density lipoprotein cholesterol (the "bad" kind) by up to 50 percent.

LDL-cholesterol is the most dangerous form of this substance in causing hardening of the arteries and in elevating triglyceride levels, they said. Garlic also inhibited the liver's ability to synthesize cholesterol and fatty acids.

"Aged garlic extract also inhibited thromboxane B2 synthesis and platelet aggregation." Dr. Lin said, "since excessive levels of serum cholesterol, triglyceride and platelet aggregation tendency are the key contributing factors to the most common cardiovascular disease, such nutritional properties of garlic are highly beneficial to cardiovascular risk reduction."

A number of the speakers reviewed garlic's anticancer properties. In laboratory studies, Drs. John A. Milner and Jinzhou Liu of Pennsylvania State

University found that aged garlic extract powder inhibited DMBA-induced mammary tumors in rats. DMBA is a potent carcinogen.

Dr. William J. Blot of the National Cancer Institute in Washington, D.C., reviewed research from abroad, showing that in northeastern China stomach cancer declined in those areas where people increased their consumption of garlic, garlic stalks, chives, scallions and onions. Garlic consumption also reduced the risk of stomach cancer in Italy, he said.

POTENTIAL AGAINST MELANOMA

Dr. David S.B. Hoon, Dr. Reiko F. Irie, Dr. Robert I. Lin and Ms. Lan Sze, all of the University of California in Los Angeles, stated that aged garlic extract has the potential for preventing and controlling melanoma, one of the fastest growing kinds of skin cancer in the United States.

Studies by Drs. Hiromichi Sumiyoshi and Michael Wargovich of the University of Texas confirmed that garlic inhibits the development of cancer caused by DMH, another powerful cancer-causing agent.

At West Virginia University, Drs. Donald Lam, Dale R. Riggs and Jean I. De Haven said that aged garlic extract reduced the incidence of cancer in mice that had been implanted with cancer cells.

In still another study, Dr. Lin suggested that garlic extract protects red blood cells from oxidation and free-radical damage.

Writing in *Nutritional Influences on Illness* (Keats Publishing, Inc., 1989), Dr. Melvyn R. Werbach reviewed the scientific literature which shows the benefits of garlic and onions in preventing hardening of the arteries and some types of cancer.

As an example, an article in the *British Medical Journal* in 1985 reported that 600 mg of garlic powder daily reduced cholesterol levels by 10 percent in the 10 patients with elevated cholesterol readings. There was also a decrease in blood viscosity, levels of triglycerides and LDL when compared with controls.

In an experimental study reported in *Carcinogenesis* in 1983, garlic oil and onion oil were equally beneficial in decreasing the number and incidence of skin tumors, he added.

"Daily intake of garlic oil (15 mg or the equivalent of eight to nine cloves of garlic) lowers total cholesterol levels, increases HDL-cholesterol and lowers LDL-cholesterol," stated Robert H. Garrison, Jr., M.A., R.Ph. and Elizabeth Somer, M.A., R.D. in *The Nutrition Desk Reference*, Second Edition (Keats, 1990).

They went on to say that studies on animals and humans show that

Allium (garlic) modifies blood lipids and reduces the risk for developing atherosclerosis and cardiovascular disease. Serum cholesterol and triglycerides are reduced in both normolipidemic and hyperlipidemic subjects when garlic or its essential oils are added to the diet.

"The reduction in serum total cholesterol ranges from 10 to 29 percent, while serum HDL-cholesterol increases as much as 31 percent, LDL-cholesterol decreases 7.5 percent, and triglycerides drop 20 percent or more," they continued. "In some cases, serum cholesterol rises initially, followed by an eventual reduction during continued use."

In an article in the February 7, 1990 issue of *The New York Times*, Molly O'Neill reported that Dr. Victor Gurewich of Tufts University, after observing a Polish folk cure, gave onions to 20 patients and found that they triggered a positive shift in cholesterol levels.

The *Times* article also said that Dr. James Duke of the U.S. Department of Agriculture became interested in the link between garlic and cancer after observing the amount of garlic eaten in certain provinces of China and the low incidence of cancer there. He is also investigating the use of garlic in reducing the incidence of blood clots.

"The National Cancer Institute plans to study garlic as a potential cancer-fighting substance this year," O'Neill continued. "Excessive amounts of raw garlic can be toxic, but when dried, extracted and aged to form a powder, its sulfur compounds can enter the body's cells and stimulate immune response, said Dr. Herbert Pierson, a toxicologist in the division of cancer prevention and control at the Cancer Institute."

With so much convincing evidence available, one cannot go wrong in using garlic in the kitchen or adding garlic supplements to the daily routine.

PART THREE

——•——

MORE ANTIOXIDANTS

THE NEW SUPERANTIOXIDANT— PLUS

The Amazing Story of Pycnogenol,
Free-Radical Antagonist and
Vitamin C Potentiator

RICHARD A. PASSWATER, PH.D.

TRIPLE ACTION ANTIOXIDANT

As an antioxidant, Pycnogenol, a blend of special bioflavonoids, reduces free-radical-caused tissue damage many times more effectively than vitamin E, potentiates the health-giving effects of vitamin C, and protects brain and nerve tissue with its nearly unique ability to penetrate the blood-brain barrier.

It also reduces inflammation and improves circulation, both relieving the distresses of arthritis, diabetes and stroke and promoting prevention of cardiovascular disease and cancer.

And its ability to bond to collagen promotes renewed youthfulness, flexibility and body integrity—even allowing it to function as an "oral cosmetic."

This chapter explains how this bioflavonoid blend works and gives you the information you need to see if it can benefit you.

A remarkable plant-derived substance has been used clinically in Europe for many years and has demonstrated apparent effectiveness in promoting longer and healthier life and in maintaining or restoring a youthful appearance. Its versatile action appears to result from its being a potent antioxidant and from its function as a unique vitamin C and bioflavonoid "helper."

This substance, Pycnogenol, (pronounced pick-nah-geh-nol) is a special blend of a type of bioflavonoid called proanthocyanidins. These flavones are also found in fruits, vegetables and other plants.[1] Pycnogenol has recently been patented in the United States and is available as a food supplement. This chapter will examine some of the research and clinical work conducted with Pycnogenol and invite you to assess its potential for benefiting your own health. As a special service to health professionals, certain sections conclude with brief extracts from the relevant professional literature.

In terms of helping vitamin C function, Pycnogenol appears to be superior to the bioflavonoids from lemons and red peppers that Dr. Albert Szent-Györgyi found potentiated vitamin C. You may recall the story about how the bioflavonoids were called "vitamin P" until it was determined that no deficiency disease could be produced when the bioflavonoids were removed from the diet. Thus, the bioflavonoids are considered "secondary food factors" rather than true vitamins, or, to put it another way, "semi-essential."

Because this bioflavonoid blend is such a strong antioxidant, it directly prevents vitamin C from being oxidized to dehydroascorbate. It is believed that another important way in which Pycnogenol helps vitamin C is by its action on the enzyme, ascorbic oxidase, that metabolizes (breaks down) vitamin C in the body. Another way it helps vitamin C is by providing hydrogen ions to reduce glutathione. The reduced form of glutathione converts oxidized vitamin C (dehydroascorbate) back into its active form (ascorbate). Other vitamin C "helper" actions have been postulated, but not fully studied as yet.

As an effective antioxidant, Pycnogenol helps our bodies resist blood vessel and skin damage, mental deterioration, inflammation and other damage caused by harmful free radicals. Free-radical damage is a common factor in a host of non-"germ" diseases, including heart disease, cancer, arthritis and accelerated aging.

Free radicals are highly reactive molecules or molecular fragments characterized by having the spin of one electron in the molecule not paired with a companion electron. This is a very unstable state, and free radicals do not persist for very long, quickly reacting with other compounds.

This reaction can set off a cascade of harmful reactions. Free radicals do a lot of damage in the body, ranging from attacking the DNA that regenerates our body to impairing cell membranes. Once free radicals are produced, they multiply geometrically in free-radical chain reactions unless they are quenched by antioxidants or other free-radical scavengers. Antioxidants are compounds that react easily with oxygen and thus protect neighboring compounds from damaging reactions with oxygen. Common protective antioxidant nutrients include vitamins A, C and E, and new evidence is mounting that the proanthocyanidin bioflavonoids may prove to be just as important as these, or even more so.

However, they do more than protect. They help repair by improving and stabilizing the skin protein collagen and improving the condition of arteries and capillaries. There are four biochemical properties of these substances that are responsible for their many benefits:

free-radical scavenging
collagen (a skin protein) binding
inhibition of inflammatory enzymes
inhibition of histamine formation

The benefits of proanthocyanidins, demonstrated in many studies and decades of clinical experience, include the following:

improves skin smoothness and elasticity
strengthens capillaries, arteries and veins
improves circulation and enhances cell vitality
reduces capillary fragility and improves resistance to bruising
    and strokes
reduces risk of phlebitis
reduces varicose veins
reduces edema and swelling of the legs
helps restless-leg syndrome

reduces diabetic retinopathy
improves visual acuity
helps improve sluggish memory
reduces the effects of stress
improves joint flexibility
fights inflammation in arthritis and sports injuries

Although the proanthocyanidin blend Pycnogenol is relatively new in North America, it has been researched extensively in Europe and has been widely available as a nutritional supplement since 1969 in Europe, Argentina, Australia, New Zealand, and the Far East (Singapore and Korea) for several years. Its safety has been well studied and its benefits documented in many European scientific and medical journals. As we will discuss in detail later, Pycnogenol is not toxic, mutagenic, carcinogenic, teratogenic or antigenic.

Continuing research presented at international symposia shows a growing interest in this class of bioflavonoids in preventing atherosclerosis, slowing cell mutagenesis (changes leading to cancer) and preventing ulcer formation.

THE DISCOVERY OF PYCNOGENOL

The story starts in the sixteenth century, after the discovery of Canada's Gulf of St. Lawrence by Jacques Cartier. During the winter of 1534–1535, ice prevented Cartier and his explorers from leaving the St. Lawrence waterways. They landed on the Quebec peninsula to hunt and trap for food as their provisions were dwindling. While on board their ship, they were subsisting mostly on salted meat and biscuits. Fresh fruits and vegetables were not to be had.

In December 1534, the explorers were struck down by scurvy. Scurvy had killed 25 of the 110-man crew, and more than 50 others were seriously afflicted. Most of the remainder were too weak to hunt or even to dig graves for their departed comrades. They could do no better than to bury their dead in the snow.

Fortunately for Cartier and those still alive, he met a Quebec Indian who told Cartier of a tea brewed from the Anneda tree that could quickly cure this deadly affliction. Cartier described the Anneda as a large tree with evergreen leaves and a bark that was easy to remove. Cartier immediately tried this remedy on two of his sailors, and they improved so much within a week that he gave the tea and poultice to all of his explorers. Indeed, feeding the crew tea from the needles and bark of Anneda pine trees cured them of scurvy, and as they say, the rest is history.[2]

The needles contained a small amount of vitamin C and the bark contained flavanols, which potentiate the antiscorbutic effect of vitamin C. The pine bark tea and its poultice were quickly effective against the horrible scurvy.

More than 400 years later, Professor Jacques Masquelier, Dean Emeritus of the Faculty of Materia Medica of the University of Bordeaux in France, was a visiting professor at Quebec University. While there, he researched the flavonols of pine bark, grape skins and various nut shells. He continued this research after he returned to France, and found that the richest source of the most bioavailable and bioactive flavonols was in the bark of the *Pinus maritima*, which is abundant in Southern France. When Professor Masquelier published his findings in 1966, he believed that the extract was one compound, a leucocyanidin.[3] He named his compound *Pycnogenol*, which means "substances which deliver condensation products." Later, improved analytical instruments showed that the extract was a defined mixture of procyanidins.

In 1982, Professor Masquelier patented his procedure for extracting the highly effective and nontoxic flavonols, as well as the use of these compounds for "preventing and fighting the harmful biological effects of free radicals."[4] In 1987, he was granted U.S. "use" Patent #4,698,360.[1] (Previously, he had been issued a "process" patent, U.S. Patent #3,436,407.) Professor Masquelier assigned his patent to Horphag Research Ltd. of Switzerland.

Although the bioflavonoids of Pycnogenol can be extracted from grapes, cranberries, beans, cola nuts and other fruits and vegetables, the patented commercial source, not unlike the source used by the

North American Indians, is the bark of the European coastal pine (*Pinus maritima* or *Pinus pinaster*).

Flavonoids are members of the flavonol family of compounds. Bioflavonoids are a group of plant substances with recognized antioxidant properties and with the ability to inhibit inflammation. There are over 20,000 bioflavonoids registered in *Chemical Abstracts*, with about 4,000 of them characterized so far. And of course, there may be others, as calculations indicate that there are over 20 million structures that fit into this classification.

Research through the years has led scientists to particular members of the bioflavonoid family that are believed to be the most effective vitamin C potentiators. This family of nontoxic, water-soluble, highly bioavailable bioflavonoids differs from other bioflavonoids, and hence has its own family name, proanthocyanidins. In man, proanthocyanidins are found in saliva within one hour after ingesting them by capsule.[5] This verifies that they are well absorbed and transported effectively throughout the body.

In foods, these desirable bioflavonoids are destroyed by storage and by many food processing procedures; but they are available in stable form as the food supplement Pycnogenol. (The patented material is also trademarked; thus Pycnogenol is capitalized and a "TM" symbol appears after the name on labels.)

There are dozens of published studies of Pycnogenol's safety and benefits. Its safety and toxicity have been fully tested, in, among many others, mutagenic and carcinogenic studies at expert centers such as the Pasteur Institute.[6,7] It has been found to be nontoxic, nonteratogenic, nonmutagenic, noncarcinogenic and nonantigenic.[1] Proanthocyanidins have been used for more than 30 years with no signs of toxicity.

I have discussed the benefits of this supplement in articles and in my book *The New Supernutrition*.[8-10] This chapter is intended to provide additional information about Pycnogenol that so many people have requested. In the next section, we will examine its power as an antioxidant and free-radical scavenger.

FOR HEALTH PROFESSIONALS

Bioflavonoids are the major sources of the blue and red pigments, and some yellows, in plants. The carotenes account for most of the yellow and orange pigments. Most bioflavonoids contain the structure 1,4-benzopyrone having a phenyl group substituted at the 2 position. The free-radical scavenging activity is primarily due to the hydroxyl groups.

Bioflavonoid nomenclature is confusing. As more is learned, their similarities and differences suggest additional classification systems. Many biochemists have been trained by Havsteen's classification system of 11 branches in the family.[10] Now many biochemists have switched to Cody's classification system of 12 branches in the family.[11] Both systems include the following seven common classifications: flavones, flavanones, flavanols, isoflavones, anthocyanidins, chalcones, and catechins.

However, this is where the common ground stops. The four remaining classifications in the Havsteen system are: isoflavanones, isoflavanols, benzo-pyrones and coumarins. The five remaining members of the Cody system are: flavans, flavanolols, leucoanthocyanidins, dihydrochalcones and aurones.

In addition, common usage before the above-mentioned approaches to systematic nomenclature only adds to the confusion. According to Haslam, the proanthyocyanidins, the family of bioflavonoids which are the precursors of blue-violet and red pigments, include: procyanidins, prodelphidins, profixtinidins, prorobinotidins and proquibourtinidins.[12]

Procyanidins are composed of various combinations of catechin and epicatechin units. In essence, procyanidins are catechin, and/or epicatechin dimers, trimers, tetramers, or oligomers. Catechin and epicatechin—the monomers that are united to form the procyanidins—are not themselves included in the procyanidin classification.

The Horphag chemists preferred to call them "monomeric substances," to emphasize their role as constituents of the dimers, trimers, tetramers and oligomers. Also, they call taxifoline, a precursor of the procyanidins, a monomeric substance.

Pycnogenol is actually a blend of oligomeric and monomeric procyanidins. About 85 percent of the compounds of Pycnogenol are identified as procyanidins. Of these procyanidins, about 60 percent are: oligomeric procyanidins—dimers, trimers, and so on; 20 percent are oligomers and phenolic acids such as gallic acid, caffeic acid and ferulic acid; 5 percent are water. The remaining 15 percent of the compounds from the bark of *Pinus maritima* in Pycnogenol have not been identified until now.

The dimeric procyanidins are more potent free-radical scavengers than the monomeric catechin or epicatechin themselves.[13] There are extensive reports of the effectiveness of catechins as antioxidants and collagen stabilizers in the scientific literature.[14,15] For more information on bioflavonoids, please consult the two-volume set entitled *Plant Bioflavonoids in Biology and Medicine*.[16]

REFERENCES

1. Plant extract with a proanthocyanadins content as therapeutic agent having radical scavenging effect and use thereof. Masquelier, Jacques. United States Patent #4,698,360 (October 6, 1987).
2. *Voyages au Canada*. Jacques Cartier.
3. Masquelier, Jacques and Claveau, Pierre. *Naturaliste Can.* 93:345–8 (1966).
4. Plant extract with a proanthocyanadins content as therapeutic agent having radical scavenging effect and use thereof. Masquelier, Jacques. French Patent #1,300,869 (July 1982).
5. Laparra et al. *Acta Therapeutica* 4:233 (1978).
6. Mutagenicity of proanthocyanidins. Yu, C. L and Swaminathan, B. *Food Chem. Toxicol.* 25 (2):135–9 (1987).
7. Cytotest Cell Research GmbH & Co, project 143010, University of Aquila Pharmaco-Toxicologica Report (Dr. G. C. Pantaleoni) and others.
8. Pycnogenol. Passwater, Richard A. *Whole Foods*.
9. *The New Supernutrition*. Passwater, Richard A. Pocket Books, NY (1991).
10. Flavonoids: A class of natural products of high pharmacological potency. Havsteen, B. *Biochem. Pharmacol.* 32(7):1141–8 (1983).

11. Substances without vitamin status. Cody, Mildred M. In: *Handbook of Vitamins*, 2nd Ed., Machlin, Lawrence J. (ed). Dekker, NY, pp. 565–82 (1991).
12. The flavonoids. Haslam, E. In: *Advances in Research*. (Harborne and Mabey, eds.) Chapman and Hall, England (1982).
13. Oligomères procyanidoliques. Masquelier, J. *Parfums, Cosmetiques, Aromes* 95:89–97 (1990).
14. *Natural Products as Medicinal Agents*. Beal, J. L. (ed.). Hippokrates Verlag, Stuttgart (Germany) (1980).
15. Collagen treated with catechin becomes resistance to the action of mammalian collagenase. Kuttan, R.; Donnely, Patricia V. and Di Ferrante, N. *Experientia* 37 (1981).
16. *Plant bioflavonoids in Biology and Medicine*. Cody, V.; Middleton, Jr., E. and Harborne, J. Alan Liss, NY (Vol. 1, 1986; Vol. 2 1988).

PYCNOGENOL, THE POWERFUL ANTIOXIDANT

Of Pycnogenol's four modes of action, its antioxidant function is the most important to our health. However, our awareness of this role is relatively new, so it is better known for its beneficial effect on blood vessels, skin and mental function.

In its antioxidant role, the supplement provides protection from the many diseases associated with free radicals. Many diseases are caused by viruses, bacteria, or fungi, but many major diseases do not involve microorganisms. Today some 50 to 60 diseases are recognized as having free radicals involved in their causes or manifestation.

When my research on slowing the aging process was reported in *Prevention* magazine in 1971, it was the first time that the public was exposed to the terms "free radicals" and "antioxidant nutrients" in terms of health and disease.[1] When my cancer research was published two years later, it was the first time that most cancer researchers had ever heard of the connection between the two.[2] It wasn't until *Supernutrition for Healthy Hearts* was published in 1977 that other nutritionists learned of the role of free radicals in heart disease.[3]

New diseases are regularly being added to the free-radical list. The research that began with the major killer diseases such as heart disease, cancer and aging, then expanded to include the major debilitating diseases such as arthritis, now surprisingly may prove to show free-radical involvement in diseases such as asthma. Now it almost seems as if hardly a day goes by that an article doesn't appear in a major newspaper or magazine about the role of free radicals in disease, and the protection offered by antioxidant nutrients. It is fair to say that these terms are now recognized concepts used in the everyday language of knowledgeable people.

It is not necessary to understand how free radicals cause diseases and how Pycnogenol protects against these diseases. The clinical evidence presented here directly shows the benefits. The remainder of this section is intended to briefly discuss the free-radical and antioxidant processes so that you can better appreciate the benefits of this remarkable substance. We only need to go a little beyond the elementary level to develop a helpful concept of the relationship between free radicals, antioxidant nutrients and disease.

FREE RADICALS

What do all these diseases have in common? How does Pycnogenol affect them? Let's begin by taking a brief look at the havoc that free radicals can inflict.

As I mentioned in the Introduction, free radicals are unstable, reactive compounds or fragments of compounds. For a more technical description of free radicals, please refer to "For Health Professionals" at the end of this section.

Compounds such as polyunsaturated fats readily become free radicals themselves when they are attacked by a free radical because some of the bonds between their carbon atoms that make them polyunsaturated are easily broken in such a way as to yield molecular fragments that are free radicals themselves.

The polyunsaturated fats stored in every cell membrane readily form free-radical chain reactions in a process that biochemists call lipid peroxidation. "Lipid" is merely the biochemists' designation for fat and oils, and "peroxidation" means a special type of reaction with oxygen.

When oxygen reacts normally with a compound, the compound becomes oxidized and the process is called oxidation. However, under certain conditions, oxygen can react in such a way that an extra oxygen atom is involved in the reaction. When this occurs, the compound becomes peroxidized and the process is called peroxidation.

Lipid peroxidation is just one example of how the oxygen reactions that we need for producing energy in our bodies can have byproducts that are harmful. There are trillions of oxygen reactions going on at any one instance in our body, and it is not surprising that some of them go astray and produce unwanted reactions. Besides lipid peroxidation, superoxides and singlet oxygen are produced, which can also be harmful. Fortunately, the good news is that certain antioxidant nutrients can quench each of the various types of free radicals.

Many antioxidants are free-radical scavengers or quenchers. These are compounds that do not regenerate the free radicals during a reaction. Antioxidants are compounds that combine readily with oxygen and neutralize oxygen radicals; the free-radical chains are thus broken and other compounds and body components are projected.

HOW FREE RADICALS CAUSE DISEASE

The first result of free-radical damage that I noticed in my 1960s experiments was a loss of healthy cells.[4,5] Free radicals can destroy cells by damaging their membranes. When the free radicals initiate the lipid peroxidation chain reaction, the excessive energy produced damages even the proteins in the membrane. As a result, the membrane does not properly function to take nutrients into the cell and to remove waste products, and so the cell cannot reproduce itself and dies due to starvation or drowning in waste products. This type of damage accelerates the aging process as tissues lose their function due to the steadily decreasing number of cells.

Another way in which free radicals decrease the number of healthy cells is by reacting with DNA in the cell interiors. DNA (deoxyribonucleic acid) is the genetic material that builds the enzymes that build the structure of the body. When DNA is damaged, it may make mutated enzymes that may not be able to function, and cells cannot be reproduced. Again, this would accelerate the aging process.

Free radicals can also weld molecules together—much like putting handcuffs on them—so they don't function properly. When free radicals weld molecules of the skin protein collagen together, the skin loses its elasticity and smoothness and becomes stiff and wrinkled. We will discuss how Pycnogenol helps keep skin young-looking in a later section.

In the early 1970s I noticed that another result of free-radical reactions in cell membranes can be the loss of the membrane's ability to recognize neighboring cells.[2] This can result in undesirable "wild" cell growth. Such wild proliferation results in tumors, either benign or cancerous. Free-radical damage to DNA can also lead to cancerous mutations.

These are just a few examples of how free radicals can cause disease, and in the next section we will discuss their role in heart disease. First we'll examine how Pycnogenol stops harmful free radicals.

PYCNOGENOL STOPS FREE-RADICAL DAMAGE

I have spent more than 30 years testing free-radical scavengers. I have several patents on synergistic mixtures of natural and synthetic free-radical scavengers.[6,7] In the 1960s and early 1970s, I found that synthetic antioxidants such as BHT (butylated hydroxytoluene) helped provide more free-radical quenching ability than the antioxidant vitamins and minerals alone. However, with synthetic antioxidants there is always the question of safety. Pycnogenol and its antioxidant partners, vitamins A, C, and E, are not only potent free-radical quenchers, but they are well proven to be safe.

Many more natural antioxidant nutrients—especially some of the bioflavonoids—have been purified enough for study as free-radical scavengers. So after 30 years, I find that the best protection against the deleterious effects of free radicals is a combination of natural antioxidant nutrients.

The various antioxidant nutrients work together. Some antioxidants can protect body components not reachable by other antioxidants. Some antioxidants protect other antioxidants, and in some cases can regenerate other antioxidants. The proanthocyanadin bioflavonoids can protect vitamin C, and vitamin C can regenerate vitamin E that has already been "spent" by sacrificing itself to free radicals.

In my opinion, this is one of the reasons that Pycnogenol is a vitamin C "helper." Some biochemists see evidence that it helps vitamin C enter cells. My experience leads me to believe that it is the protective effect on vitamin C that results in more vitamin C being available to enter cells. In any event, it is a proven fact that proanthocyanadins potentiate vitamin C.

In the section on heart disease, we will look at how these substances protect vitamin C and beta-carotene, which in turn protect the vitamin E in cell membranes. The fact is that we need all of those potent antioxidants to obtain optimal protection from free radicals.

Some studies show that these bioflavonoids are more potent free-radical scavengers than either vitamin C or vitamin E, but this is less relevant than it might seem. It is not a matter of potency only, but of complete protection, safety and stability. You need all the important antioxidant nutrients. It would be foolish to rely on vitamin E or vitamin C or bioflavonoids alone. The combination is needed for synergism.

The great free-radical scavenging power of Pycnogenol is why the Horphag Research scientists patented it. This free-radical scavenging property is prominently featured in the patent's title.[8] Although Professor Masquelier was the first to actually verify the free-radical scavenging effect of proanthocyanidins, in retrospect, this property shouldn't have been surprising.

The biological precursors of the oligomeric procyanidins such as catechin and taxifoline (which are also in the Pycnogenol mixture) are effective free-radical scavengers. Professor Masquelier measured the ability of the individual components of the mixture to quench free radicals with a test that used the disappearance of the color of a dye, the NBT test.[9,10] He found that the most potent compounds were the dimeric procyanidins B-3, B-2 and B-1. Epicatechin and catechin, both contained in the formula, inhibit the formation of oxygen radicals less than the dimeric procyanidins, but they are clearly more potent than vitamin C.

As biochemists became more interested in free radicals, they verified the free-radical scavenging effect of these compounds. In 1980, Dr. Joachim Baumann and colleagues reported that several flavonoids inhibited the cyclo-oxygenase reaction that produces the inflammatory prostaglandins.[11] They also found that some flavonoids were strong scavengers for peroxide anion radicals and others were not.

Researchers at the Department of Pharmacy of Nagasaki University School of Medicine determined that the bioflavonoids of Pycnogenol were very effective, as measured by a standard chemical test.[12] These bioflavonoids proved to be fifty times more powerful than vitamin E in a test that measures the ability of compounds to scavenge free radicals such as DPPH. "Among the various [bioflavonoids] tested, procyanidin was the most potent scavenger of the DPPH radical. The concentration of this [bioflavonoid] required for 50% inhibition was 50 times more effective than that of vitamin E. Making use of Electron Spin Resonance analysis with a spin trapping agent, we found that these [bioflavonoids] had a potent scavenging action toward active oxygen free radicals such as superoxide anion, hydroxyl, and peroxide radicals. . . . The [bioflavonoids] that we investigated warrant further study as a promising alternative in the prevention and therapy of several diseases attributed to reactions of oxygen free radicals."[12]

The researchers demonstrated that the formulation was also a potent scavenger of oxygen free radicals such as superoxide, hydroxyl and peroxide radicals. In these standard *in vitro* tests, Pycnogenol proved to be 20 times more powerful than vitamin C.

Another French study utilizing the inhibition of peroxidation caused by microsomes and leading to the formation of malondialdehyde was measured under the influence of different bioflavonoids. Taxifoline and catechin, both components of Pycnogenol, and cyanidine, which is formed from dimeric procyanidins in gastric juice, all inhibited the peroxidation to a considerable extent.[13]

FOR HEALTH PROFESSIONALS

Free radicals are unstable, highly reactive compounds or molecular fragments. Compounds consist of two or more elements held together by a chemical attraction called a "bond." The bonding involves negatively charged parts of the atoms called "electrons." The arrangement of the electrons determines the stability of the compound.

A stable compound has electrons that are in pairs. It's like a buddy system. It is a state of lower energy as the electrons spin in opposite directions. In nature, all systems seek the lowest energy level. However, if an electron is not paired with another, it becomes very reactive and unstable. It will seek out another electron to pair with. In the process of grabbing a partner, a reaction between compounds occurs, and the other compound can become a free radical and perpetuate the process. One free radical can damage a million or more molecules by this self-perpetuating process. The process can be stopped by compounds called "free-radical scavengers." Most antioxidants are good free-radical scavengers.

Do not confuse free radicals with ions. Ions are formed when electrons are removed, and an electrical imbalance results in the atom or molecule having a positive or negative charge. Neutral atoms and molecules can be free radicals, as can ions.

REFERENCES

1. Don't age too fast. Anon. *Prevention* 23(12):104–10 (December 1971).
2. Cancer: New directions Passwater, Richard A. *Amer. Lab.* 5:10–22 (1973).
3. *Supernutrition for Healthy Hearts*. Passwater, Richard A. Dial Press, NY (1977).
4. Plans for a large-scale study of a possible retardation of the human aging process. Passwater, Richard A. *Gerontology* 10(3):28 (1970).
5. Slowing the aging process. Passwater, Richard A. and Welker, Paul American Laboratory.
6. U.S. Patent no. 39,140 (1970).

7. Patents: U.S. 97,011, U.S. 271,655, U.S. 398,596, U.S. 481,788, U.S. 593,812, U.S. 613,420, U.S. 718,469, U.S. 806, 535, U.S. 930,657.

8. Plant extract with a proanthocyanidins content as therapeutic agent having radical scavenging effect and use thereof. Masquelier, Jacques. United States Patent #4,698,360 (October 6, 1987).

9. Oligomères procyanidoliques. Masquelier, J. *Parfums, Cosmetiques, Aromes* 95:89–97 (1990).

10. Radical scavenger effect (RSE) of proanthocyanidins. Masquelier, J. and Laparra, J. *Proanthocyanidine et radicaux libres* (1985).

11. Hemmung der prostaglandinsynthetase durch flavonoide und phenolderivative im vergleich mit deren O_2-radicalfanger-eigenschaften. Baumann, Joachim,; Wurm, Gotthard and Bruchhausen, Franz. *Arch. Pharm.* 313:330–7 (1980).

12. Condensed tannins scavenge active oxygen radicals. Uchida, Shinji; Edamastu, Rei; et al. *Med. Sci. Res.* 15:831–2 (1980).

13. Siess, M. H. and Barbe, P. Station de recherches sur la qualite des ailments de l'homme. INRAAA, Dijon, France.

PREVENTING HEART DISEASE

When Dr. David White of the Faculty of Medicine at the University of Nottingham, England, gave his lecture at the International Conference on Pycnogenol Research in 1990, he may have provided the final clue needed to solve the heart disease mystery.[1]

It had long been known that the one common factor shared by all of the populations having the lowest death rate from heart disease was that of significant wine consumption.[2] It was not known if this was a cause-and-effect relationship or merely coincidental. As early as 1957, it had been shown that wine protected animals on a high-cholesterol diet.[3] It was believed that the bioflavonoids in wine provided the protective effect, rather than the alcohol.

In the 1980s, several researchers were independently becoming aware that antioxidant nutrients were reducing the risk of heart disease. In 1990, Dr. Charles Hennekens of Harvard reported that beta-carotene reduced the incidence of heart attacks in half in a double-blind, placebo-controlled clinical trial.[4]

Dr. Ishwarlal Jialal of the University of Texas Southwestern Medical Center in Dallas showed that antioxidant vitamin E could block the adverse changes to low-density lipoprotein (LDL) that leads to plaque formation and blockages in arteries.

Dr. Jialal explained that "researchers are now of the opinion that fats in the bloodstream become lodged in artery walls and begin to clog arteries *only* when their transporters, the lipoproteins, have chemically combined with oxygen to turn rancid."

Smoking promotes the oxidation of lipoproteins, as do fats when they are not protected from oxidation by antioxidant nutrients such as Pycnogenol, vitamins C and E, and beta-carotene.

Beta-carotene and vitamins C and E have previously been shown to block the oxidation of LDL in the test tube. Dr. Jialal said that his is the first study to demonstrate that an antioxidant nutrient can actually prevent LDL oxidation in the body.[5]

Dr. Hermann Esterbauer's group at the University of Graz in Austria has reported that the "oxidation of polyunsaturated fatty acids in LDL is preceded by a sequential depletion of antioxidants."[6] Oxidation of LDL can begin only when these antioxidants have been depleted. Various antioxidant nutrients have their specific place in their affinity for oxygen-free radicals. This "pecking order" results in various antioxidant lines of defense against these reactive agents.

What we now know is that vitamin E is the last defense against the oxygen-free radicals that damage the cholesterol carriers. The carriers, low-density lipoproteins, normally contain vitamin E, which protects them from oxidation. However, the vitamin E can be quickly destroyed during exposure to many oxygen molecules or oxygen-species free radicals. Vitamin C can help by regenerating this "spent" vitamin E.

THE ATHEROSCLEROSIS ANTIDOTE

Now you can see the importance of Pycnogenol. Its compounds protect vitamin C; thus, they become the body's first line of defense against heart disease. Other antioxidant nutrients such as beta-carotene and selenium contribute to this defense as well.

Now that Dr. White and others have shown that the antioxidant nutrients are major protectors against heart disease, the public can pay better attention to the most important factor instead of being sidetracked by lesser ones.

Most of us should be paying more attention to our intake of antioxidant nutrients. If you are one of those affected by cholesterol as well, then you can watch your cholesterol *and* antioxidants both. My point is that even in cholesterol-sensitive people, *antioxidant protection is more important than cholesterol level*. Don't concentrate on the minor problem and ignore the major factor.

Dr. JoAnn Manson of Brigham and Women's Hospital in Boston studied the diets of 87,245 nurses over more than eight years. She found that women who take supplements of more than 100 International Units of vitamin E daily have 36 percent fewer heart attacks than those who consume less than 30 IU daily.

Dr. Manson also found that women who consumed 25,000 IU of beta-carotene daily had 40 percent less stroke and 22 percent fewer heart attacks than those women who consumed less than 10,000 IU of beta-carotene daily. She did not study Pycnogenol, but the point is that the antioxidant protection of LDL is critical in preventing heart disease, and that this bioflavonoid blend is synergistic with the other antioxidant nutrients and has been shown to be a very powerful and effective antioxidant in its own right.

Other supporting evidence comes from the fact that vitamin E has been shown to be protective against heart disease in epidemiological studies. Dr. Fred Grey showed that vitamin E deficiency is the single most important risk factor in predicting heart disease incidence.[7]

My study of 17,894 persons between the ages of 50 and 98 showed that heart disease dropped dramatically among those taking vitamin E over a long period of time. I found that the length of time vitamin E was taken was more important than the amount. This trend was especially apparent above nine years of usage.

The First Stage of Protection.   The path to a heart attack is a two-step process. First "foam cells" (macrophages filled with oxidized LDL) adhere to the artery lining. These cells promote the infiltration of various substances through the artery wall into its middle layer. Now the artery can be said to be diseased, as a plaque is formed in the artery interior. As the plaque expands, the wall is pushed out and the opening where the blood flows through is narrowed, and blood flow to the heart disease is decreased. The narrowed artery also damages the blood platelets passing through, making the blood "sticky" and encouraging clot formation at the plaque site.

Until recently, most of the emphasis in vitamin E research has been on its ability to safely prevent clots from forming. Now many researchers are looking at how antioxidant nutrients such as Pycnogenol prevent the first steps in this process from occurring as well.

The Second Stage of Protection. These natural antioxidants protect us against heart disease in several other ways as well. They protect the artery lining against injury and keep the blood platelets from clumping, so that clots are not formed. They reduce the adhesion of platelets to collagen surfaces which may be present in the lining of the blood vessels.

The anti-clotting factor is especially important. The first action most cardiologists take today is to prescribe aspirin. Aspirin doesn't lower cholesterol or blood pressure, but studies show that it reduces heart attacks by 30 to 50 percent by reducing blood clotting. Unfortunately, aspirin affects the clotting process too much, and some people develop serious gastrointestinal bleeding.

Pycnogenol does not interfere with the enzyme that aspirin interferes with, which results in a longer time required to form a clot. It protects the blood platelets and also prevents the platelets from adhering to the artery walls. Both of these actions reduce the risk of forming deadly clots.

We will discuss the beneficial effects of the proanthocyanidin bioflavonoids on collagen more fully in the section on skin.

Two Approaches, Two Goals. Thus, we have two distinct approaches and goals in preventing heart disease: the cholesterol approach, which produces limited results; and the antioxidant approach which produces many major health benefits. This does not mean that the two approaches are mutually exclusive—it is not a case of one approach or the other. Dietary cholesterol and fats are certainly not causes of heart disease, but they are significant factors for the approximately 20 percent of people lacking adequate lipoprotein compensatory mechanisms.

The classical risk factors all together—smoking, high blood pressure and high blood cholesterol—still account for less than half of heart disease deaths. I suggest that concentrating on the minor factors exposes you to risk from the *major* cause of heart disease, antioxidant deficiencies. Keep in mind that Pycnogenol is an extremely safe and efficacious nutrient.

FOR HEALTH PROFESSIONALS

When LDL particles become oxidized, we have an entirely different situation than with healthy nonoxidized LDL. Oxidized LDL is taken up by LDL receptors uncontrollably and contributes to invasive foam cell production. Thus, oxidized LDL becomes a major cause of plaque buildup, independent of the otherwise prerequisite damage to the artery lining.

The collagen-rich connective tissue in artery walls is protected and stimulated for repair by Pycnogenol.[8] Studies show that Pycnogenol is protective against early atherosclerosis.[9-12] Pycnogenol reduces histamine production, thereby helping artery linings resist attack by mutagens, oxidized LDL-cholesterol and free radicals.

As discussed earlier, recent research by Dr. David White of the University of Nottingham shows that Pycnogenol reduces oxidized-LDL and foam cell formation and is thus an "atherosclerosis antidote."

The initiation of atherosclerosis is thought by many researchers today, including Dr. White and myself, to result from injury to the layer of endothelial cells which normally form the luminal surface of blood vessel walls. Such injury disturbs local vascular homeostasis, resulting in platelet deposition, aggregation and release of factors which promote smooth muscle proliferation and eventual fibrosis. The damaged endothelium also becomes permeable to lipoproteins, particularly low-density lipoproteins (LDL) and macrophages, which invade the site of injury, accumulate cholesterol as cholesterylester, and develop into foam cells.

Eventually, a rather complicated structure, the atherosclerotic plaque, develops consisting of lipids (fats) complex and carbohydrates, blood, blood products, fibrous tissue and calcium deposits. A raised blood LDL-cholesterol concentration has been recognized by man as a major risk factor for heart disease because it appears to be the donor of cholesterol deposited in the atherosclerotic plaque.

The accumulation of LDL-borne cholesterol by macrophages is something of a paradox, however, since the cell has few LDL-receptors and is able to down regulate the receptor number when the LDL-cholesterol concentration is increased. The resolution of this paradox may lie in the observation that certain modifications of LDL produce a molecule which is no longer recognized by the LDL receptor but by a nonregulated scavenger receptor. Macrophages can then accumulate cholesterol from this modified LDL.

REFERENCES

1. Cholesterol and foam cell control with Pycnogenol: The atherosclerosis antidote. White, David. The International Conference on Pycnogenol Research, Bordeaux, France (October 4–6, 1990).
2. Eighteen country study of mortality due to ischemic heart disease. St. Leger, A. S.; Cochrane, A. L. and Moore, H. *Lancet* 1017 (May 12, 1979).
3. Protective effect of wine in laboratory animals fed a cholesterol-enriched diet. Fay-Morgan, A.; Brinner, L.; Plaa, C. B. and Stone, M. M. *Amer. J. Physiol.* 189:290 (1957).
4. Beta-carotene reduces heart risk in the Physicians Health Study: Preliminary data. Hennekens, Charles Amer. Heart Assoc., 63rd Sci. Sess., Dallas (November 14, 1990).
5. Baracco et al., *Gaz Med. de France* 88:2035 (1981).
6. The role of vitamin E and carotenoids in preventing oxidation of low-density lipoproteins. Esterbauer, Hermann, et al. In: Vitamin E: biochemistry and Health Implications, Diplock, A., et al., eds., *Ann N. Y. Acad. Sci.* pp. 254–67 (1989).
7. Inverse correlation between plasma vitamin E and mortality from ischemic heart disease in cross-cultural epidemiology. Gey, K. Fred; Puska,

Pekka; Jordan, Paul and Moser, Ulrich K. *Amer. J. Clin. Nutr.* 53:326S–334S (January 1991).

8. Effet protecteur des oligomeres procyanidoliques sur le lathyrisme experimental chez le rat. Gendre, Philippe M. J., Laparra, J. and Barraud, E. *Annales pharmaceutiques francaises* 43(1):61–71 (1985).

9. Variations in rabbit aortic endothelial and medical histamine synthesis in pre- and early atherosclerosis. Markle, Ronald A. and Hollis, Theodore M. *Proceed. Soc. Exper. Biol. Med.* 155:365–8 (1977).

10. Relationship between aortic histamine formation and aortic albumin permeability in atherosclerosis. Hollis, Theodore M. and Furniss, John V. *Proceed. Soc. Exper. Biol. Med.* 165:271–4 (1980).

11. Shear stress and aortic histamine synthesis. DeForrest, Jack M. and Hollis, Theodore M. *Amer. J. Physiol.* 234(6) H701–5 (1978).

12. Rabbit aortic endothelial and medial histamine synthesis following short-term cholesterol feeding. Markle, Ronald A. and Hollis, Theodore M. *Exp. Mol. Path.* 23:417–25 (1975).

BLOOD VESSEL HEALTH AND CIRCULATION

As important as protection against free radicals is, the proanthocyanidin bioflavonoids are better known for their beneficial effects on the blood vessels and circulation. Knowledge of the great effectiveness of Pycnogenol against free radicals and free-radical diseases is relatively new, but it has been used in Europe for more than two decades to strengthen blood vessels—including the capillaries—and to reduce edema (swelling due to water retention) and arrest varicose veins.

The bioflavonoids adhere to the collagen protein fibers in the blood vessels, which restores resilience and flexibility to them, but their greatest effect on the circulatory system is strengthening the capillaries. In other words, Pycnogenol restores the elasticity of collagen, and in so doing, restores the impermeability of blood vessel walls.

The "strength" or integrity of our capillaries is a major factor in health, but few people think anything at all about the importance of capillaries. Occasionally we hear of someone who has been told something like "Your blood system is old and weak and your organs are beginning to fail." What is happening in such cases is that their capillaries are too porous—permeable—and water and small molecules from the blood leak through the capillaries. The tissues are filling up with this fluid, which makes it harder for the heart to pump blood through the organs. In addition, the tissues are not receiving the nutrients they need and are not able to rid themselves of wastes.

There are other consequences of capillary leaking that are not so dramatic, but serious nonetheless. Before we examine them, we will briefly consider the basic role of the capillaries.

THE BLOOD VESSEL SYSTEM

Most people think of the blood vessel system as arteries and smaller arterioles that carry blood from the heart to the organs, veins and smaller venules that carry blood back to the heart from the organs, and capillaries that link arteries and veins together. This view is essentially correct but misleading. Arteries and veins are merely pipes or tubes through which blood flows. Capillaries, on the other hand, are where all the action takes place. While it is necessary to transport blood to where it is needed, it does no good unless the blood components can reach the cells.

The sole function of the circulatory system is to exchange nutrients for waste products. The heart merely pumps the blood and the arteries, and veins merely carry the blood. What is important—but usually overlooked—is that the capillaries allow the cells to live by exchanging nutrients for wastes.

Pycnogenol protects the capillaries in three ways. Capillaries, unlike the multilayered arteries and veins, are composed of a single cell layer. These cells are reinforced with collagen, a somewhat elastic protein fiber. Also, the "intercellular cement" or ground substance—the material that fills the space between cells—consists largely of collagen. Vitamin C is needed for the production of collagen so that vitamin C's helpers, the bioflavonoids, are also important. In the Introduction, three ways they help protect vitamin C were discussed. Protecting vitamin C is the first way in which Pycnogenol helps maintain a healthy capillary system. The bioflavonoids have a second function, adhering to collagen to offer additional protection.

If the intercellular substance is damaged, there is a microscopic hole in the capillary which becomes a channel for a leak. The thin wall of cells can be damaged by free-radical attack and also leak. The third way in which Pycnogenol protects capillaries is by guarding cells against free-radical attack.

Capillary resistance and permeability are improved by administration of proanthocyanidins.[1] Several European medical studies show that this improves peripheral circulation, restores lost capillary activity, and strengthens weak blood vessels.[2-6] By reducing capillary fragility, these substances help prevent bruising and improve varicose veins.[7,8] In addition, they reduce venous insufficiency, reduce the severity of restless legs and diminish lower leg blood volume.[9,10]

They also protect the membranes of red blood cells so that they remain flexible and easily squeeze through the very narrow capillaries, one at a time.

CAPILLARY RESISTANCE

Scientists measure capillary integrity directly by measuring the permeability according to the amount of dye that leaks through the capillary. This leakage can also be measured by placing a constriction around a part of an extremity and taking blood samples from both sides of the constriction over a period of time. The blood samples are then analyzed for proteins that have leaked and accumulated.

Or the capillaries' integrity can be determined indirectly by measuring the resistance of the capillary to leakage when suction is applied.

The first two methods are not often preferred, because they require that a dye be injected into the blood system and/or blood samples taken. The third procedure, involving an instrument called an angiosterrometer, is comparatively easy because it is noninvasive. A measured suction—partial vacuum—is applied to the skin and the suction force is increased until red spots (purpura) appear on the skin surface.

This test has shown that Pycnogenol produces a greater and longer improvement in capillary resistance (resistance to leakage) than most bioflavonoids. Nearly all bioflavonoids produce a moderate, short-term improvement, or monophasic effect. However, Pycnogenol produces an additional effect which is stronger and longer-lasting, termed diphasic. This longer effect has been measured as lasting up to 168 hours, and is thought to be due to Pycnogenol's sparing effect on vitamin C and its adherence to collagen. Citrus bioflavonoids and hesperidin do not produce the diphasic effect.

In one study by Professor Henri Choussat, University of Bordeaux, 47 persons, aged 37 to 85, were given a single 100-milligram supplement of Pycnogenol and 72 hours later were found to have increased capillary resistance by 140 percent. In the placebo group, no change was seen during the same time.[8]

In another study by Professor Leng-Levy, University of Bordeaux, 31 persons were given 90 milligrams of Pycnogenol daily for two months. Their capillary resistance improved markedly, and ecchymosis disappeared. The study subjects reported that their edema had vanished and their legs felt invigorated.

In a study performed at the University of Aquila, involving guinea pigs (which, like humans, are one of the few animals who do not produce vitamin C in their bodies) under scorbutogenic diet, 5 milligrams of Pycnogenol per kilogram of body weight increased their survival time relative to the control group with scorbutogenic diet only.

A study by the Institute of Bio-Research, Hanover, Germany, measured capillary resistance in guinea pigs after 10 days of oral administration of 1500 milligrams of Pycnogenol daily. There was nearly a 300 percent improvement, which was highly statistically significant.

VARICOSE VEINS AND VENOUS INSUFFICIENCY

After the blood is collected by the capillaries and returned to the veins, it must be pumped back to the heart. But by now, the pressure of the heartbeat has been diminished as the blood diffuses through the capillaries. The veins have a built-in pump powered by the action of our skeletal muscles.

The large muscles of the legs help power the blood the long way through the veins. This system is called the muscle-vein pump. Every time we use a large muscle, that muscle simultaneously presses on veins, which helps push the blood along. The veins have one-way valves, which prevent the blood from being pulled back by gravity when there are no muscle contractions.

When we are inactive for long periods of time, the muscle-vein pump is not active, blood volume increases in the veins and the pressure rises. The one-way valves can give in, allowing gravity to pull the blood. This results in edema, swelling and pain. Over time, this produces varicose veins and/or hemorrhoids.

Dr. G. Feine-Haake, a specialist in internal medicine in Hamburg, Germany, studied the benefit of 90 milligrams of Pycnogenol daily on 110 persons having varicose veins. Seventy-seven percent showed a clear improvement. In addition, among the 41 individuals in that group who had nightly calf cramps, 93 percent had an improvement in symptoms.

EDEMA

Italian scientists from the University of Florence studied the effect of Pycnogenol on venous congestion in the legs—leg edema. The study involved 40 subjects consisting of 13 men and 27 women between the ages of 34 and 74, having an average age of 60 years. The subjects were randomly divided into two groups. One group served as the control group and received a placebo supplement that appeared identical to the Pycnogenol supplement but contained an inactive substance. The other group received 300 milligrams of Pycnogenol daily for 60 days.

All of those taking the Pycnogenol had relief from at least some of the symptoms. There was a decrease in the feeling of heaviness in lower limbs in 11 percent of those receiving Pycnogenol after 30 days, and in 33 percent after 60 days.[11]

The swelling disappeared in 26 percent of those taking the Pycnogenol after 30 days, and in 63 percent after 60 days (circumference measured above the ankle before and after test). Pain in the lower limbs was totally relieved in 38 percent of those taking Pycnogenol after 30 days, and in 67 percent after 60 days.

REFERENCES

1. Etude de L'administration d'oligomeres procyanidoliques (OPC) chez le rat. Cahn, J. and Borzeix, M. G. *Extrait de La Semaine des Hopitaux de Paris* 59 (27–28 2031–4 (1983).
2. Dartenus et al., *Bordeaux Med.* 13:903 (1980).
3. Beylot et al., *Gaz. Med. de France* 87:2919 (1980).
4. Biard et al., *Medicine Prat.* 786:62 (1980).
5. Baracco et al., *Gaz Med. de France* 88:2035 (1981).
6. Laparra et al., *Expertise Pharmacologique* (1978).
7. Lagru et al., *Vie Med.* 1299 (1980).
8. A new therapy for venous diseases. Feine-Haake, G. *Zeitschrift für Allgemeinmedizin* 51:7 839 (June 30, 1975).
9. Oedema-inhibiting effect of procyanidin. Blazso, G. and Gabor, M. *Acta Physiologica Scientiarium Hungaricae,* Tomus 56(2) 235–40 (1980).
10. Das hydrostatische odem and seine medikamentose beeinflussung. Schmidtke, I. and Schoop, W. Schweizerische gesellschaft fur phebologie. Jahrestagung 1984. "Die Objektivierung der Wirkung von Venepharmaka." Lenzerheide (January 19/21, 1984).
11. Report of Prof. Arcangeli, University of Florence (June 16, 1989).

THE SKIN COSMETIC IN A CAPSULE

Skin is considered to be the body's largest organ, consisting of about 10 percent of normal body weight. A piece of skin the size of a quarter has one yard of blood vessels, four yards of nerves, hundreds of nerve endings, and 100 sweat glands, 10 hair follicles, 15 sebaceous glands and more than 3 million cells.

Skin consists of the epidermis, which is the outer layer, and the dermis, which lies underneath. There is also a fatty subcutaneous layer that helps insulate the body and absorb shocks. The epidermis is constantly renewing itself, and with a turnover rate of about three to four weeks. Millions of epidermal cells are formed daily just above the dermis, and they in turn are pushed upward toward the outside by new cells as they form. As the epidermal cells migrate upward, they change from round cells having a jellylike consistency to flatter and harder cells. These cells die as they near the harsh environment of the outside world, and they slough off.

Aging causes the skin to become thinner and more transparent. The subcutaneous layer loses fat and the skin sags. And, unfortunately, elastic skin fibers lose their resilience.

Collagen, one of the body's most widespread proteins, is the primary component of the dermis. An interlacing of collagen fibers with a fine net of elastin (an essential component of connective tissue) gives skin its strength, elasticity and smoothness.

There is no blood supply in the epidermis, so cell nourishment depends on diffusion from the dermis. The combination of bioflavonoids in Pycnogenol reactivates damaged collagen and elastin and protects them against further attack by free radicals and the degrading enzymes, elastase and collagenase.[1-4]

These bioflavonoids bind to collagen fibers and realign them to a more youthful, undamaged form. This protective action helps to prevent early facial wrinkles that occur due to skin inelasticity. Pycnogenol therefore is an oral cosmetic to help keep skin smooth and elastic. Actually, it was dermatological and phlebological disorders that started Dr. Jacques Masquelier of Bordeaux University on the research that led to the formulation of Pycnogenol. He treated 45 patients having eczema, ulcerated varicose veins and related disorders.

When collagen fibers are soaked in water for 24 hours with a weight attached, their strength can be measured relative to the length that the fiber is stretched. When Pycnogenol is added to the water, the collagen fibers decrease in length proportional to the amount added. This decrease represents an increase in collagen strength. The weight of the collagen fibers also increases after incubation into the solution. Bioflavonoids such as rutin and hesperidin do not have this strengthening effect on collagen.

The fragmentation of elastin fibers during aging can be attributed to an imbalance between the elastase enzyme and its natural inhibitors. When the enzyme elastase is introduced into the dermal layer of skin in laboratory animals, the degradation of the elastin fibers can be observed with a microscope. If the animals are given Pycnogenol first, this degradation is reduced by up to 70 percent.[1,2]

Studies at Baylor College of Medicine show that the catechin bioflavonoids bind tightly with skin collagen to prevent enzyme degradation.[3]

Besides the protection provided when the bioflavonoids bind to collagen and elastin, additional protection is provided by its free-radical quenching ability. Healthy skin needs to be protected against damaging ultraviolet radiation from the sun. External sunscreens are your first line of protection, but the skin also needs free-radical fighters in your skin to protect against the UV-released radicals from the UV that does penetrate the sunscreen.

Pycnogenol makes an excellent external and internal sunscreen. Dr. Antti Holevi Arstila, Chairman of the Department of Cell Biology at the University of Jyvaskyla in Finland, reported that in an in vitro (test tube) experiment in which human skin cells were exposed to UV energy, Pycnogenol provided excellent protection, clearly better than equal amounts of vitamin E. Vitamin E's protection leveled off, whereas Pycnogenol's protection remained dose-dependent over a wider range. In typical experiments of this type, sunlight will kill about 50 percent of the skin cells. When adequate Pycnogenol is added, about 85 percent of the skin cells survive. To measure the effect of Pycnogenol as an external sunscreen, Dr. Arstila exposed skin having various concentrations of Pycnogenol ointment to 30 minutes of controlled UV energy. The results compared favorably to those of other sunscreens.[5]

Well-nourished, healthy skin is radiant and youthful. Pycnogenol is an important part of optimal nourishment for your skin. It isn't an essential nutrient for skin, but it does offer important protection and revitalization. It will not make old skin new, but it will improve the elasticity and appearance of your skin.

REFERENCES

1. Stabilisation du collagene par des oligomeres procyanidoliques. Masquelier, J., Dumon, M.C., and Dumas, J. *Acta Therapeutica* 7:101–5 (1981).
2. Evidence by in vivo and in vitro studies that binding of Pycnogenol to elastin affects its rate of degradation by elastases. Tixier, J. M.; Godeau, G.; Robert, A. M. and Hornebeck, W. *Biochem. Pharmacol.* 33(24) 3933–9 (1984).
3. Collagen treated with catechin becomes resistance to the action of mammalian collagenase. Kuttan, R., Donnelly, Patricia V. and Di Ferrante, N. *Experientia* 37:221–3 (1981).
4. Kakegawa, H., et al. *Chem. Pharm. Bull.* 33:5079 (1985).
5. Pycnogenol seminar Arstila, Antti Holevi. Natural Foods Expo, Anaheim, CA (April 11, 1992).

OTHER IMPORTANT RELATIONSHIPS

There are many other important ways in which Pycnogenol helps maintain optimal health. There is preliminary evidence that it improves mental function, reduces the risk of stroke, protects against the effects of stress, reduces inflammation of hay fever and sports injuries, reduces some of the side effects of diabetes and possibly may improve vision. There is even a suggestion that it may protect against cancer, beyond its cancer-protective antioxidant function. The strength of the evidence varies from laboratory studies to anecdotal, but since the mechanism believed to be involved has been proven in other studies, these relationships should be considered.

BRAIN FUNCTION

Pycnogenol is important to brain function, not only because it protects blood vessels, but also because it is one of the few dietary antioxidants that readily crosses the blood-brain barrier to protect brain cells. The blood-brain barrier protects the brain from compounds that normally circulate in the blood. Brain cells are very sensitive to some compounds, even though they may not damage other cells in the body or even be needed by other cells.

Protection of brain cells will help memory and reduce senility. There are indications that even sluggish memories are improved, perhaps due to better circulation and cell nourishment.

Strokes are the result of brain cells being damaged either by not receiving blood or by excessive pressure from blood pooling in brain tissue. The former is caused by blood clots that block flow, while the latter is caused by arteries bursting or leaking.

The strengthening of capillaries and other blood vessels helps protect against stroke. In earlier sections, I discussed how Pycnogenol increases capillary resistance and strengthens blood vessels. It has significantly increased the life span of rats that are genetically hypertensive and prone to early death from stroke.[1]

In laboratory experiments in which blood is rapidly injected into brain blood vessels, dramatically increasing the blood pressure within those vessels for a brief time, Pycnogenol shows a significant protective effect.[2] First, the amount of blood that bleeds into the brain when the "extra" blood is injected into the brain blood vessels is measured in animals not protected with the proanthocyanidin mixture. Then the experiment is repeated in animals receiving various amounts of Pycnogenol prior to the injections. Increasing amounts of bioflavonoids yield greater reductions in bleeding.

STRESS

Acute hemorrhagic ulcers of the esophagus, stomach and duodenum are common today. They can result in serious gastrointestinal bleeding and death. Histamine is believed to be involved in the pathogenesis of stress ulcer disease. Pycnogenol inhibits the enzyme histidine decarboxylase and thus lowers histamine levels.

Because it prevents excessive histamine release, it has been shown to reduce stress ulcers in the stomach and intestine by 82 percent.[3] This has been confirmed by Dr. Duncan Bell of Ipswich Hospital in England and reported at the 1990 International Symposium on

Pycnogenol.[4] Dr. Bell, a gastroenterologist, reported on its antistress action and how it prevents ulcer formation.

INFLAMMATION, HAY FEVER AND SPORTS INJURIES

Allergy has been described as "a process of inflammation now known to be a disorder of the immune system, which is made up of cells with the capacity for recognizing, evaluating and neutralizing or eliminating alien material."[5]

Inflammatory diseases include allergies or sensitivities, rheumatoid arthritis, osteoarthritis, hepatitis, Crohn's disease, lupus erythematosus and ulcerative colitis.[5] They all involve free radicals, and, of course, Pycnogenol quenches free radicals and inhibits the inflammatory enzymes.

Hay fever is a common allergy disease. In Finland, Pycnogenol is very popular for alleviating hay fever symptoms. As mentioned previously, histamine is one of the more important mediators in allergic reactions. At the 1990 International Symposium on Pycnogenol, Dr. D. White of the University of Nottingham reported that it greatly reduces the formation of histamine, and thus, reduces inflammation.[6]

It also inhibits the degranulation of mast cells. Mast cells are large cells with coarse granules that contain histamine. The connective tissue is well supplied with mast cells. Mast cells are mediators of inflammation upon contact with antigens. When mast cells are degranulated, all mediators of the allergic reaction, including histamine, are liberated from the stock inside the mast cell, the granula. Thus Pycnogenol prevents the liberation of the allergic mediators and the production of one of the brain mediators, histamine.[7]

The ability of this bioflavonoid blend to improve joint flexibility and repair the collagen in connective tissue should be of interest to athletes. In addition, it reduces inflammation due to injury. Many bioflavonoids inhibit the enzymes (elastases) and prostaglandins that lead to inflammation, but this formulation is particularly effective.[8] However, it also inhibits histamine release, which further reduces inflammation.

I advise athletes to take Pycnogenol regularly in order to minimize inflammation and swelling in case an injury does occur. Controlling swelling has a significant effect on how soon you will be able to return to action.

DIABETES

Pycnogenol reduces vascular fragility, to which diabetics are prone. Its protective effect on capillaries extends to the fragile capillaries of the eyes. The damage to the retina caused by the microbleeding of the eye capillaries due to diabetes is one of the more common causes of blindness in adults.

Pycnogenol has been licensed in France for years for treating diabetic retinopathy. This use was first based on clinical studies of 40 patients by Dr. G. Maynard and colleagues. The patients were given 80 to 120 milligrams of Pycnogenol daily for a week and then maintained on 40 to 80 milligrams daily for 1.5 to 4 months. The microbleeding of the capillaries decreased remarkably in 90 percent of the patients, and their eyesight improved noticeably.

Professor Saracco of the Clinic for Ophthalmology in Marseille studied 60 patients and confirmed that Pycnogenol improved diabetic retinopathy and hypertensive retinopathy, as well as reduced loosening of the retina.

German medical researcher Professor H.C.W. Leydhecker found that Pycnogenol compares favorably with any other current treatments for diabetic retinopathy.[9]

Dr. Leydhecker, Director of the University Eye Clinic in Wurzburg at the time, compared the effectiveness of Pycnogenol with the drug Dexium (calcium dobesilate). Dexium is routinely used to suppress the progress of diabetic retinopathy. There were 16 patients in each group, but it was impractical to assign a placebo group because the patients were referred to the study from private practice. Seven university professors evaluated the photographs of the patients' retinas, before and after treatment, without being aware of which patients were taking which compound. After six months of treatment, both compounds were found to be effective, and equally so.

EYESIGHT

In the study just described, many patients also experienced improved visual acuity. Similarly, a small-scale clinical experiment designed to study diabetic retinopathy was conducted by Dr. Emilio Balestrazzi of the University of Aquila. He concluded: "The overall clinical judgment on Pycnogenol, compared with the control groups treated with placebo, and taking account of all the clinical and instrumental tests and the absence of side-effects, is to be considered beneficial, inasmuch as all patients benefited to a varying degree from the treatment. In fact, the effects on the resistance and peripheral capillary permeability of the vessels have shown themselves to be positive in improving the functioning of the retina."

CANCER

Pycnogenol also has been shown to inhibit tumor production in the skin.[10] Recent research by Dr. Stewart Brown of the University of Nottingham shows that its radical scavenging effect slows cancer mutagenesis.[11] At the same international symposium on Pycnogenol, Dr. D. White of the University of Nottingham reported that it inhibits the enzyme monooxygenase, thereby preventing the formation of the highly carcinogenic diole epoxide of benzopyrene.[6] This protective action may be very important to smokers. Tobacco smoke contains significant amounts of benzopyrene.

ARTHRITIS

Several anecdotal reports claim that arthritics feel improvement overnight with a bedtime dose of 120–150 milligrams of Pycnogenol. Both osteoarthritis and rheumatoid arthritis are inflammatory diseases. Pycnogenol may help by quenching some of the free radicals that are involved in the inflammatory process.

REFERENCES

1. Condensed tannins scavenge active free radicals. Uchida, S., et al. *Med. Sci. Res.* 15:831–2 (1987).
2. Etude de l'administration d'oligomeres procyanidoliques (OPC) chez le rat. Cahn, J. and Borzeix, M. G. *Extrait de La Semaine des Hopitaux de Paris* 59 (27–8):2031–4.
3. Histamine and acute hemorrhagic lesions in rat gastric mucosa: Prevention of stress ulcer by catechin. Reimann, H. J.; Lorenz, W.; Fischer, M.; Frolich, R.; Meyer, H. J. and Schmal, A. *Agents Actions* 7(1):6972 (1977).
4. Bell, Duncan. International Symposium on Pycnogenol, Bordeaux, France (October 1990).
5. Inflammation and nutrition. Anon. *Medical Nutrition* 42–5 (Autumn 1989).
6. White, D. International Symposium on Pycnogenol, Bordeaux, France (October 1990).
7. Kakegawa, H.; et al. *Chem. Pharm. Bull.* 33:5079 (1985).
8. Evidence by in vivo and in vitro studies that binding of Pycnogenols to elastin affects its rate of degradation by elastases. Tixier, J. M.; Godeau, G.; Robert, A. M. and Hornebeck, W. *Biochem. Pharmacol.* 33(24):3933–9 (1984).
9. Scientific report on effectivity and tolerance of Pycnogenol in treating diabetic retinopathy, based on clinical comparative test. Leydhecker, H.C.W. University Eye Clinic, Wurzburg.
10. U.S. patent 4,698,360 (October 6, 1987).
11. Brown, Stewart. International Symposium on Pycnogenol, Bordeaux, France (October 1990).

PYCNOGENOL'S OUTSTANDING SAFETY

Pycnogenol has been taken in Europe under medical supervision for decades with no reports of adverse effects. More than 4 million capsules and tablets are taken every day at this writing. More importantly, Pycnogenol has been tested and tested again by conventional tests of safety at expert centers including the Pasteur Institute in Lyon,

France and Cytotest Cell Research (CCR) in Darmstadt, Germany.[1,2] Pycnogenol has been found to be nontoxic, nonteratogenic, nonmutagenic, noncarcinogenic and nonantigenic.[3-6]

The safety of Pycnogenol was reviewed in depth by Dr. Peter Rohdewald of the Pharmacology Institute of the University of Munster in Germany during the October 1990 International Pycnogenol Symposium in Bordeaux. Dr. Rohdewald stated that Pycnogenol is a safe natural product with no adverse effects whatsoever.

The LD^{50}—the dose lethal to 50 percent of animals tested—is 3 grams per kilogram of body weight. Nutritional supplementation is usually 30 to 150 milligrams daily. This safety range precludes any risk of acute or chronic toxicity.

Several researchers report recommending that people start with 100 to 150 milligrams of Pycnogenol daily for one to several weeks, and then switch to a maintenance level of 50 milligrams per day.

As previously mentioned, Pycnogenol is absorbed into the bloodstream in about 20 minutes (depending on tableting and capsule factors) and can be detected in saliva within one hour. Once absorbed, the maximum protective effect lasts about 72 hours. Then the protective effect will begin to fall as it is excreted in the urine. Thus, for optimal protection, Pycnogenol, like other water-soluble nutrients, should be taken daily.

Although we have traced the history of Pycnogenol through more than 450 years, and although it has been used for decades, it seems destined to wider popularity and utility as researchers understand more about it. We have just scratched the surface.

REFERENCES

1. Mutagenicity of proanthocyanidins. Yu, C. L. and Swaminathan, B. *Food Chem. Toxicol.* 25(2) 135–9 (1987).
2. Pantaleoni, G. C. & Quaglino, D. University of Aquila Pharmaco-Toxicologica Report.
3. Laparra et al. *Acta Therapeutica* 4:233 (1978).

4. Mutagenicity of proanthocyanidins. Yu, C. L. and Swaminathan, B. *Food Chem. Toxicol.* 25(2) 135–9 (1987).
5. Micronucleus assay in bone marrow cells of the mouse with Pycnogenol. Volkner, Wolfgang and Muller, Ewald Cytotest Cell Research GmbH & Co, project 143010 (February 1989).
6. Acute and Chronic Toxicity tests. International Bio-Research, Inc., Hannover, Germany.

Amazing Antioxidant Derived from Plants Has Triple Action Against Free Radicals

Used Around the World for 20 Years, Pycnogenol
Is Now Available in U.S.
by Richard A. Passwater, Ph.D.

Pycnogenol (pronounced pic-nah'-je-nol) is a remarkable plant-derived substance that has been used clinically in Europe for many years. A blend of special bioflavonoids, this potent antioxidant reduces free radical-caused tissue damage many times more effectively than vitamin E, potentiates the health-giving effects of vitamin C, and protects the brain and nerve tissue with its nearly unique ability to penetrate the blood-brain barrier.

It also reduces inflammation and improves circulation, both relieving the distresses of arthritis, diabetes and stroke and promoting prevention of cardiovascular disease and cancer. Moreover, its ability to bond to collagen promotes renewed youthfulness, flexibility and body integrity—even allowing it to function as an "oral cosmetic."

COMMON FACTOR

As an effective antioxidant, Pycnogenol helps our bodies resist blood vessels and skin damage, mental deterioration, inflammation and other damage caused by harmful free radicals. Free-radical damage is a common factor in a host of non-"germ" conditions, including heart disease, cancer, arthritis and aging.

Free radicals are highly reactive molecules or molecular fragments characterized by having the spin of one electron in the molecule not paired with a companion electron. This is a very unstable state, and free radicals do not persist for very long, quickly reacting with other compounds.

This reaction can set off a cascade of harmful reactions. Free radicals do a lot of damage in the body, ranging from attacking the DNA that regenerates our body to impairing cell membranes. Once free radicals are produced, they multiply geometrically in free-radical chain reactions unless they are quenched by antioxidants or other free-radical scavengers. Antioxidants are compounds that react easily with oxygen and thus protect neighboring compounds from damaging reactions with oxygen. Common protective antioxidant nutrients include vitamins A, C and E, and new evidence is mounting that Pycnogenol, the trade name for the proanthocyanidin bioflavonoids, may prove to be just as important.

MANY BENEFITS

Antioxidants do more than protect. They help repair by improving and stabilizing the skin protein collagen and improving the condition of arteries and capillaries. There are four biochemical properties of these substances that are responsible for their many benefits:
* free-radical scavenging
* collagen (a skin protein) binding
* inhibition of inflammatory enzymes
* inhibition of histamine formation

The benefits of proanthocyanidins, demonstrated in many studies and decades of clinical experience, include:
* improves skin smoothness and elasticity
* strengthens capillaries, arteries and veins
* improves circulation
* reduces capillary fragility and improves resistance to bruising and strokes
* reduces risk of phlebitis
* reduces varicose veins
* reduces edema and swelling of the legs
* helps restless-leg syndrome
* reduces diabetic retinopathy
* improves visual acuity
* helps improve sluggish memory
* reduces the effects of stress
* improves joint flexibility
* fights inflammation

Although the proanthocyanidin blend Pycnogenol is relatively new in North America, it has been researched extensively in Europe and has been widely available since 1969 in many countries. Pycnogenol is not toxic, mutagenic, carcinogenic, teratogenic or antigenic. ❏

RICHARD A. PASSWATER, PH.D.

FROM PINE BARK TO GRAPE SEED

Pycnogenol was originally isolated in 1951 from the bark of the French maritime pine tree. The term "pycnogenols" actually describes an entire complex of plant flavonoids or proanthocyanidins all with exceptional antioxidant activity.

These compounds are found in various plants including grape seed, lemon tree bark, peanuts, cranberries and citrus peels. Both grape seed and pine bark are excellent sources of proanthocyanidins. Some studies indicate that the grape seed extract may be more potent and effective since it contains chemical forms of proanthocyanidins not present in pine bark extracts.

It is also more economical to extract these compounds from grape seeds than from pine bark. Regardless of the source, these protective antioxidants can be used to maintain good health and prevent free radical damage.

COENZYME Q-10

Is it our New Fountain of Youth?

William H. Lee, R.Ph., Ph.D.

FROM HEART TO MOUTH

The amazing nutrient coenzyme Q-10 has been shown to be helpful in such disparate conditions as life-threatening cardiomyopathy and periodontal disease. Because of its antioxidant effect and its role in the production of cellular energy, it is also often effective in managing diabetes and obesity, in detoxification and longevity, and in sustaining the immune system. With virtually no side effects reported in international studies, and with many verified remarkable health benefits, coenzyme Q-10 should be investigated by all concerned with maintaining or regaining good health.

INTRODUCTION

The body is a collection of systems working together for the good of the whole. The body cannot function at its best unless all systems are performing at peak efficiency. We usually think of this collection in terms of the individual systems, such as the digestive system, the respiratory system, the reproductive system, and so forth. Such a perception is adequate for most purposes, but, unfortunately, it does not go far enough for the purposes of this book.

Each system has an effect on other systems. Mental stress can cause digestive problems, sexual problems and headaches. Eating the wrong foods can cause lethargy, lack of concentration and loss of energy. Constipation can cause nausea, dizziness, lack of appetite and lack of energy. What bothers any one system ends up disrupting all of the other systems in one way or another.

When we think of systems, we usually think of them as wholes rather than their components. We should think of a system as a collection of individual cells that, together, make up the system. Each cell is a miniature body. It carries on all of the functions of the body including ingestion, digestion, waste removal and reproduction. It is the individual cell's health that is vitally important to the total health of the body. If the individual cell is kept supplied with adequate nutrition and if it functions as it should, then the system functions, and the body functions. But should the individual cell falter, it is the beginning of problems for the entire body structure and, perhaps, the disease we call aging!

All systems, internal or external, run on energy. Food is the important source of energy to the body and to the individual cell. Each cell has a miniature engine within it that converts the nutrients it receives into the energy it must have to carry on its activities. If a cell does not receive nutrients, it will not be able to carry on its functions and to reproduce itself as a perfect cell. The production of imperfect cells can be called aging, and is detected by wrinkles, sagging skin, loss of hair, loss of memory, and other consequences. A starved cell will not perform as a perfect part of the whole body. Nutritional deficiency will affect muscle status, circulation, cardiovascular health, blood pressure, and the immune system.

Because coenzyme Q-10 is found in every cell in the body, it is the key to the process that produces 95 percent of cellular energy.

Without coenzyme Q-10, we wouldn't have enough energy to stay alive! Coenzyme Q-10 may be the ultimate antidote to aging, the life-force your body produces to stay alive and healthy . . . and it can be taken as a nutritional supplement!

Coenzyme Q is also known as ubiquinone. The name was formed from the word *ubiquitous* and the coenzyme *quinone*, because coenzyme Q is found in virtually every cell in the body.

Ubiquinone is a naturally occurring substance with a molecular structure that is similar to vitamin K. It is found in humans, animals, and plants. The form naturally present in plants is known as plasta-quinone. Animals and humans have a variety of molecular formations ranging from coenzyme Q-6 to coenzyme Q-10. The difference in the numbered designations refers to the number of isoprene units in the molecular chain. Coenzyme 6 to coenzyme 10 are found in animals, while only coenzyme Q-10 is found in humans. Although coenzyme Q-10 is the form utilized by the body for its energy function, the animal forms can be raised to the Q-10 position when ingested as part of the diet.

The richest source of the coenzyme for supplemental purposes is beef heart. Although initial investigations were carried out using this source, the expense of extracting the coenzyme made general use prohibitive. The Japanese later discovered a fermentation process and have mass-produced it at affordable levels.

Although this substance shows remarkable promise and safety in its ability to normalize many critical body situations such as cardio-vascular disease, hypertension, and periodontal disease, it has not been approved by the Food and Drug Administration as anything but a food supplement. Karl Folkers, biomedical researcher at the University of Texas at Austin, holds the Food and Drug Administration permit to test the substance as a treatment for heart problems.

One of the basic precepts of nutritional healing is illustrated by coenzyme Q-10. If the enzyme is low or deficient in the body, coenzyme Q-10 therapy is likely to be rewarding. If the level of coenzyme Q-10 is normal, the addition of supplemental coenzyme Q-10 will usually have little or no effect.

ENZYMES AND COENZYMES

Enzymes are protein substances found in plants, animals, humans, and all living things. They are necessary for the building and rebuilding of tissues and cells. Enzymes are catalysts that influence all life systems from our heads to our toes. They are produced by living cells but are capable of acting independently. They are complex proteins that can induce chemical changes in other substances without being changed themselves. Enzymes are specific in their action; they will act only on a certain substance or a group of closely related substances and no others.

Enzymes consist of at least two parts: the protein portion and the cofactor portion. The specific amino acids that compose the protein portion of the enzyme are determined by the genetic code. Either mineral ions (such as calcium, magnesium and zinc) or vitamins, or both in some instances, make up the cofactor portion of the complete enzyme. The vitamin portion is usually called the coenzyme.

Most people know a little about the workings of a car engine. To help us understand the way energy is used in the body, it may be useful to use the analogy of the automobile. The individual cell, of course, is far more complex than the gasoline engine in a car, but they are analogous.

In an automobile engine, the proper mixture of gasoline with oxygen ignites to provide the necessary energy to drive the pistons. Various gears and linkages harness this energy to turn the wheels. Within this framework energy can be viewed as the capacity or ability to do work. Increasing or decreasing the energy supply either speeds up or slows down the engine. Similarly, the human body must continuously be supplied with its own form of energy to perform its many complex operations. Aside from the energy needed for work performed by the muscle system, there is a considerable demand for energy by other forms of biologic work. This includes the energy for digestion, absorption and assimilation of the food nutrients. It also includes energy for the functioning of various glands that secrete special hormones, for the establishment of the proper electrochemical gradients along the cell membrane to permit transmission of brain signals through the nerves to the muscles, and for the building of new chemical compounds such as protein. *All of this energy begins in the individual cell.*

ATP, THE ENGINE'S FUEL

The cell's engine is called the *mitochondria*. The enzyme that makes it all work is succinate dehydrogenase-co-Q-10 reductase. The cells do not use the nutrients consumed in the diet for their immediate supply of energy. Instead, they prepare an energy-rich compound called *adenosine triphosphate*, or simply ATP.

ATP is the "fuel" used for *all* the energy-requiring processes within the cell. In turn, the energy in food is extracted to build more ATP. The potential energy stored in the ATP molecule represents chemical energy made in the cell as it is needed.

Molecules are composed of atoms held together by bonds. It is the breaking of the ATP molecule's bonds that releases energy. ATP consists of one molecule of adenine and ribose called *adenosine,* combined with three phosphates and oxygen atoms. A considerable amount of energy is stored in the ATP molecule at the bonds that link the two outermost phosphate groups with the remainder of the molecule. When the outermost bond is broken, it releases an amount of energy equivalent to approximately 7000 calories.

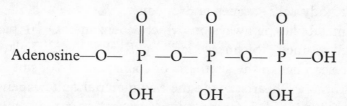

This equation is the chemical reason for 95 percent of the energy required for the operation of the body.

Although ATP serves as the energy current for *all* cells, its quantity is limited. In fact, only about three ounces of ATP are stored in the body at any one time! This would provide only enough energy to sustain strenuous activity, such as running as fast as you can, for 5 to 8 seconds. Therefore, ATP must be constantly synthesized to provide a continuous supply of energy. If it were not constantly produced, our "fuel tanks" would read "empty" and all movement would cease. The foods we eat and store in ready access within the body provide the basic raw material to change into ATP with the help of coenzyme Q-10.

The body extracts the potential energy stored within the structure of carbohydrate, fat and protein molecules consumed in the diet or stored in the body. This energy is harnessed for one major purpose, to combine adenosine and phosphate to form the energy-rich compound ATP.

COENZYME Q-10

Ubiquinone, another name for coenzyme Q-10, was formed from the word *ubiquitous* because the enzyme was found in all of the cells of the body. It is a naturally occurring molecule that resembles the chemical structure of vitamin K in molecular appearance. It is the cofactor in the electron transport chain, the biochemical pathway in cellular respiration from which ATP and most of the body's energy are derived.

Because the body must have available energy to carry on the simplest operation, for example, breathing in oxygen and breathing out carbon dioxide, coenzyme Q-10 is considered essential for the health of all the body cells, tissues and organs.

The metabolic pathways in which coenzyme Q-10 participates have been termed "bioenergetics" by Karl Folkers. Folkers was a pioneer researcher in the synthesis of coenzyme Q-10, since its initial source, from beef hearts, made the raw material quite expensive. The Japanese have used a fermentation process to produce coenzyme Q-10 for the mass market for several years. This has enabled six million Japanese to use this unique supplement on a daily basis at a low cost. Although the body can produce this substance, deficiencies have been reported in a wide range of clinical conditions. We will go into the individual diseases associated with coenzyme Q-10 deficiency a bit later in this chapter.

Animal studies have shown that the decline in coenzyme Q-10 levels that occur with age may be partly responsible for age-related deterioration of the immune system. In one animal study, E. Z. Bliznakov (1978) found that coenzyme Q-10 declined by 80 percent in the course of normal aging. A decline of this magnitude in a human being would be fatal, but deficiencies approaching this have been observed in aged humans and are associated with grave heart disease.*

*References to the published reports on this substance are given in the Bibliography at the end of this chapter.

Human cells contain coenzyme Q-10, while animal cells have co-enzyme Q-6 to Q-10. Plants, algae and the photosynthetic bacteria contain a substance that is similar to the enzyme. The plant substances are called plastaquinones. Although the animal structure can be raised from coenzyme Q-6 to coenzyme Q-10 in the body, there is some question whether plastaquinones could act as a supplement if coenzyme Q-10 is required. Synthesis of the enzyme from plant sources through chemical modification is, however, entirely possible.

COENZYME Q-10 SUPPLEMENTS

A need for supplemental Q-10 could arise for several reasons:

1. Impaired coenzyme Q-10 synthesis due to nutritional deficiencies
2. Genetic or acquired defect in coenzyme Q-10 synthesis
3. Increased tissue needs resulting from a particular medical condition

Because of its role in energy production, a deficiency of the enzyme could cause or aggravate many medical conditions.

If taken orally, coenzyme Q-10 can be taken up and utilized by the body. Because coenzyme Q-10 plays such an important role in energy production and can be administered orally, it is possible to correct a deficiency of the enzyme and the metabolic associated consequences by supplementing with it.

The early research done with coenzyme Q-10 used the Q-7 form, which the body converted to the Q-10 form. Although the body is capable of converting Q-7 into the natural form, coenzyme Q-10 is now commercially available from a number of companies.

DEFICIENCY DOCUMENTATION

Coenzyme Q-10 participates in the Krebs (citric acid) cycle enzyme system known as succinate dehydrogenase-CoQ10 reductase. In order to detect a deficiency in this enzyme, an assay of its activity is performed. If the enzyme is fully saturated with coenzyme Q-10, then supplementation will not increase the activity. If, on the other hand, tissue levels are shown to be low, the use of supplemental coenzyme Q-10 will increase the activity appreciably.

COENZYME Q-10, MEDICINE AND LONGEVITY

Coenzyme Q-10 is present in all body cells. Within the cells it is found in the cytosol (soluble cell fraction) and in the mitochondria (a cellular organelle). The major portion of cellular coenzyme Q-10 is present in the mitochondria as part of the electron transport system. It is in this system that oxidative phosphorylation, a critical link to life itself, and the rate of oxidation of nutrients are regulated. Thus, the heart and the liver, which are both central to this process, contain the largest number of mitochondria per cell and the greatest amount of coenzyme Q-10.

CARDIOVASCULAR DISEASE

In the heart, cellular mitochondria provide energy for the intake of nutrients and for the constant pumping action. The heart muscle utilizes triglycerides prepared by the liver as fuel to generate its energy; thus the heart is entirely dependent on mitochondrial phosphorylation to generate the energy needed for nonstop action.

The action of promoting better functioning of the myocardial tissue is one component of an overall treatment program for cardiovascular disease. Frequently, however, it is overlooked by the profession. The pumping function can be impaired by degenerative lesions. These lesions can be found in most types of cardiovascular problems such as hypertension, atherosclerosis, valvular heart disease and primary cardiomyopathy.

It is possible that the lesions result from repeated insults to the cardiac tissue from a variety of reasons. They can include ischemic events, inflammation, the release of catecholamines in greater than normal amounts due to stress (emotional or physical), as well as other factors.

If optimum nutrition is supplied at the cellular level, which means diet, vitamins and minerals, as well as coenzyme Q-10, it appears that degeneration may be delayed or forestalled and that the mechanical action of the heart may be improved.

Animal studies and human tests have clearly shown the results of the supplementation with coenzyme Q-10. In animals, coenzyme Q-10 reduced the infarct size resulting from acute coronary occlusion and protected the myocardium against experimentally induced cardiomyopathy and myocarditis.

A deficiency of coenzyme Q-10 is common in cardiac patients. When it was looked for, myocardial biopsies done on patients with various cardiac diseases showed that there was a deficiency of the enzyme in 50 to 75 percent of the patients studied.

Because the heart is so metabolically active and needs the constant supply of usable fuel for its constant contraction and pumping action, it may be unusually susceptible to the effects of coenzyme Q-10 deficiency. Conversely, coenzyme Q-10 has shown to be a supplement of great promise in the treatment of heart disease.

ANGINA PECTORIS

According to *Taber's Cyclopedic Medical Dictionary*, angina pectoris causes severe pain and feeling of pressure in the region of the heart. It is accompanied by great anxiety, fear of approaching death, sweating and an ashen or livid face. Attacks may be brief or last for a considerable period. The prognosis may be grave. Attacks may be intermittent, and with proper rest and care, recovery is possible.

A small study, at least in the number of patients involved if not in importance, was done on 12 patients with stable angina pectoris (Kamikawa, 1985). They were given 150 milligrams of coenzyme Q-10 daily for four weeks. The patients being given the supplement were compared to a second group receiving a medication that looked like coenzyme Q-10 (a placebo) but was really only milk sugar. Neither the patients nor the doctors knew who was receiving what. At the end of the test, results were compared.

Compared to the placebo patients, the patients receiving the real supplement had a reduced frequency of anginal episodes of 53 percent. There was also a significant increase in treadmill exercise tolerance (time to onset of chest pain) during the treatment.

Since there have been no side reactions to the use of coenzyme Q-10 in the dosages prescribed, the results suggest that coenzyme Q-10 might be a safe and effective treatment for angina pectoris under the supervision of a competent health practitioner.

CONGESTIVE HEART FAILURE

Several studies were run concerning the use of coenzyme Q-10 and congestive heart failure.

In one study, 17 patients suffering from mild congestive heart failure (CHF) were given 30 milligrams of coenzyme Q-10 daily. After four weeks results were tabulated. All patients improved, and nine of the patients no longer showed any symptoms of the disease. In other words, 53 percent of the patients treated were asymptomatic in four weeks.

Another study included 20 patients with congestive heart failure due either to ischemic (local or temporary deficiency of the blood supply due to obstruction of the circulation to the heart) or hypertensive heart disease. Treatment included 30 milligrams of coenzyme Q-10 every day for one to two months. Fifty-five percent of the patients reported subjective improvement. Fifty percent showed a decrease in New York Heart Association classification, a measure of heart disease severity. Thirty percent showed a "remarkable" decrease in chest congestion as proven by chest x-rays. The milder the disease, the greater the improvement, although those patients with a more severe problem showed improvement as well.

The patients who had reported subjective improvement were given a series of tests to bear out their reported findings. The researchers tested stroke volume, cardiac output, cardiac index and ejection fraction. Test results showed the improvement in cardiac function consistent with the patients' reports.

Results were consistent with a positive inotropic effect of coenzyme Q-10, although the effect was not as powerful as that of the cardiac drug digitalis. In addition, coenzyme Q-10 prevented the negative effect of beta-blocker therapy without reducing the beneficial effects of the beta-blockers on myocardial oxygen consumption.

Digitalis has been used in severe cases of congestive heart failure, but the chance of digitalis toxicity at the dose necessary to attempt to correct the problem is always present. There is a possibility that a combination of digitalis and coenzyme Q-10 might reduce the needed dosage of digitalis and the accompanying risk.

The remarkable safety of coenzyme Q-10 and the almost total lack of toxicity at the dosages prescribed appear to suggest that it might possibly replace conventional therapy and become the treatment of choice for mild congestive heart failure. Coenzyme Q-10 might also be an adjunctive therapeutic agent to be used along with beta-blockers to prevent the impairment of cardiac functions that sometimes appear during this therapy.

Since coenzyme Q-10 is a natural substance produced within the body, and since the body also responds to it as a supplement, and it appears to be effective in treating mild cases of congestive heart failure by increasing the intrinsic strength of the heart muscle, it would appear to be a subject for very close scrutiny by the medical community. However, at this time it is sold only as a nutritional supplement in the United States, to maintain health.

CARDIOMYOPATHY

Cardiomyopathy is a term which usually refers to a disease of the heart muscles of obscure etiology. The diagnosis of cardiomyopathy is difficult, but doctors believe this disease is killing thousands of patients yearly. The substance coenzyme Q-10, still not accepted by the FDA, offers the promise of being the first substance effective for the disease.

According to an article in the *Miami Herald* for December 19, 1985, Earl Weed of Temple, Texas, was so sick with a diagnosed case of cardiomyopathy that it was all he could do to sit up. Weed began taking treatments of synthetic coenzyme Q-10, a lab copy of the natural substance needed by the heart to convert food and oxygen into life-giving energy. The results were remarkable; the 61-year-old man recalled: "I've been painting my house inside and out. If I can do that, I can do most everything."

Deficiency of coenzyme Q-10 has been uncovered in the myocardial tissue and in the blood of patients suffering from severe cardiomyopathy. Where there was evidence of a deficiency, supplementation of the enzyme was begun on patients with diagnosed cardiomyopathy. Oral supplementation for two to eight months increased the level of the enzyme in the myocardial tissue in the patients. In some, the increase was greater than in others. In a double-blind study with the use of 100 milligrams of coenzyme Q-10 daily for 12 weeks, it was determined that shortness of breath and increased cardiac muscle strength showed the benefits of supplementation. These shown improvements lasted as long as three years in patients treated continuously. In contrast, when use of the supplement was discontinued, the cardiac function deteriorated.

There are no firm statistics on deaths due to cardiomyopathy because of the difficulty in diagnosis, but Dr. Eugene Morkin, professor of medicine at the University of Arizona Health Science Center, where almost 100 heart transplant operations have been performed, said that cardiomyopathy was a major problem for about one-third of the patients. He also said that those suffering from the disease do not respond well to conventional therapy.

Dr. Per Langsjoen of Scott & White Memorial Hospital in Tempe, Arizona, when reporting on his research done in Tokyo, Japan, was supportive of coenzyme Q-10 therapy. He said that cardiomyopathy patients steadily worsening and expected to die within two years under conventional therapy generally showed an extraordinary clinical improvement when given coenzyme Q-10, indicating that the supplemental therapy might extend their lives (Judy, 1984).

In an open trial, 34 patients with severe congestive cardiomyopathy were given 100 milligrams of coenzyme Q-10 daily. Eighty-two percent of the patients improved with the supplement. The two-year survival rate increased to 62 percent compared to less than 25 percent for a similar group of patients treated by conventional methods but without added coenzyme Q-10.

In Japan, coenzyme Q-10 is used to treat several cardiac diseases.

Eisai Co. Ltd., of Tokyo, has been marketing it under the trade name Neuquinon since 1974. Neuquinon is also sold in Korea, Taiwan and Italy.

HYPERTHYROID HEART FAILURE

Overstimulation of the thyroid gland and excess thyroxin secretion can cause huge problems to the body. The symptoms include exophthalmia (bulging of the eyes), weight loss, heat intolerance, excessive nervousness, irritability, elevated heart rate, elevated blood pressure and muscle weakness.

Serum coenzyme Q-10 levels appear to be significantly lower than normal levels in patients with hyperthyroidism. Because congestive heart failure may occur as a result of the thyroid condition or as a result of the decreased amount of the enzyme, 120 milligrams of coenzyme Q-10 daily were given for one week to 12 hyperthyroid patients. The patients' hearts, already stimulated by the condition far past the normal action, responded with augmented performance (Suzuki, 1984).

It is possible that coenzyme Q-10 has a therapeutic value for congestive heart failure induced by thyrotoxicosis. This area is one which should be investigated further by qualified researchers. A book by Stephen E. Langer, M.D., *Solved: The Riddle of Illness,* Keats Publishing, New Canaan, Conn., attributes many of the health problems suffered by people to the thyroid gland.

MITRAL VALVE PROLAPSE

A cardiac evaluation was made of 194 children with symptomatic mitral valve prolapse using the standard isometric hand grip test (Oda, 1984). All of the tested patients showed an abnormal response to hand grip previous to supplementation.

Eight of the children were given 2 milligrams per kilogram of body weight of coenzyme Q-10 every day for eight weeks while a control group of eight children were given placebo tablets of milk sugar that physically resembled the tablets of coenzyme Q-10. At the end of the eighth week, all of the children were tested again. The hand grip test became normal for seven of the eight children who received the coenzyme Q-10, but none of the children who had received the placebo tablet showed any improvement.

Relapse to the former condition was frequently noted in those patients who discontinued using the supplement within one year to 17 months, but rarely occurred in those patients who continued to use the coenzyme Q-10 for 18 months or longer.

HYPERTENSION

Systolic pressures of 140 to 150 mm Hg(mercury) and diastolic pressures of 90 to 100 mm Hg are generally regarded as the upper limits of normal to slightly high blood pressure. Sustained elevation of systolic pressure, diastolic pressure, or both, above these limits is termed hypertension.

If a cause of the hypertension can be determined, the hypertensive state is called secondary hypertension. That is, it occurs secondary to some other demonstrable disorder. If no specific cause for the hypertension can be discerned, the hypertension is designated as essential or primary hypertension.

Among the causes of secondary systolic hypertension are increased cardiac output, the rigidity of the walls of the aorta and main arteries (arteriosclerosis).

Diastolic hypertension appears to be particularly dangerous and can result in vascular damage that may affect the operation of the organs that the affected vessels serve. Vessels serving the kidneys, liver, pancreas, brain and retina appear to be particularly prone to damage.

When 59 patients with hypertension were tested for the presence of coenzyme Q-10, 39 percent showed a deficiency. As a control, 65 people with normal pressure were also tested for coenzyme Q-10. Of this group, only 6 percent showed a deficiency (Yamagami, 1977).

Twenty-five patients suffering from essential hypertension were given supplemental coenzyme Q-10, 60 milligrams a day for eight weeks. The results showed a highly significant decrease in blood pressure in the group as a whole. The results also showed that 54 of the test group had a mean blood pressure drop greater than 10 percent less than the pressure at the start of the test (Yamagami, 1974).

Thus, coenzyme Q-10 is not a typical antihypertensive drug but a natural substance that appears to correct some metabolic abnormality, which, in turn, has a favorable influence on blood pressure.

The effect of the supplement is not instantaneous. Results are not usually seen until after therapy has been continued for anywhere from four to twelve weeks. This delay in perceptible results is consistent with the gradual buildup in enzyme activity that has appeared in other coenzyme Q-10 therapy.

In animal studies of experimental hypertension, it was found that induced hypertension led to a deficiency of coenzyme Q-10, which was then corrected by addition of the supplement. Whether coenzyme Q-10 deficiency is a cause or an effect of hypertension, correction of the deficiency may improve the blood pressure in selected cases.

Coenzyme Q-10 has reduced aldosterone secretion in dogs and inhibited the sodium-retaining effect of aldosterone and angiotensin in rats. Other animal tests involving spontaneously hypertensive rats and experimentally hypertensive dogs have also shown response to oral coenzyme Q-10.

COENZYME Q-10 AND BETA-BLOCKERS

Prescription drugs are frequently prescribed for hypertension, and they do a marvelous job in preserving life. However, some of the drugs have side effects which, if controlled, would enable the drug to do an even better job. Propanolol and metoprolol, two of these drugs, have been found to inhibit coenzyme Q-10-dependent enzymes. It is also likely, but as yet not investigated, that many other drugs in this class have the same inhibitory effect.

In the long run, the benefits of the use from these antihypertensive agents may be compromised by the development of a coenzyme Q-10 deficiency. Therefore, supplementation with the enzyme may help to prevent a shortage of coenzyme Q-10 and may actually improve the drug's ability to help the patient.

Coenzyme Q-10 may also help to prevent other common side effects of beta-blockers, such as their reduction of cardiac contractility, or fatigue and malaise. Medical authorities should investigate the possible combination of coenzyme Q-10 and beta-blockers.

COENZYME Q-10 AND LONGEVITY

According to nutritional science, we should live to the ripe old age of 125 or more. We, all of us, are being cheated out of many enjoyable and productive years because of degenerative diseases common to aging.

Who wants to grow old the way that degeneration has made old age in the commonest sense? Who wants the sagging skin, the wrinkles, the bulges of fat that appear as if by magic one day and refuse to leave us?

Who wants a menu restricted to the blandest of foods and a life dependent on the vicinity of the nearest bathroom?

Failing memory, indigestion, constipation or diarrhea on a regular basis—who wants these? Who wants just enough energy to get us through the day. And sex—did it leave with the failing memory? Tooth troubles, gum trouble, bone troubles . . . trouble everywhere . . . are the too-common companions of aging.

We can assume that aging is the way nature limits the number of lives on earth to make room for new generations, and that it is impossible to leave this earth alive. But why be cheated out of up to 50 years of life that is available to us according to the laws of nature?

LONGEVITY AND NUTRITION

For a longer life, nutritional intervention can be an answer. The biogenic potential for a longer life is a possibility for those who decide to take matters into their own hands and investigate the body and its systems: energy, digestion, assimilation and elimination.

The average American diet will do little to extend life. If it did, there wouldn't be millions of Americans suffering from cardiovascular disease; diabetes, cancer, hypertension and a host of other degenerative ailments. About two-thirds of our people are suffering from chronic malnutrition, leading to obesity and to the killer diseases from failing livers and failing kidneys.

It should be obvious that changing one's diet will contribute to a longer life. Switching over to complex carbohydrates, raw fruits, raw or lightly steamed vegetables, fish and fowl will help. Eliminating canned, processed and refined foods, and eating foods in season will also improve the body systems. But there are also "uncommon" supplementary suggestions which can help to ward off the insults the body has to endure.

As you have read, this chapter has to do with coenzyme Q-10 and its involvement with the generation of essential energy. The heart and the liver contain the largest number of mitochondria (fuel cells) per tissue concentration, and therefore, the greatest amount of coenzyme Q-10 and the greatest need for the enzyme.

The mitochondria contain a large number of enzymes organized and grouped together according to their function, for example, electron transport enzymes, citric acid cycle enzymes and fatty acid alteration enzymes.

These enzyme systems require coenzymes, which, in many cases, are derived from vitamins, in particular, the B-complex family of vitamins such as vitamin B3 (niacin) and vitamin B2 (riboflavin). Niacin is involved in the production of nicotinic acid-nicotinamine adenine-denucleotide (NAD), and riboflavin in riboflavin-flavineodenine dinucleotide (FAD).

The important cofactor in the electron transport chain and the mitochondria is coenzyme Q-10. It plays the critical role in the pumping of protons across the mitochondrial membrane. As we age, the amount of coenzyme Q-10 in the body declines.

In humans, coenzyme Q-10 serves the following purposes that may be connected to the aging process:

1. Increases energy and exercise tolerance. Most aging people claim they do not have the energy to exercise or even to do more moder-

ate amounts of walking. This may be the result of a deficiency of the enzyme or may be a sedentary habit.

2. Corrects age-related declines in the immune system which can leave the body easy prey to bacterial and viral infection. Mouse experiments have shown that coenzyme Q-10 is able to partially correct declines in the immune system of mice related to age. It is possible that coenzyme Q-10 is a significant immunologic stimulant.

3. Has considerable healing effect on age-related periodontal disease. When people can keep their teeth longer, they can eat better and keep their nutrition at peak level. (More will be said about coenzyme Q-10 and periodontal disease later in this chapter.)

4. Defuses peroxides from within and without the body. The antioxidant action of certain nutrients has been shown to exert an important influence on longevity. Free radicals, highly reactive particles, damage the cells and the cell nucleus. The damaged cell cannot reproduce an undamaged cell because the blueprint for cell-building has been harmed. As a result an inefficient cell is formed with the potential for building another damaged cell, and so on. Antioxidant nutrients such as vitamin E react with the free radicals to render them harmless. Coenzyme Q-10 has a chemical structure that is similar to that of vitamin E, which may account for its potent antioxidant ability. Coenzyme Q-10 is able to inhibit lipid peroxidation in the membrane of the mitochondria, peroxidation which would attack the cell membrane and severely limit its energy-making potential.

It is strange but true that the very process of producing energy also generates free radicals. Coenzyme Q-10, when it is present in sufficient quantities, is in a perfect position to squelch these overactive molecules as soon as they are formed.

COENZYME Q-10 AND DETOXIFICATION

In addition to the direct anti-aging effects shown by this enzyme, it also appears that it is able to act against the possible toxic side effects of some prescription drugs used to treat older people for common illnesses of aging. (More will be said about this later in connection with adriamycin.)

One of the least discussed and most important of all of the body systems for promoting long life and health is the liver. The liver is responsible for nutrient assimilation and storage as well as detoxifying the body system and eliminating poisons that might accumulate in the body. The liver is the largest solid organ in the body and weighs about four pounds. It is a chemical plant that can modify almost any chemical structure.

A powerful detoxifying organ, it can break down a variety of toxic molecules, rendering them harmless. It is a storage organ and a blood reservoir. It stores vitamins A and D, digested carbohydrates and glycogen, which is released to sustain blood sugar levels. The liver manufactures enzymes, cholesterol, proteins, and blood coagulation factors.

One of the prime functions of the liver is to produce bile which promotes efficient digestion of fats. It synthesizes amino acids used in building tissues, it breaks up proteins into sugar and fat when they are needed as such, it produces urea, and it is closely connected with normal calcium metabolism.

Studies have shown that the aging liver is often operating at less than peak efficiency. Although the liver employs several pathways for energy generation, mitochondrial oxidative phosphorylation is the major pathway for generating energy. As we have read throughout this chapter, this pathway requires quantities of coenzyme Q-10.

Life extension requires many nutrients, among them the essential mineral selenium. Selenium is a potent anti-cancer agent and an antioxidant. There is some evidence that the use of selenium as a supplement also elevates the coenzyme Q-10 content in the tissues of laboratory rats. Magnesium, another necessary mineral, also appears to stimulate the production of the enzyme within the body.

It is remarkable that many diverse dietary and hormonal alterations that can promote longevity also elevate coenzyme Q-10 levels.

Nevertheless coenzyme Q-10 levels are depressed by interventions that adversely affect health and longevity. For example, increased dietary cholesterol lowers coenzyme Q-10 levels. The level is also decreased by cortisone, suggesting that stress is a factor in lowering the enzyme value.

In view of the foregoing, it is interesting to speculate that coenzyme Q-10 might play a fundamental role in decelerating aging.

PERIODONTAL DISEASE

"Your teeth are good but, your gums will have to come out" is an old joke that's all too true. Gum disease affects nine out of ten Americans in the course of a lifetime. At least one out of four people will lose all their teeth by the time they reach age 60 to gum disease. Gum disease accounts for 70 percent of all lost teeth.

More than 30 million Americans have gum disease in such an advanced state that they will lose tooth after tooth unless they get immediate dental help. Periodontal disease affects 60 percent of the young and 90 percent of all individuals over the age of 65.

This doesn't have to be!

Dr. Edward G. Wilkinson, periodontal specialist and dental researcher, investigated some of the causes of gum disease while on duty with the United States Air Force. He and his co-researchers found that diseased dental tissue showed a remarkable deficiency in coenzyme Q-10. By supplementing patient with daily doses of the natural enzyme, Dr. Wilkinson and his team were able to reverse the gum conditions that were threatening the life of the teeth. Even in cases that appeared to be hopeless with no other choice but to remove the teeth to treat the gums, the use of coenzyme Q-10 showed great promise.

Proper oral hygiene and the services of a thorough dentist are helpful in every case, but healing and repair of periodontal tissue require efficient energy production.

Many studies have pointed out the deficiency of coenzyme Q-10 in gum tissue. The frequency of a deficiency ranged from 60 percent to 96 percent. Periodontitis may itself lead to a localized enzyme deficiency. However, studies have shown that 86 percent of the patients also had low levels of coenzyme Q-10 in white blood cells, indicating the presence of a systemic imbalance.

The use of supplemental coenzyme Q-10 is safe, as shown by its daily use in Japan for conditions ranging from heart disease to dental protection to life extension. As mentioned earlier, in the United States coenzyme Q-10 is available as a food supplement. The Food and Drug Administration forbids it to be advertised as anything else until its medical properties are approved.

Dr. Karl Folkers holds an FDA permit to test the substance. He has to prove it is safe and effective and, according to him, the proof is there! (Wilkinson, 1976, 1977)

Clinical studies on 18 patients with periodontal disease were performed in the classic double-blind test where neither the doctors nor the patients knew which patients had received a placebo capsule and which had received a capsule containing coenzyme Q-10.

The patients took their capsules for three weeks in a row. The results were calculated according to a periodontal procedure that took into account a number of factors including gingival pocket depth, swelling, bleeding, redness, pain, exudate, and looseness of teeth.

All eight patients receiving coenzyme Q-10 showed real improvement. The healing was considered to be very impressive by a group of outside dentists who had no knowledge that a test was being run. In fact, one prosthodontist remarked that the healing seen in three weeks would usually take about six months!

In an open trial, coenzyme Q-10 produced postsurgical healing that was two to three times faster than usual in seven patients suffering from advanced periodontal disease (Wilkinson, 1975). Coenzyme Q-10 may act by improving the energy-dependent processes of healing and tissue repair. It also tends to help improve abnormal citrate metabolism frequently found in many patients with periodontitis.

DIABETES MELLITUS

Diabetes is a general term for diseases characterized by excessive urination. In the form called diabetes mellitus, it is considered to be a disorder of carbohydrate metabolism characterized by hyperglycemia and glycosuria. It is the result of inadequate production or utilization of insulin.

In most instances diabetes mellitus is the result of a genetic disorder, but it may also result from a deficiency of beta cells caused by inflammation, surgery, malignancy, or other unknown problems. It is currently thought that insulin acts primarily at the cell membrane facilitating transport of glucose into the cells. Recent studies have given glucose tolerance factor (GTF) chromium a functional role in the process.

Since it is a multifactorial illness and is associated with a number of different metabolic abnormalities, it is prudent to examine the role coenzyme Q-10 plays in this illness.

Coenzyme Q-10 is intimately involved in the metabolism of carbohydrates. Studies of diabetic rats in laboratory circumstances have shown those rats to be deficient in the enzyme. During the laboratory tests, coenzyme Q-7, which is normally present in rats as coenzyme Q-10 is normally present in humans, was administered on a supplemental basis. It was found that supplementation partly corrected abnormal glucose metabolism in alloxan-induced diabetes in the rats.

A human study of 120 diabetic patients showed that 8.3 percent were deficient in coenzyme Q-10 compared to 1.9 percent of a group of healthy people used as controls (Kishi, 1976).

When a group of diabetics using a variety of oral hypoglycemic drugs to control their diabetes were tested for coenzyme Q-10 levels, the deficiency rate was much higher. It amounted to around 20 percent, apparently because oral hypoglycemics interfere with the metabolism of the enzyme.

When the supplement was given to a group of 39 diabetics, who were in a stabilized condition, for periods ranging from two weeks to 18 weeks, the fasting blood sugar was found to be reduced by at least 20 percent in 14 of the subjects and by at least 30 percent in 12 of the subjects (Shigeta, 1966). The dosage was 120 milligrams a day.

In some cases, when the test period was over and the supplement was withdrawn, there was an increase in blood sugar or blood ketone bodies. One of the group who had difficulty controlling his condition on 60 units of insulin showed a marked fall in fasting blood sugar after supplementation.

The above studies were done with coenzyme Q-7, since coenzyme Q-10 was not available at that time. Since the Q-7 form is upgraded to Q-10, there is no reason to suspect that Q-10 will not have the same results.

We do not know how coenzyme Q-10 helps to improve diabetic control. Perhaps it induces the body to synthesize more of the enzyme itself, or perhaps it helps to enhance carbohydrate metabolism. In any event, more work is necessary to pin down the effective action, although supplementation can be done even if the mechanism is unknown.

COENZYME Q-10 AND THE CARDIOTOXICITY OF ADRIAMYCIN

Chemotherapy against malignant disease has certain drawbacks in the way the chemotherapeutic agents interfere with normal body activities. We are all aware of the accompanying falling hair, swelling, and bone and blood problems.

One particularly effective chemotherapeutic agent is called adriamycin. It has been used against certain tumors, but because it has a serious effect on the heart, particularly after treatment has gone on for some time, the use of this effective agent has been limited (Folkers, 1980).

When it was discovered that adriamycin inhibited coenzyme Q-10 dependent enzymes in tests on 11 cancer patients being treated with this drug, it was decided to use supplemental coenzyme Q-10 to see the effect (Judy, 1984). One group of seven patients received 100 milligrams of coenzyme Q-10 daily beginning three to five days before treatment with adriamycin was started. Another group of seven patients were given adriamycin but were not given any coenzyme Q-10.

The group that had received the enzyme along with the anti-tumor agent did not suffer the increase in cardiac problems that occurred in the group not given the supplement.

This conclusion was even more astounding since the group receiving the coenzyme Q-10 received a cumulative dosage of adriamycin about 50 percent greater than the control group. It should be noted that coenzyme Q-10 did *not* appear to protect patients with impaired cardiac function prior to adriamycin treatment.

WEIGHT LOSS

When you take in more calories than you burn, the excess calories are stored in the form of fat. Obese people may be able to reduce the amount of stored fat by a number of methods, including reducing the intake of food, increasing the output of energy through exercise, or increasing the efficiency of their cellular respiration and caloric output.

Certain individuals do not produce as much heat energy as others. The tendency to become overweight can, in some cases, be connected to faulty metabolic activity. Some subjects with a family history of obesity show only half the thermogenic response to food of the average person. This suggests that there is a factor in obesity that is a result of poor energy production. Since coenzyme Q-10 is an integral part of energy production on the cellular level, it is possible that a deficiency of this enzyme may play a part in some cases of obesity.

When some very obese individuals (27 subjects in all) were examined for a deficiency of coenzyme Q-10, over 50 percent or 14 of the 27 were found to be deficient (Val Gaal, 1984).

As a test, five subjects with low levels of the enzyme, and a control group of four people with normal enzyme levels, were given 100 milligrams of coenzyme Q-10 daily along with a restricted diet. After nine weeks, the mean weight loss for the group that was initially deficient in coenzyme Q-10 was 13.5 kg (a kg is equal to 2.2 pounds) compared to a weight loss of only 5.8 kg in the control group.

The study suggests that some individuals, perhaps up to 50 percent of really obese persons, may be deficient in coenzyme Q-10. A combination of a low-calorie diet and supplementation with the enzyme may result in a weight loss superior to that obtained by a restricted diet alone.

ATHLETIC PERFORMANCE

Another area where the concept of "bioenergetics" supplementation might enhance aerobic capacity and muscle performance is athletic performance.

A study of six healthy men not used to doing any type of exercise, sedentary in the fullest sense of the word, involved working out on a stationary bicycle (Vanfrachem, 1981). The first test was performed before taking any coenzyme Q-10 and the comparison test was done four and eight weeks after taking the supplement. The dose was 60 milligrams a day. The second test showed improved performance parameters in several areas including work capacity at submaximal heart rate, maximal oxygen consumption and oxygen transport. The improvements ranged from 3 to 12 percent.

Although much work remains to be done, the study does suggest that the use of supplementary coenzyme Q-10 could improve the physical performance of sedentary individuals.

It is also suggested that trained athletes might benefit from supplementation with improved performance and/or the relief of chronic fatigue. This possibility has yet to be investigated.

It should be pointed out that most supplements on the market are in the form of 10-milligram capsules, with a suggested regimen of one capsule three times a day.

COENZYME Q-10 AND THE IMMUNE SYSTEM

The immune system of the body is generally thought to consist of the thymus gland, the lymphatic system, the long bones of the body, the spleen and the various products they manufacture.

Many illnesses are associated with abnormalities of the immune system. Attempts to improve the immune function of the body are standard therapy in the treatment of cancer, chronic infections, candidiasis and acquired immune deficiency syndrome (AIDS). Just as important but seldom thought about is the energy needed by these factors to perform their jobs! Since immunity demands a constant supply of first-grade energy, coenzyme Q-10 must be in constant and adequate supply.

There have been a number of studies concerned with the immune-enhancing effect of coenzyme Q-10 in animals (Bliznakov, 1970). Studies on mice have shown that supplementation with the enzyme increased phagocytic activity of macrophages, the germ-killing ability of the white blood cells. Also, supplementation increased the number of granulocytes (other killer cells) in response to experimentally induced infection.

Coenzyme Q-10 prolonged the survival of mice which had been infected with a number of pathogenic organisms including *Pseudomonas aeruginosa, Staphylococcus aureus, Escherichia coli, Klebsiella pneumoniae* and *Candida albicans*. Two out of ten mice were able to survive a massive dose of *E. coli* which killed all ten of the control group.

In some human studies, eight patients with various diseases including diabetes, cancer and cardiovascular problems were given coenzyme Q-10 over a long period of time. The dosage was 60 milligrams daily (Folkers, 1982).

Significant increases in the level of immunoglobulin G (IgG) were found in the serum of these patients after three weeks to twelve weeks of supplemental treatment. This increase could represent a correction of the immunodeficiency or an increase in immunocompetence.

Immune function appears to decline with advancing age. Older mice show thymic atrophy and a marked deficiency of the enzyme. Along with that is a pronounced depression of the immune system. This depression was partially reversed when the enzyme was given on a supplemental basis, so it is possible that regular supplementation with coenzyme Q-10 may help to prevent or even to reverse age-related immunosuppression.

ANTIOXIDANT POWER

Free radicals occur within and without the body. The damage caused to tissues and cells by these highly reactive particles is believed to contribute to aging and to disease. Cancer, arthritis, autoimmune disease, cardiovascular disease and other diseases are initiated or exacerbated by these free radicals.

A number of papers reveal the research done on antioxidant therapy and the way antioxidants can reduce the damaging effects of these articles. Research suggests that nutrients such as selenium, zinc, vitamin E, vitamin C, and B-complex vitamins, L-cysteine, L-methionine and others may reduce the pathological effects of free radicals.

Coenzyme Q-10, in addition to its role in energy production, also functions in a similar manner. In laboratory experiments, rats given the enzyme via injection had significantly fewer lipid peroxides (free radicals) in the heart and liver than a control group of animals not given the enzyme. Coenzyme Q-10 appeared to be as effective as vitamin E in the area of the heart but less effective in the liver.

The study suggests that any antioxidant program using conventional nutrients as mentioned above should also include coenzyme Q-10.

SAFETY

Coenzyme Q-10 has been used for a dozen years in Japan. Millions use the enzyme on a daily basis, usually in dosages of 10 milligrams, three times a day.

It is generally well tolerated, and no serious adverse effects have been reported even over long-term use. It should not be used during pregnancy or lactation, not because there have been any reported problems, but simply because its safety during these periods has not yet been proven. It is contraindicated in cases of known hypersensitivity.

When a series of patients (5,143) being treated with 30 milligrams a day of coenzyme Q-10 were studied for adverse effects, the following side effects were reported:

epigastric discomfort	0.39 percent
loss of appetite	0.23 percent
nausea	0.16 percent
diarrhea	0.11 percent

This indicates the safety and tolerance this supplement offers.

Because the synthesis of new coenzyme Q-10-dependent enzymes is a slow process, response should not be expected until at least eight weeks after supplementation is started.

BIBLIOGRAPHY

Bliznakov, E.G., et al. Coenzyme Q: stimulants of the phagocytic activity in rats and immune response in mice. *Experientia* 266:953, 1970.

———, et al. Coenzyme Q deficiency in aged mice. *J. Med.* 9:337, 1978.

Folkers, K. and Y. Yamura, eds. *Biomedical and Clinical Aspects of Coenzyme Q*, Vol. 2. Amsterdam: Elsevier/North Holland Biomedical Press, 1980, pp. 333–347.

Judy, W.V. et al. Coenzyme Q-10 reduction of adriamycin cardiotoxicity. In: Folkers and Yamura, Vol. 4, 1984.

Kamikawa, T., et al. Effects of coenzyme Q-10 on exercise tolerance in chronic stable angina pectoris. *Am. J. Cardiol.* 56:247, 1985.

Kishi, T., et al. Bioenergetics in clinical medicine. XI. Studies on coenzyme Q-10 and diabetes mellitus. *J. Med.* 7:307, 1976.

Mayer, P., et al. Differential effects of ubiquinone Q-7 and ubiquinone analogs on macrophage activation and experimental infections in granulocytopenic mice. *Infection* 8:256, 1980.

Oda, T. and K. Hamamoto. Effect of coenzyme Q-10 on the stress-induced decrease of cardiac performance in pediatric patients with mitral valve prolapse. *Jpn. Circ. J.* 48:1387, 1984.

Shigeta, Y., et al. Effect of coenzyme Q-7 treatment on blood sugar and ketone bodies of diabetics. *J. Vitaminol.* 12:293, 1966.

Suzuki, H., et al. Cardiac performance and coenzyme Q-10 in thyroid disorders. *Endocrinol. Japan.* 31:755, 1984.

Vanfrachem, J.H.P. and K. Folkers. *Coenzyme Q-10 and Clinical Aspects of Coenzyme 9.* Amsterdam: Biomedical Press, 1981.

Van Gaal, L., et al. Exploratory study of coenzyme Q-10 in obesity. In: Folkers and Yamura, Vol. 4, 1984, pp. 369–373.

Wilkinson, E. G., et al. Bioenergetics in clinical medicine. II. Adjunctive treatment with coenzyme Q in periodontal therapy. *Res. Commun. Chem. Pathol. Pharmacol.* 12:111, 1975.

————, et al. Bioenergetics in clinical medicine. VI. Adjunctive treatment with coenzyme Q in periodontal therapy. *Res. Commun. Chem. Pathol. Pharmacol.* 14:715, 1976.

————, et al. Treatment of periodontal and other soft tissue diseases of the oral cavity with coenzyme Q. In: Folkers and Yamura, Vol. 1, 1977, pp. 251–265.

Yamagami, T., et al. Reduction by coenzyme Q-10 of hypertension induced by deoxycorticosterone and saline in rats. *Internat. J. Vit. Nutr. Res.* 44:487, 1974.

———— et al. Correlation between serum coenzyme Q levels and succinate dehydrogenase coenzyme Q reductase activity in cardiovascular disease and the influence of coenzyme Q administration. In: Folkers and Yamura, Vol. 1, 1977, pp. 251–265.

BIOFLAVONOIDS

The Friends and Helpers of Vitamin C in Many Hard-to-Treat Ailments

Jeffrey Bland, Ph.D.

UNBEATABLE TEAMWORK

Viral infections, vascular troubles, allergies, diabetic cataracts and many other serious disorders have been found to be helped by the powerful combination of vitamin C and the bioflavonoids which are found in the white lining of citrus-fruit rinds and other plants. Like C, they increase the immune defense against disease; together they provide much more strength against inflammation than each does separately. For half a century, research and clinical data have recorded the good work of the bioflavonoids. Now they are beginning to receive the attention they deserve—and Jeffrey Bland is the nutrition expert who can tell their story.

One of the most exciting chapters in the history of nutrition and medicine is the story of a pioneer investigator, Dr. Albert Szent-Györgyi, who was able in the 1930s to isolate from vegetable and fruit products a chemical substance capable of treating the disease scurvy. This antiscorbutic factor was named ascorbic acid and became known as vitamin C. Once isolated and chemically identified, it opened the door for the development 40 years later of what is called orthomolecular medicine—the use of substances that are natural to the human body for the enhancement of physiological function.[1] Szent-Györgyi's work provided an explanation for the observation made almost two hundred years previously by Dr. James Lind, a British naval surgeon who found that scurvy could be prevented or treated in seamen if citrus fruits or juices were added to their diet on long voyages.

In a way, Dr. Lind was performing early orthomolecular therapy by using a natural substance, ascorbic acid, to treat a health problem related to a specific derangement in the body's metabolism. The term "orthomolecular" was coined by Dr. Linus Pauling to describe the use of natural substances—vitamins, minerals and other accessory nutrients—to help regulate metabolism and improve health. A key principle of orthomolecular therapy is to recognize each patient's biochemical individuality and to administer therapeutic nutrients on the basis of that individuality. It has to do not only with the use of vitamin C, but all other necessary nutrients, as well as natural substances found in the body, to help augment and support biochemical individuality. Vitamin C, as found in whole foods, is associated with many other natural products that may be considered orthomolecular substances.

Dr. Szent-Györgyi made one other important observation when working with natural products with antiscorbutic properties. He found that there were synergistic substances in these foods that tended to potentiate the action of vitamin C. These substances, which were extracted from red pepper and lemon, were shown by later chemical analysis to be members of a class of compounds called flavones or flavonols. When tested, they were found to decrease the breakage of small blood vessels, to prolong life in guinea pigs that had been deprived of vitamin C and to overcome small hemorrhages in human subjects who were vitamin C-deficient.[2]

This group of substances was later called vitamin P, referring to their effect on preventing small vessel or capillary permeability. None of them was later shown to have a true vitamin effect, however, in that deficiencies of them in the diet did not lead to an overt or diagnosable deficiency disease; and the designation of vitamin P was dropped in 1950 on the recommendation of the American Society of Biological Chemists and the American Institute of Nutrition.[3] Since that time, these substances—citrin, hesperidin, rutin, flavones and flavonols—

have been termed *bioflavonoids* and have been found by a number of investigators, including Dr. Z. Zloch of Charles University in Czechoslovakia, to enhance the antiscorbutic activity of ascorbic acid.[4] According to Zloch, when bioflavonoids are administered with vitamin C, there is an increased uptake of the vitamin into the liver, kidney and adrenal glands, and protection of the vitamin C by the bioflavonoids, which seem to work as antioxidants—that is, preventing the destruction of C by its conversion to a less active form called dehydroascorbate. He also reported a greater decrease in blood cholesterol than in tests in which animals were treated with vitamin C alone.

Bioflavonoids are water-soluble substances associated with colored materials that often but not always appear in fruits and vegetables as companions to vitamin C. Bioflavonoids were first found in the white segments of citrus fruits; there is ten times the concentration of bioflavonoids in the edible part of the fruit as is in the strained juice. Major natural sources of bioflavonoids include lemons, grapes, plums, black currants, grapefruit, apricots, buckwheat, cherries, blackberries and rose hips. Commercial methods of extracting bioflavonoids from the rinds of oranges, tangerines, lemons, limes, kumquats and grapefruits include those employing hot water or isopropanol. The antioxidant activity of bioflavonoids which protects vitamin C seems to result from their unique chemical structure; they act as reducing agents which are transported to the site where vitamin C is to be stored in the cell.[5]

BIOFLAVONOIDS–WHAT AND WHERE?

RUTIN AND HESPERIDIN

Rutin is found in many plants. Buckwheat contains about 3 percent dry-basis rutin when the plant is starting to bloom. The rutin molecule is made up of a sugar half that makes the compound water-soluble and an antioxidant flavone half.

Hesperidin is the predominant flavonoid in lemons and sweet oranges. It is reasonably soluble in water and, like rutin, is made up of a sugar half attached to a flavone half. The chemical similarity of rutin and hesperidin indicates that both have a similar mode of action. Rutin is a slightly better reducing reagent than hesperidin.

Because bioflavonoids have not been identified as actual vitamins or essential nutrients, there is no Recommended Dietary Allowance (RDA) for them. This places the bioflavonoids in a class of substances known as accessory nutrients—nutrients which are therapeutically valuable for those whose biochemical individuality makes them essential.[6]

Since bioflavonoids occur with vitamin C only in natural food sources, synthetic vitamin C does not contain them unless they have been added by the manufacturer. Bioflavonoids have been found to be virtually nontoxic, because they are eliminated rapidly from the body by excretion after breakdown. Also, they will not cause yellowing of the skin, as does a high intake of carotene pigments from carrots and other red/orange-colored vegetables, even with consumption of fairly high doses.

QUERCETIN AND EPICATECHIN

Two flavonoids not found in foods but which have similar chemical structures to rutin and hesperidin are quercetin, which is derived by steam distillation of quercitrin bark, and epicatechin. These materials are also widely distributed in the plant kingdom, especially in the rinds and barks of wild fruits and trees, in clover blossoms and in ragweed pollen. They have been isolated from rhododendron, forsythia, hydrangea, pansies and eucalyptus. Considerable pharmacological research has been done on the use of these substances in the treatment of various medical problems. Doses of between 10 and 20 milligrams per day of quercetin have been used on patients who experience capillary fragility, easy bruising and small pin-point hemorrhages called petechiae. Quercetin has also been found to be a very powerful inhibitor of an enzyme called aldose reductase. The medical implications of this relationship will be discussed in a later section of this chapter dealing with bioflavonoids and diabetic cataracts.[7]

All these bioflavonoids have a very bitter taste and are therefore generally taken as supplements in timed-release tablets or in capsules that will not dissolve readily in the mouth.

BIOLOGICAL AND CLINICAL
INVESTIGATIONS

Although a tremendous amount of work has been done with bioflavonoids, no deficiency state has ever been proven in animals or discovered in humans. Quercetin has been reported to have an inhibitory effect not only on aldose reductase, but also on other enzymes such as histidine decarboxylase.[8] A number of reports have not shown any relationship between oral ingestion of the bioflavonoids and diminishment of capillary fragility. It is possible that the compound used in some of these experiments may not have been adequately absorbed from the intestinal tract. This seems to be one of the major problems with bioflavonoid preparations—inappropriate processing of the bioflavonoid can make it virtually unabsorbable. One of the major questions that needs to be asked about the therapeutic usefulness of bioflavonoids for nutritional supplementation is whether the supplement to be used has truly been demonstrated to be absorbable into the blood across the intestinal barrier. In the absence of such proof, the substance employed may do nothing but color the stool.

Work has been done to try to determine whether a bioflavonoid supplement is useful in preventing hemorrhages in the eye and in reducing the risk of stroke in susceptible patients. One report indicates a decreased incidence of hemorrhages of the retina and stroke in individuals who have taken bioflavonoid supplements,[9] although some other reports have not confirmed this observation.[10]

Beardwood and his associates have claimed that bioflavonoids are useful for preventing retinal damage in diabetics and for preventing bruising; however, these reports have not been confirmed by other investigators.[11]

It is clear from this brief summary that the history of the clinical and biological usefulness of bioflavonoids is clouded. There are many advocates of the therapeutic usefulness of bioflavonoids; others challenge their effectiveness. A review by Shils and Goodhart was published in 1956, discussing the pros and cons of bioflavonoid supplementation in nutritional medicine and confirming the controversial aspect of their usefulness.[12]

The following table lists the purported applications of bioflavonoid supplementation in the improvement of human functioning.

PURPORTED USEFULNESS OF BIOFLAVONOIDS
AS FOOD SUPPLEMENTS

Prevention of retinal hemorrhages
Reduction of capillary fragility (bruising)
Reduced risk of stroke in high blood pressure patients
Increased protection against arthritis, rheumatic fever
Reduced risk of arteriosclerosis
Decreased menopausal symptoms
Increased protection against oral herpes infection
Decreased risk of diabetic cataract
Decreased histamine response to allergen exposure
Prevention of habitual abortion
Reduction in ulcer problems
Treatment of dizziness due to inner ear problem
Decreased symptoms of asthma
Protection against radiation damage
Decreased inflammation after injury

RECENT DISCOVERIES ABOUT THE BIOFLAVONOIDS

Much of the history of the use of bioflavonoids as nutritional supplements has rested on their apparent ability to improve capillary wall integrity. The capillaries, or small blood vessels, must maintain a barrier between blood plasma and cells and the cellular environment.

When the capillaries lose their integrity and become weakened, materials from the blood can penetrate into tissues, leading to easy bruising or hemorrhages, or substances can penetrate from the external environment through the intestinal tract or respiratory tract into the blood. When there is increased penetration of environmental substances into the body the symptoms of allergy or immune sensitivity can develop and the body's immune system can become sensitized to environmental agents. This may be the reason bioflavonoids have been suggested as useful in the management of asthma and stomach ulcers, as well as intestinal problems and some food allergies. The supplemental dose used in many of these clinical trials is between 500 and 3000 milligrams a day of the citrus or buckwheat bioflavonoid complex, along with vitamin C at the same level. A stronger capillary wall prevents the invasion of the blood by foreign substances or the leakage of blood cells and plasma materials into tissues.

The role bioflavonoids play as protectors against vitamin C destruction may account for the way they guard capillaries against damage. The capillary walls are made up of a protein called collagen, which requires vitamin C for its synthesis; if the vitamin C in these cells is converted by oxidation to the dehydroascorbate, it is less active in its ability to stimulate the synthesis of collagen, which is used as the connective tissue to manufacture the capillary walls. Bioflavonoids seem to protect vitamin C from being converted to dehydroascorbate, and therefore may be very important in stimulating collagen synthesis and capillary wall integrity.

This favorable effect on collagen of the C-bioflavonoid complex has led to its suggested use for preventing viral infections or treating some forms of such infections. One relevant study deals with the common virus *herpes labialis,* which produces cold sores. These are generally self-limiting and tend to get better by themselves in about nine and a half days. When only vitamin C was supplemented at 1000 mg per day, there was a slight reduction in the duration of the cold sores to approximately seven days. However, when vitamin C and bioflavonoids were administered together at levels of 1000 mg each, the length of time dropped from nine and a half to about three and a half days, which indicates that the vitamin C-bioflavonoid complex was extremely useful in helping the body defend itself against infection by the *herpes labialis* virus and was more effective than vitamin C by itself. This may be the result of the stimulating effect of the complex on collagen synthesis, which provides better protection against the infiltration of viruses.[13]

Another interesting study has demonstrated that vitamin C in combination with bioflavonoids and an oral proteolytic enzyme preparation containing chymotrypsin was more effective than nonsteroidal antiinflammatory drugs in reducing inflammation.[14] This may also be the result of strengthening the cells against agents which cause inflammation, or of some yet-to-be understood role that bioflavonoids play in the immune mechanism. The level of bioflavonoids, vitamin C and proteolytic enzymes given to animals in this study is equivalent to a human dose of approximately 1000 mg of vitamin C, 500 mg bioflavonoids and 25,000 units of chymotrypsin administered orally.[14]

A recent review of the physiological action of flavonoids shows a favorable effect on white blood cells in increasing immune defense, which may account for the antiinflammatory activity resulting from the oral supplementation.[15]

The past 15 years have witnessed a rekindled research interest in the bioflavonoid family of accessory nutrients. The citrus industry has long recognized the uniquely high concentrations of potassium, folic acid and vitamin C in citrus juice products but has only recently turned its attention to exploration of the biochemical functions of the concentrate of the white, soft, fleshy part of the fruit inside the rind, which is rich in bioflavonoids. This research has reconfirmed the value of bioflavonoids in the prevention of capillary fragility, and in the prevention of abnormal platelet adhesion ("sticky" blood cells) and reduction of inflammation.[23] The renewed interest in bioflavonoids by nutritional investigators will, we hope, delineate further the mechanisms of action of this family of accessory nutrients and will put their use on a more scientifically supportable basis.

Much of our present understanding of the role that therapeutic nutrition plays in improving health was born out of the clinical observations of practitioners. An example of this was the interesting observation made by John Ellis, M.D., practicing in a small Texas community, who reported that vitamin B6 in large quantities (10 to 20 times the Recommended Dietary Allowance) cured some patients with painfully swollen hands. It took some ten years to confirm this association by detailed scientific studies.[24]

This situation is like that of the bioflavonoids, where clinical associations have been made for years, but only in the last few years have definitively controlled scientific studies been done to examine these observations critically. The preliminary data from these studies are most exciting, as they seem to confirm much of what has been previously observed as successful in bioflavonoid therapy.

USES OF BIOFLAVONOIDS

DUODENAL ULCERS

Thirty-six cases of bleeding duodenal ulcers have been studied in relation to treatment with bioflavonoids and a low-acidity diet, compared to a group of patients on the same diet with no bioflavonoid supplementation. In the group given the supplements—500 mg of citrus bioflavonoids every six hours—the bleeding ceased on the fourth day. Continued supplementation with bioflavonoids and the bland diet led to healing of the intestinal mucosa and a normal duodenal contour after 12 to 22 days. There was no recurrence of bleeding after two years in 23 of the 31 cases. Twelve cases remained ulcer-free for one year or more, and the remaining cases were successfully treated with a second course of bioflavonoids; they were ulcer-free for four months. In the group that used the diet without bioflavonoids, less than 50 percent remained ulcer-free with continuation of the diet, and their improvement was much slower than it was in those who took the bioflavonoid supplement.[16]

PREVENTION OF DIABETIC CATARACT

One of the major complications of diabetes is a change in the opacity of the eye, leading to cataract. The mechanism by which cataract is generated in the eye has been studied extensively over the last few years and seems to relate to the activity of an enzyme in the eye called aldose reductase.[17] This enzyme is able to convert glucose in the eye into sugars such as sorbitol, which remain in the eye and crystallize out into the lens. In diabetics, this sorbitol attains a dangerously high level in the lens, which results in a change in the ability of the eye to transmit light and also produces excessive water retention, or what is called osmotic pressure, causing tissue damage. The sorbitol deposited in the eye does not come from dietary sources, but rather from the action of the enzyme aldose reductase converting blood sugar (glucose) to sorbitol. The reason the eye of the diabetic attracts a tremendous amount of sugar and activates this enzyme is that the lens, the nerves and the kidneys are insulin-insensitive tissues, which means that they take up sugar from the blood without the need of insulin. When the diabetic is unable to secrete enough insulin to take up more sugar from the blood into the other cells of the body such as muscle cells, the sugar is then driven into the eye by its high concentration in the blood and produces a significant elevation of its level in the lens, where it is converted from glucose to sorbitol by aldose reductase.

If this is the reason why diabetics get cataracts, then anything that can be done to either inhibit the aldose reductase or decrease the flow of sugar from the blood into the eye would help prevent them. One method of prevention is to regulate the blood sugar level of the diabetic through diet. This means using a higher-complex carbohydrate, lower-sugar and higher-fiber diet than is standard for the management of the diabetic patient.

Inhibition of aldose reductase would also prevent the buildup of sorbitol in the lens of the eye. A number of enzyme inhibitors have been studied in animals, and it has been found that they effectively delay the onset of cataract of diabetic subjects.[18]

It has also been found that oral administration of quercetin, a known inhibitor of aldose reductase, leads to a significant decrease in the accumulation of sorbitol in the lens of diabetic animals, resulting in a delay in the onset of cataract if the bioflavonoid administration is continued.[19] The level of bioflavonoid given as an oral supplement in this study was very high—in human equivalents approximately 3000 to 7000 mg per day. The firm conclusion investigators made from their animal studies was that aldose reductase initiates the formation of cataract in diabetics and that the bioflavonoid aldose reductase inhibitor when given orally may be an effective preventive agent for cataract.

Studies are being continued to determine which flavonoids are most useful for the prevention of cataract and at what dose they would be most successful.[20] It is clear that when bioflavonoids are used for their pharmacological function as enzyme inhibitors, very high doses are required. These doses, on the order of thousands of milligrams per day, are far higher than normal dietary levels.

BIOFLAVONOIDS AS NUTRITIONAL SUPPLEMENTS: THE CONTROVERSY

It is apparent that bioflavonoids are not really a family of essential nutrients (substances required by all people on a daily basis, as are vitamins). The reason for this is that there are no acute deficiency symptoms when bioflavonoids are not included in the diet.

Their role is evidently that of accessory nutrients which potentiate the action of the antioxidant vitamin C and may have other potentiating effects. An accessory nutrient is a substance not considered essential for all individuals, but which may be required by some individuals to promote optimal function. Some examples of these are carnitine, taurine, octacosanol and dimethylglycine.

Bioflavonoids seem to fit this definition, since many individuals respond favorably to bioflavonoid supplementation, but not everyone requires them to maximize performance. Because of the controversy surrounding the use of nutrients as therapeutic agents, bioflavonoids have been discredited by many standard nutritionists as having no effective action. It should be recalled that many times the end of a story depends on its beginnings, and such may be the case with those who claim that bioflavonoids are not useful. If one assumes that the only use of trace nutrients such as vitamins and minerals is to prevent specific, definable deficiency diseases that occur in the absence of those nutrients, then it is true that bioflavonoids are not required in the diet. However, if one extends the definition of what is to be considered an important nutrient to include substances that enhance performance instead of simply preventing a deficiency disease, then bioflavonoids may be quite important for some individuals to achieve their best health.

There are still many nutritionists and medical people who believe that nutritive items are not useful in therapeutic doses, and therefore not needed as supplements beyond the average daily intake, particularly such substances as bioflavonoids, which have not been found useful as essential nutrients. There is a different, rapidly emerging school of thought which recognizes that many nutrients may be used as pharmacological agents. In amounts exceeding those which one would normally get in the diet, they may have profound, positive influences on physiological function that can help normalize people who have certain types of illness.[21]

This certainly seems to be the case with bioflavonoids; a wealth of clinical information and experimental data indicates their pharmacological impact in facilitating better vitamin C utilization and their roles in the reduction of capillary fragility, protection against viral infections, decreased inflammatory response and protection against diabetic cataracts. It is obvious that much more work needs to be done to identify the action of these substances in controlled human studies and to verify their clinical usefulness, but it is important to recognize that the therapeutic effectiveness of bioflavonoids has been reported for over sixty years, and as we learn more about their chemical structure and physiological action, it appears that the clinical testimonies have scientific foundation.

One other interesting reported use of bioflavonoids is in the amelioration of the symptoms of menopause, such as flushing or hot flashes and heart palpitations. Bioflavonoids have been reported at doses of 500 to 3000 mg per day, along with magnesium, vitamin B6 and vitamin E to control these menopausal symptoms successfully; however, no definite study has yet appeared as proof. Clinical observation precedes scientific investigation, so because it hasn't been proven doesn't necessarily mean it isn't correct. Future exploration of the relationship of bioflavonoid supplementation to the reduction of menopausal symptoms should settle the matter.

A very important characteristic of bioflavonoids is that they are naturally occurring substances with virtually no toxicity and can thus be used safely. Dietary intake of bioflavonoids is quite high in those who eat oranges or grapefruit, including the white part next to the rind. Individuals who drink fruit juice and do not eat the whole fruit may get fair amounts of vitamin C, but not adequate levels of bioflavonoids. This would argue once again for eating foods that are as little processed as possible and as much in the natural state as possible.

It is also interesting to note that the amount of bioflavonoids required for optimal benefit in controlled studies seemed to be about equal to the amount of vitamin C used. This would mean that balances of bioflavonoids to vitamin C in therapeutic trials should be on the order of 1000 mg of the citrus or rutin bioflavonoids to 1000 mg of vitamin C. At this level there need be no worry of toxicity from either bioflavonoids or vitamin C, and therefore the risk of a clinical trial of these substances is negligible, while there is significant potential benefit, such as improvement of capillary-wall integrity and other positive physiological effects.

Given these controversies, how might supplementation with bioflavonoids be considered clinically justifiable? There is uncertainty about the role bioflavonoids play in promoting health, and whether they are required nutrients in some individuals. It appears that the best way of identifying the therapeutic value of bioflavonoids and vitamin C is a clinical trial where there is no risk of toxicity and there is a potential significant benefit. Suitable subjects for such a clinical trial, in which vitamin C and bioflavonoids would be taken concurrently daily for two weeks to a month to see if any benefit results, would include individuals who bruise easily, have extensive muscle pain after contact sports, or those individuals who are at risk of stroke because of high blood pressure or of arteriosclerosis because of high blood cholesterol levels. It also would be indicated as a clinical trial for people who have symptoms of arthritis or significant allergies with advanced histamine response, including asthma. The literature is rich in reports of bioflavonoids and vitamin C being useful in wound healing, in protecting against various viral infections, including oral herpes, and in reduction of duodenal ulcer problems. Bioflavonoids have also been shown in a few clinical studies to help reduce the symptoms of menopause and prevent problems of habitual spontaneous abortion.[22]

Lastly, individuals who have diabetes and who should be protecting their eyes against cataract formation may want to use a clinical trial of vitamin C and bioflavonoids, as well as dietary modification to improve the management of blood sugar.

This range of clinical impacts of the use of bioflavonoids in conjunction with vitamin C indicates the potential therapeutic usefulness of this family of accessory nutrients. Because the benefits are potentially so significant and the toxic reactions negligible, it seems that the risk/benefit trade-off in a clinical trial of these substances would weigh heavily on the side of benefit for people displaying one or more of the symptoms discussed.

There is hope that in the future much more research will utilize the bioflavonoid complex and identify more completely the role of these substances at the cellular and physiological levels, so that their usefulness can be substantiated. Until then we must regard the bioflavonoid–substance P family as being an accessory group of nutritional substances which may in some individuals have very powerful therapeutic effects, and whose function appears to be protective against the cellular destruction of vitamin C, and which would therefore be suitable in a whole vitamin C complex supplementation program.

NATURAL VERSUS SYNTHETIC NUTRIENTS

One topic that has generated considerable controversy in the nutritional supplement field is the difference between natural and synthetic nutrients. In general, there is no chemical difference between a naturally derived vitamin B1 from yeast and a synthetically derived vitamin B1 from petrochemical starting materials. They have the same chemical structure, and they have the same physiological effects in the prevention of beri-beri. The same is true for all the other B-complex vitamins and vitamin C, but not for such nutrients as vitamin E, where there is a difference in chemical structure between the natural and synthetic forms of the vitamin.

The most interesting question is not the chemical structure of the nutrient in question but whether there is a difference between the benefits obtained from naturally derived nutrients and those derived from a synthetic source. In a nutrient from a natural source, such as yeast or rose hips, there is a whole array of substances; some of them are known nutrients, such as vitamin C, and others may be trace substances of unknown chemical structure or physiological nature. This is certainly the case with vitamin C extracted from the whole grapefruit compared with synthetic vitamin C manufactured by chemical modification of corn sugar. Extraction from the whole grapefruit would not only provide ascorbic acid but might also provide a myriad of other substances, some of which may potentiate the activity of vitamin C. This is the case with the bioflavonoids, which are reported to potentiate the activity of vitamin C and would be found only in a naturally derived vitamin C product (unless added to synthetically derived vitamin C).

VITAMIN C METABOLITES AND BIOFLAVONOIDS

An exciting new suggestion has been made within the past few years concerning the therapeutic role that vitamin C may play in the activation of the immune system and in the prevention of such diseases as cancer. This suggestion is that vitamin C itself may not be the sole activating substance and that some of the metabolites of vitamin C, such as dehydroascorbate, isoascorbic acid, and other chemical substances that are derived from vitamin C in the human body, are involved.

Observations made by a number of investigators, and research by

Dr. Constance Tsao at the Linus Pauling Institute of Science and Medicine in Palo Alto, California, have confirmed the fact that there are a number of trace metabolites of vitamin C present in biological samples and that some of these may actually have a more profound effect upon intracellular function than vitamin C itself. This may be the reason why some individuals, when given a large oral dose of vitamin C, excrete almost all of it unchanged in the urine, while others excrete only a small amount. Those people who have great need for vitamin C metabolites may actively convert the vitamin C itself into other substances which have profoundly beneficial cellular effects.

One of the metabolites of vitamin C which is known *not* to be beneficial is oxalic acid. It has been suggested that high-dose vitamin C therapy can increase urinary oxalate excretion and the consequent risk of kidney stones; however, work done several years ago indicates that consumption of up to 10,000 milligrams of vitamin C a day by normal individuals on ordinary diets leads to no significant increase in oxalate output in the urine and, therefore, that the risk of kidney stones from vitamin C is minimal to nonexistent.

Bioflavonoids may play a role in this whole story of vitamin C metabolites because they are known to have an effect on the rate at which C is converted into its various metabolites; bioflavonoids are chemical reducing agents. If bioflavonoids do in fact help divide vitamin C into its metabolites in the tissues of the body, this would profoundly affect the cellular role of vitamin C in activating the immune system or repairing cells.

This may explain at the molecular level what is observed clinically: that bioflavonoids have been shown to improve the therapeutic action of vitamin C in some areas. It is exciting, since these observations of the effects of vitamin C metabolites on cellular function have opened the door to new types of studies which will examine the biochemical individualities of people in terms of their metabolism of vitamin C and relate that to their needs and functional capacities. Bioflavonoids deserve study in terms of the effect they may have on facilitating the metabolism of vitamin C and the improvement of health.

It is known that, in vitamin C-treated mice, the metabolite isoascorbic acid may have a different effect on cancer risk than vitamin C itself.[52] If bioflavonoids have an influence on the dissolution of vitamin C into its metabolites, then it is possible that these nutrient substances serve as potentiating agents for the effective functioning of vitamin C. This suggestion awaits further proof by detailed studies, but is certainly an interesting hypothetical explanation of the observed clinical benefits of bioflavonoids.

It is not clear whether everyone would benefit from taking bioflavonoids along with vitamin C for their synergizing ability. It is possible that certain individuals do not need the reducing-action effects of bioflavonoids for optimal activity for vitamin C as a nutrient, but in those individuals who may have specific cellular functional capacity which requires the bioflavonoids for protection of ascorbic acid and delivery of ascorbic acid metabolites in proper levels to tissues, this accessory nutrient would prove very useful.

If clinical symptoms of easy bruising, lowered immune defense or cataract formation continue while supplementing with straight vitamin C as ascorbic acid or ascorbate, it might be worthwhile to consider taking bioflavonoids along with the vitamin C.

It is important to recognize that the mention of bioflavonoids on the label of a supplement container does not guarantee that the product was from natural sources. Read the label carefully, keeping in mind that whatever is not clearly specified as being in the product probably is not. Also check the label for the bioflavonoid content, given in milligrams; the nearer to the vitamin C (ascorbic acid) content it is, the more natural the supplement's formulation is likely to be.

Also remember that some bioflavonoid preparations have been found to be virtually unabsorbable due to the way in which they were extracted from the natural product. Studies which demonstrate that the product that you are going to purchase has absorbable bioflavonoids are very important in helping you to determine the potential biological effects of the preparation. Manufacturers should be prepared to provide information concerning the absorbability and assimilability of bioflavonoids in their products.

CONCLUSION

It can be said that there is some apparent difference between natural and synthetic nutrients, taking into account the complex of accessory substances that result from the extraction of a natural product and the specific single nutritive substance resulting from manufacture from an isolated, purified starting material.

It is clear that bioflavonoids as a family come only from the extraction of natural products, and may be found either in the complex of naturally derived vitamin C or added to the synthetically derived vitamin C. Either of these preparations would provide therapeutically useful supplementation as long as the bioflavonoids were biologically absorbable.

The future of bioflavonoids as nutritional supplements depends upon the quality and direction of future research, but at this point it can be said that, from the clinical information available over the past 40 years, vitamin C, administered with bioflavonoids, appears to have therapeutic benefit above and beyond that of vitamin C by itself in many areas pertaining to capillary fragility and cellular function.

REFERENCES

1. Rusznyak, D., and Szent-Györgyi, A., *Nature* 138: 27 (1936).
2. Armentuno, P., Bentsath, M., Beres, B., and Szent-Györgyi, A., *Deut. Med. Wchnschr.* 62: 1325 (1936).
3. Joint Committee on Nomenclature: *Science* 112: 628 (1950).
4. Zloch, Z. *International J. Vit. Res.* 39: 269 (1969).
5. Scarborough, S. and Bacharach, T. *Vitamins and Hormones* 8: 1 (1949).
6. Bland, J., *Choline, Lecithin, Inositol, and Other "Accessory" Nutrients.* New Canaan, CT: Keats Publishing, 1982.
7. Underhill, L. *Can. J. Biochem. Physiol.* 35: 219 (1957).
8. Smyth, S., Lambert, M., and Martin, S. *Proc. Soc. Exp. Biol. Medicine* 116: 593 (1964).
9. Griffith, G., Krewson, L., and Naghiski, N. *Rutin and Related Flavonoids.* Easton, PA: Mack Publishing Co., 1955.

10. Schweppe, S. and Barker, T. *Amer. Heart J.* 35: 393 (1948).

11. Beardwood, A., Roberts, T., and Trueman, M. *Proc. Amer. Diabetes Assoc.* 8: 243 (1948).

12. Shils, S. and Goodhart, H. *The Flavonoids in Biology and Medicine.* New York: The National Vitamin Foundation, Inc. (1956).

13. Tengherdy, T. *Nutrition Reviews* 36: 10 (1978).

14. ———, *Arzneim-Forsch. Drug Res.* 27: 6 (1977).

15. Review: "Action of Flavonoids on Blood Cells," *International J. Vit. Res.* 44: (1974).

16. Weiss, S., Weiss, J., and Weiss, B. *Amer. J. of Gastroenterology* 34: 726 (1958).

17. Kinoshita, J. H. *Opthalmol.* 13: 713 (1974).

18. Dvornik, D., Krami, M., and Kinoshita, J. H. *Science* 182: 1146 (1973).

19. Varma, S.D., Mixuno, A., and Kinoshita, J.H. *Science* 195: 205 (1977).

20. Varma, S.D. and Kinoshita, J.H. *Biochim. Biophys. Acta* 338: 632 (1974).

21. Spiller, A. *Nutritional Pharmacology.* New York: A.R. Liss, 1982.

22. Jacobs, A. *Surg. Gynec. and Obstet.* 103: 233 (1956).

23. Robbins, R.C. "Medical and Nutritional Aspects of Citrus Bioflavonoids in *Citrus Nutrition and Quality,* F. Nagy and J.A. Attaway, eds. Washington, DC: Symposium Series 143, American Chemical Society, 1980.

24. Ellis, J., Folkers, K., Watanabe, T., and Wood, F.F. "Clinical Results of a Cross-over Treatment with Pyridoxine and Placebo of the Carpal Tunnel Syndrome." *Amer. J. Clin. Nutr.* 32: 2040 (1979).

25. Tsao, C., and Pauling, L. "The Effect of Isoascorbic Acid-Treated Mice." *International Journal for Vitamin and Nutrition Research,* accepted for publication.

The Bioflavonoids-Vitamin C Partnership—
How They Work to Promote,
Improve Your Health

Scientist's "Accidental" Discovery Provided Key to Blood
Vessel Strength and Suppleness; Citrus Fruits,
Supplements Are Best Source

Accidents are not unusual in the field or in the laboratory, but when an accident is followed by careful observation and a momentous discovery, we are reminded of Freud's remark that "there is no such thing as an accident."

Consider the unlooked-for discovery of penicillin by Fleming, or a chemist absentmindedly putting one finger in his mouth after an experiment, resulting in the artificial sweetener Aspartame—or Dr. Albert Szent-Györgyi giving peppers to some of his guinea pigs and ending up with an unknown nutrient he called vitamin P, the permeability factor.

Szent-Györgyi's discovery was followed by intensive analytical work and strong disagreement among scientists until they found that vitamin P was not a vitamin—or in fact any one thing—but rather a group of biologically active substances. The scientific community finally settled on the term bioflavonoids, which are compounds from different fruits, all biologically active and all synergistically active with vitamin C.

The bioflavonoids include eriodictyol, hesperitin, hesperidin, rutin, quercetin, quercetrin, citrin, narigen and esculin; and they are found in peppers, buckwheat, the leaves of many plants and in fruits, particularly citrus fruits. In these, they are concentrated in the white fibrous material just under the peel. At first they were thought to be a natural means by which pigmentation was provided to plants and flowers. They were named "flavonols" from the Latin word meaning yellow, and were divided into hundreds of different classes, such as blues, reds, ambers and yellows.

When Szent-Györgyi demonstrated the ability of these "pigments" to decrease capillary fragility, something that vitamin C alone could not do, the color elements assumed a new importance. When they were combined with pure vitamin C they greatly increased the effectiveness of the vitamin. Hundreds of "pigments" combined with vitamin C were tested on thousands of lab animals. Diets containing both nutrients were found to prolong the animals' life and to reduce hemorrhage.

The flavonols, now officially known as bioflavonoids, were originally classified into two main groups, the citrus bioflavonoids (hesperidin, hesperitin, narigen, lemon bioflavonoid complex, calcium flavonate) and the non-citrus bioflavonoids (esculin, quercetin, rutin). Modern nutrition has simplified the classification even further. There are five recognized categories: citrin, hesperidin, rutin, flavones and flavonals. The first three are of more substantial nutritional interest than the last two (however, see the chapter on Pycnogenol in this book).

RUTIN, THE AGE FIGHTER

Rutin, derived from buckwheat leaves, appears to be the flavonoid of choice to be combined with vitamin C when a decrease in the permeability of tiny blood vessels is desired. Rutin with vitamin C has been shown to help prevent recurrent bleeding, to assist in the reduction or control of hemorrhoids, and to delay the onset of capillary fragility—one of the symptoms of old age.

Citrin and hesperidin exist commonly in the white pith of lemons, grapefruit and oranges and provide most of the dietary bioflavonoids, although some are also provided by grapes, plums, black currants, apricots, cherries, and rose hips.

Like vitamin C, the bioflavonoids are water-soluble, easily absorbed from the digestive tract and easily lost through the regular avenues of excretion (perspiration and urination). A deficiency of either can produce identical results, the most prominent being subcutaneous bleeding and bruising, sometimes known as "devil's pinches."

C complex, as the combination of vitamin C and the bioflavonoids is sometimes called, has been found to be more useful in stress management than either used alone. We know that vitamin C is stored in the adrenal glands so it will be available for use when the body is subject to stress, but it is the C complex that provides much of the power in this biochemical reaction. Without both nutrients on call, the permeability of the blood vessels is increased, the adrenal cortex is less able to cope with the stress reaction and many body functions lose efficiency.

C complex is also important for balance since capillary resiliency enhances the fragile function of the inner ear. Ménière's syndrome, a malfunction of the inner ear, is often coupled with capillary problems.

NOT BY ORANGES ALONE

It is not wise to depend on foods for your complete supply of Vitamin C and the bioflavonoids. Unless you have the good fortune to live in an area where citrus fruits grow and can eat them from the tree, you can't be sure of the nutritional content. Fruit begins to lose its vitamins within hours after picking. If it has to travel a great distance to reach your local store, the exposure to air and the time spent standing around in a warehouse and finally in the store may result in as much as a 90 percent loss of nutritional content. You may therefore want to consider supplements. Supplements are also useful for people allergic to raw fruit.

Ideally, a combination of food and supplements should be used to insure a complete supply of C complex. Although dosages vary according to individual biochemistry, supplements should contain about five times as much vitamin C as bioflavonoids. If the supplement you are using does not have that proportion, add vitamin C or bioflavonoids until you reach the correct proportion and then take them all together. If you are using megadoses of vitamin C, purchase tablets of bioflavonoids alone and adjust the dosage.

We also are in a race against debilitating old age. Vitamin C and the bioflavonoids—the C complex—along with suitable amounts of vitamins, essential amino acids, proteins, carbohydrates, fats and minerals, can help assure that our later years are not endured but enjoyed to the fullest.

A NEW GENERATION OF PHYTOMEDICINES

Plant Antioxidants

J. Auguste Mockle, D. Pharm.

BENEFICENT BOTANICALS

More and more, plant extracts are coming to be seen as medicines of astounding versatility and effectiveness, with far fewer and milder side effects than synthetic drugs. Dr. J. Auguste Mockle discusses the properties of three major medicinal plants, ginkgo, bilberry, and garlic, and their therapeutic influences on blood vessel and heart problems, free-radical damage, eye disorders, immune system deficiency, cancer and many other conditions.

PHYTOMEDICINES

The plant kingdom is made up of thousands of plants (ca. 300,000), some of which are used as decoration, others in day-to-day nutrition and many for the treatment of human ailments.

From time immemorial, in every corner of the world, we have tried to cure ourselves by using local plants. By trial and error, we have acquired the knowledge of the healing powers of certain plants, or their parts, such as leaves, bark, and roots. This knowledge has been passed down from one generation to another until today.

Many manuscripts bear evidence of the use of plants as a remedy.

The *Pen Ts'ao,* written by Shen Nung in 2800 B.C., lists more than 350 plant drugs. The *Papyrus Ebers,* named after their discoverer, the German Egyptologist George Ebers, reveals that the Egyptians had a thorough knowledge of the medicinal properties of many plants. Written in 1550 B.C., it contains an impressive list of drugs derived from plants. The treatises of Hippocrates (460–370 B.C.), known as the *Corpus Hippocraticum,* note a plant remedy for each disease described. Dioscorides, a Greek physician for the first century B.C., wrote *De Materia Medica,* in which he listed some 600 plants with medicinal properties, some of which are still in use today, for example, opium, hyoscyamus, ergot, and squill.

Galen (A.D. 131–200) described a method of preparing formulas with plant drugs. His work led to the widespread use of preparations such as extracts, tinctures and the like, referred to thereafter as "galenicals." Much later, a Swiss physician and pharmacist, Paracelsus (1490–1541), forged the path of medicinal chemistry through his challenge to the alchemists to prepare medicines. (He is also the one who created the "Doctrine of Signatures," stating that God, in His kindness, put a sign in each plant indicating its use.)

At the beginning of the eighteenth century, the emerging botanists made a great contribution to the classification of plants. Carl von Linné (Linnaeus) (1707–1778), a Swedish physician, is the most notable, for he established a binomial nomenclature system for plants which was universally accepted. His *Species Plantarum,* published in 1753, sanctions the classification of plants based on two components, the "genus" and the "species." Garlic, for instance, is classified as *Allium sativum L.*

For all their knowledge of botanical drugs, however, it was still necessary for the botanists to find their "quintessential" principle, that is to say, the substance(s) that give each plant its therapeutic qualities. The attempt to isolate these principles began in the beginning of the nineteenth century. Some notable discoveries of this period include:

• Morphine from opium by Sertürner in 1803.
• Emetine from ipecac by Pelletier and Caventou in 1817.

- Strychnine from nux vomica by Pelletier and Caventou in 1818.
- Quinine from cinchona bark by Pelletier and Caventou in 1820.
- Physostygmine from calabar bean by Jobst and Hesse in 1864.
- Digitalin from foxglove leaves by Nativelle in 1869.

These substances and their source plants are still in use today. Synthetic drugs came along in the twentieth century with various scientific and chemical advancements, and moving on rather slowly up until the Second World War. Botanical drugs, on the other hand, have held on tenaciously, taking a dominant place in phytotherapy. Many of them have been listed in the world's official pharmacopeias.

The World Health Organization (WHO) has estimated that 80 percent of the world's population relies chiefly on traditional medicine and that a major part of traditional therapies involve the use of plants in entirety, their parts, their galenical preparations or their active principles.[1] Notwithstanding the advent of numerous synthetic drugs since World War II, there has remained a great demand for botanical drugs in various cultures around the world, especially during the last 30 years. In fact, medicinal plants have always played a key role in world health. They are commonly available at fairly low prices, and they offer the population access to generally safe and effective products. Today, we can rely on data from published literature, as well as information supplied by practicing physicians, reports from patients, pharmacological investigations and clinical studies.

The effects of botanical drugs are based mainly on the subtle and hard-to-quantify "sum of their parts," rather than on their isolated components. The American botanist/physician Andrew Weil, author of a book on natural medicine,[2] believed that whole plants have different effects than those of their isolated active principles and that the beneficial effects of botanical remedies are likely to represent synergistic and holistic interactions of all the active components.[3]

Many books, treatises, compendiums, periodicals, review articles and even pharmacopeias are devoted to the study of "plant drugs," "botanical drugs," "herb drugs" or remedies—whatever we may wish to call them—thus illustrating the vitality of these phyto-therapeutic agents. The prefix "phyto-" means plant. It has been pointed out that scientists are entering into an era in which research on botanical drugs can be expected to occupy a dominant place in the national priorities of developing countries.[4]

During the last few years, a tendency has developed to use crude drugs, or their galenicals, now called "phytomedicines," in high-quality standardized preparations. Such a tendency should be encouraged. These can be considered the New Generation of Phytomedicines. This is particularly the case with the following herb drugs: ginkgo, bilberry, ginseng and garlic.

GINKGO *(Ginkgo biloba L.)*

Ginkgo biloba L. is a popular ornamental tree, considered a living fossil as it is the remaining species of its group. Native to Asiatic countries, ginkgo is now cultivated in other countries, mainly in Europe and North America.

While traditional Chinese medicine uses both seeds and leaves, modern Western medicinal use of ginkgo is limited exclusively to its leaves. They are harvested while green, dried under controlled temperatures and prepared as a dry extract. This extract is standardized to a fixed percentage of its naturally occurring flavonoids and lactonic terpenes.

The flavonoids in ginkgo consist of a complex mixture of quercetin, kaempferol and isorhamnetin glycosides. Lactonic terpenes refers to a mixture of diterpenes and ginkgolides, along with the sesquiterpene bilobalide.[5] The standardized dry extract—24 percent w/w (i.e., by weight) of Ginkgoflavonoids and 6 percent w/w of lactonic terpenes—is usually cited by the following acronyms: GBE, GBx or EGb. This extract is the most important phytomedicine to be marketed in Europe during the last decade and has gained wide acceptance.

What makes this phytomedicine so interesting is its effectiveness in the treatment of ailments associated with vascular problems. Pharmacological and clinical studies with GBE[6-10] indicate positive effects:

• Increase in vasodilatation and blood flow rate in the vessels—capillaries and end-arteries—thus benefiting various circulatory disorders, such as chronic cerebrovascular insufficiency, obliterative arterial diseases of the lower limbs, varicose conditions, post-thrombotic syndrome, etc.

• Decrease in blood clotting, which is very important in thrombotic disorders.

In a review article[9] some 20 clinical trials done with GBE were summarized. These included eleven double-blind studies, eight open studies and one open-multicenter. The effectiveness of GBE was demonstrated in various vascular disorders, bringing the author to conclude that many categories of elderly patients could benefit from this phytomedicine. The author also believes that it could be used at the onset of symptoms associated with cerebrovascular insufficiency, resulting in a better quality of life and possibly avoiding hospitalization. In another review article,[8] some 40 different studies are described showing the effectiveness of GBE, increasing blood flow in the capillaries and decreasing blood clotting.

A double-blind placebo-controlled study has also shown that GBE significantly improves long-distance vision in humans suffering from macular degeneration.[11]

The beneficial actions of GBE in various vascular disorders, as stated above, is the result of both the free-radical scavenging properties of the flavonoids principles[12] and the effects of the lactonic terpenes as selective antagonists of platelet aggregation induced by the platelet-activating factor.[13] These are very important actions, since:

• Free radicals are highly reactive molecules that damage, by deprivation of oxygen, the membrane of the blood vessels and also essential biochemicals, such as DNA. Their neutralization helps maintain the integrity and permeability of the cell walls. The prevention of free-radical damage is considered important to life extension, since they play a significant role in the aging process and in degenerative conditions such as atherosclerosis and cancer.

• Platelet aggregation is responsible for the formation of clots and thrombi in veins and arteries, leading to various thrombotic situations. The inhibition of blood clotting is important in preventing these situations and the recovery from strokes and heart attacks.

There is also evidence concerning the vascular effects of GBE within the nervous system, as a regulatory action due to, on the one hand, the stimulation of neurotransmitter (catecholamine) release into the synaptic ends and, on the other, the release of endogenous relaxing factors (prostacyclins) in the arterial endothelium.[14]

These results strongly suggest a certain pharmacological synergism between the various active principles within GBE (a synergy that is not found when tested separately).

The basic therapeutic property of GBE is to increase blood flow into deprived areas, as well as to prevent its clotting. GBE should then be considered beneficial to central and peripheral vascular disorders, such as chronic cerebrovascular insufficiency, arterial insufficiency in the lower limbs, obstructive arteriopathies, varicosis, diabetic angiopathy, vascular disturbances of the inner ear and macular degeneration.

It may also be of some help in lessening the development of Alzheimer's disease.

Let us recall the main symptoms involved in chronic cerebrovascular insufficiency: absentmindedness, anxiety, confusion, decreased physical performance, depression of mood, difficulty with concentration and memory, dizziness, headache, lack of energy, tinnitus (ringing in the ear) and tiredness.

No toxicity has been reported in the various clinical tests; only rare minimal and reversible side effects were mentioned, namely, gastrointestinal troubles (nausea, vomiting), headaches and skin allergies. We can summarize by saying that GBE improves memory and brain function, protects the heart, facilitates blood circulation, benefits hearing and vision problems, and helps preserve general health and vitality.

The recommended dosage for the standardized *Ginkgo biloba* dry extract, GBE, is up to 120 mg daily. It is used for the prevention or treatment of vascular problems or disorders described above as well as in senile dementia. It is also a general tonic for the maintenance of health and vitality. For an in-depth discussion of *Ginkgo biloba*, see page 281.

BILBERRY *(Vaccinium myrtillus L.)*

Vaccinium myrtillus L. is a perennial shrub that grows in the woods and forest meadows of Northern Europe and in the sandy areas of North America. The plant is cultivated in these countries. The parts used are the ripe fruits, which are deep-blue colored berries. They are prepared as a dry extract, standardized to a fixed percentage of their naturally occurring principles, the anthocyanoids. These are a complex mixture of five anthocyanidine glycosides and lucoanthocyanins (catechins).[15]

The standardized dry extract is regulated at 25 percent w/w of bilberryanthocyanosides. This phytomedicine has gained in popularity in the European countries during the past few years.

The berries of *Vaccinium myrtillus L.* have been used in nutrition for many years, but it is only recently that interest in their potential use as a phytotherapeutic agent has arisen, owing to the empirical experience of Royal Air Force pilots during World War II. It was determined that Allied pilots had better sight in twilight than the enemy. As bilberry jam was part of their diet, it was believed that this could explain their better vision.

Preliminary studies with an extract of the berries of *Vaccinium myrtillus L.* showed some positive results in visual function and disorders.[16]

Additional pharmacological and double-blind clinical studies have demonstrated the effectiveness of the bilberry extract in the treatment of eye diseases of vascular origin, such as retinopathies and macular degeneration.[17-20] Some other double-blind and open studies showed positive results in peripheral vascular disorders, including chronic venous stasis in the lower limbs.[21,22]

The anthocyanoids, which are chemically similar to flavonoids, are very active free-radical scavengers and antioxidant agents. This leads to a vasoprotective action of the capillaries and end-arteries. These anthocyanoids also possess an antiplatelet activity, which inhibits blood clotting.[23,24]

The main applications of the standardized extract of the berries of the bilberry herb include disorders of the peripheral venous circulation (venous insufficiency, i.e., varicose veins), telangiectasia, and intermittent claudication, as well as visual disturbances, such as poor vision, retinopathies and macular degeneration.

No toxicity has been reported, and the tolerance was excellent, even after prolonged treatments.[25]

The recommended dosage for the standardized 25 percent w/w Bilberryanthocyanosides dry extract is up to 480 mg daily.

GARLIC *(Allium sativum L.)*

Garlic is the result of thousands of years of cultivation. Its origins are in central Asia, and it has spread worldwide, used predominantly as a nutritional seasoning.

The bulbs of garlic have been used either as part of an individual's diet or as a remedy, from time immemorial. Many consider garlic the "quintessential medicinal food."

Over the past ten years, an impressive number of scientific articles and books have been published concerning the chemistry, pharmacology and clinical uses of garlic. While dozens of chemical substances have been identified, the active principles are sulphur compounds which derive from alliin, the odorless precursor of allicin and other allylsulphides, responsible for the characteristic pungent odor.[26,27] The alliin content has been estimated at 0.25—1.15 percent, but, if the bulbs are carefully dried in order to avoid the enzymatic action of alliinase on alliin, this figure could reach 0.7–1.7 percent.[38] The market offers different galenical preparations, some of which are dry extract, standardized in the alliin or allicin content.[29] The main transformation products of allicin, which is unstable, are diallyl di and tri-sulphides, ajoenes and vinyldithiins.[30]

The pharmacological action of garlic on the cardiovascular system has only been known for some ten years, and recent research has indicated anticancer activity.

Several clinical studies concerning the cardiovascular effects of garlic, among which double-blind placebo-controlled tests were included, have shown:[31–45]

• a lowering of blood cholesterol and low-density lipoproteins (the bad cholesterol), while the high-density lipoproteins (the good cholesterol) increased;

• a lowering of blood pressure;

• an inhibition of platelet aggregation and an enhancement of the fibrinolytic activity.

A meta-analysis of placebo-controlled tests indicates a significant reduction of plasma cholesterol in adults having a high rate of cholesterol.[44]

The anticancer activity of garlic has been demonstrated in many studies. Garlic reduces the risk of stomach cancers[46] and inhibits the growth of tumors due to the effects of metabolically activated monoalkylating carcinogens on the gastrointestinal tract.[47] Eating garlic on a regular basis results in a significant lowering of the incidence of gastric cancers.[46]

The cardiovascular and anticancer activities are due to allicin and its transformation products. Allicin increases the levels of two important antioxidant enzymes in the blood, catalase and glutathione peroxydase. This confirms the antioxidant and free-radical scavenging actions of garlic.[48] The diallyl polysulphides resist the damaging effects of free radicals on the cellular membrane and inhibit the platelet aggregation.[49] Ajoenes also reversibly inhibits platelet aggregation.[42] The anticancer properties belong to the diallyl sulphides and to the ajoenes.[47–54] It is reported that the ajoenes are twice as toxic to malignant cells as they are to normal cells, which greatly increases the potential therapeutic applications of garlic.[51]

This is very important in the formation of blood clots, for example, caused by mildly or severely damaged vessels. Turbulence in the arteries can cause platelet aggregation and clot formation, which can result in heart attack and stroke. On the other hand, the stimulation of the immune system enhances the macrophages and the T lymphocytes, which destroy tumoral cells.

Garlic, then, with such a beneficial effect on blood lipids, blood coagulation and blood vessels, is used in hypertension and in lipid disorders, such as atheroma, hyperlipidemia, atherosclerosis and thrombosis. It may also be of some help in the prevention and alleviation of gastrointestinal cancer.

Garlic is, for the most part, recognized as safe. However, occasional gastrointestinal disturbances or allergic reactions may occur. It is also generally agreed that garlic is best administered in enteric-coated dosages, and, preferably, in high-quality standardized preparations, in order to obtain maximum results. A standardized 4 percent w/w alliin dry extract may be taken up to 150 mg daily.

Garlic is listed in both the British Herbal Pharmacopeia and the British Herbal Compendium.[55]

SUMMARY

Ginkgo leaves dry extract, standardized at 24 percent w/w of ginkgo-flavonoids and 6 percent w/w of ginkgolactonicterpenes and bilberry fruits dry extract, standardized at 25 percent w/w of bilberry anthocyanosides, both possess, in various intensities, free-radical scavenging and antiplatelet aggregation properties.

The anti-free-radical action results in a vasoprotective effect on the blood vessels and increased blood flow rate in the capillaries and end-arteries, with apparent beneficial therapeutic applications in both cerebral and peripheral circulatory disorders, such as:
• chronic cerebrovascular insufficiency, characterized by absentmindedness, anxiety, confusion, decreased physical performance, difficulty of concentration and of memory, lack of energy, dizziness, headaches, tinnitus and tiredness;
• arterial insufficiency in the lower limbs, for example, varicose veins, intermittent claudication, and
• vascular disturbances of the inner ear as well as visual disturbances (retinopathies and macular degeneration).

The antiplatelet aggregation action results in decreased blood clotting, which is helpful in the prevention of clot formation in veins and arteries, as well as in the treatment of thrombotic situations, like cerebrovascular accident and post-thrombotic recoveries.

Garlic bulb dry extract, standardized at 4 percent w/w alliin, lowers blood pressure and has a very beneficial effect on serum cholesterol. In fact, it has been shown to lower low-density lipoproteins, referred to as "bad cholesterol," and raise high-density lipoproteins or "good cholesterol." This explains why it may be helpful in the prevention or treatment of lipid disorders, such as hyperlipidemias and atherosclerosis. This phytomedicine also stimulates the body's immune system, resulting in an improved resistance to infections. Garlic standardized dry extract has also shown anticancer properties which could reduce the risk or the incidence of gastric cancers.

No significant toxicity has been reported with the standardized dry extract. The following side effects, rare and reversible, may occur: gastric troubles (e.g., nausea, vomiting), headaches, dizziness and skin allergies. Garlic odor on the breath may occur, even with preparations using deodorized bulbs marketed in enteric-coated dosage forms. To minimize this, as well as the side-effects, this phytomedicine should be taken during mealtime.

CONCLUSION

In using these phytomedicines, one has to take into account the daily recommended dosage. They can also be used in several combinations, depending on the desired result. In these combinations, however, the synergism derived from the similarities in the properties of some active principles, as well as their complementary actions, have to be taken into consideration. No matter what their intended uses, either separately or in appropriate combinations, it would be wise to compound a dosage form with the minimum effective dose of the standardized dry extracts in order to allow for a daily intake of one to three doses. This will also give the opportunity to use a low-dosage form for prevention purposes or a higher one for alleviation, taking into account the severity of the symptoms.

It is highly recommended that one maintain a supporting diet, consisting of yellow vegetables, blue and red berries, and fruits rich in vitamin C.

REFERENCES

1. Akerlee, O. WHO Guidelines for the Assessment of the Herbal Medicines, *Fitoterapia*, 1992, 63, 99–110.
2. Weil, A. *Natural Health, Natural Medicine,* 1990, Houghton Mifflin Co. Boston, Mass, U.S.A.
3. Weil, A. A new look of botanical medicine. *Classic Botanical* Reprint, number 210, American Botanical Council.
4. Farnsworth, N. R., et al. Medicinal plants in therapy. *Bulletin of the World Health Organization,* 1985, 63, 965–981.
5. Sticher, O. Quality of ginkgo preparations, *Planta medica,* 1993, 59, 2–11.
6. Bauer, U. Six-month double-blind randomized clinical trial of *Ginkgo biloba,* Extract versus placebo in two parallel groups in patients suffering from peripheral arterial insufficiency. *Arzneim. Forsch.,* 1984, 34, 716–721.
7. Vorberg, G. *Ginkgo biloba* extract: a long-term study of chronic cerebral insufficiency in geriatric patients. *Clin. Trials J.,* 1985, 22, 149–157.
8. Kleijnen, J., & Knipschild, P. *Ginkgo biloba* for cerebral insufficiency, *Br. J. Clin. Pharmac.,* 1992, 34, 352–358.
9. Warbuton, D. M. Psychopharmacologie clinique de l'extrait de *Ginkgo biloba. Presse Médicale,* 1986, 15(31), 1595–1604.
10. Taillandier, J., et al. Traitement des troubles du vieillissement cérébral par l'extrait de *Ginkgo biloba.*-Etude longitudinale multicentrique à double-insu face au placébo. *Presse Médicale,* 1986, 15(31), 1583–1587.
11. Lebuissen, D. A., et al. Traitement des dégénérescences maculaires séniles par l'extrait de *Ginkgo biloba.*-Etude préliminaire à double-insu face au placébo. *Presse médicale,* 1986, 15(31), 1556–1558.
12. Pincemail, J., & Deby, C. Propriétés anti-radicalaires de l'extrait de *Ginkgo biloba, Presse médicale,* 1986, 15(31), 1475–1479.
13. Braquet, P. BN 52021 and related compounds: a new series of highly specific PAF-acether receptor antagonists isolated from *Ginkgo biloba. Blood Vessels,* 1985, 16, 559–572.
14. Auget, M., et al. Bases pharmacologiques de l'impact vasculaire de l'extrait de *Ginkgo biloba. Presse médicale,* 1986, 15(31), 1524–1528.

15. Baj, A., et al. Qualitative and quantitative evaluation of *Vaccinium myrtillus* anthocyanins by HRGC and HPLC. *J. Chromatography,* 1983, 279, 365–372.

16. Jayle, G. E., & Aubert, L. Action des glucosides d'anthocyanes sur la vision scotopique et mesopique du sujet normal. *Thérapie,* 1964, 19, 171–185.

17. Scharrer, A., & Ober, M. Anthocyanosides in the treatment of retinopathies. *Klin. Monatsbl. Augenheilkd,* 1981, 178, 386–389.

18. Caselli, L. Clinical and electrotetinographic activity of anthocyanosides. *Arch. Med. Int.,* 1985, 3, 29–35.

19. Perossini, M., et al. *Ann. Ottalm and Clin. Ocul.,* 1987, 112, 1173.

20. Repossi, R., et al. *Ann. Ottalm. and Clin. Ocul,* 1987, 113, 357.

21. Neumann, L. Long-term therapy of vascular permeability disorders using anthocyanosides. *Munch. Med. Wochenschr.* 1973, 115, 952–954.

22. Spinella, G. Natural anthocyanosides in treatment of peripheral venous insufficiency. *Arch. Med. Int.,* 1985, 9, 21–29.

23. Zarogoza, F., et al. Comparison of thrombocyte antiaggregant effects of anthocyanosides with those of other agents. *Arch. Pharmacol. Toxicol.,* 1985, 11, 183–188.

24. Bottechia, D., et al. Preliminary report on the inhibitory effect of *Vaccinium myrtillus* anthocyanosides on platele aggregation and clot retraction. *Fitoterapia,* 1987, 48, 3–8.

25. Eandi, M. Post-marketing investigation on Tegens preparation with respect to side-effects. Instituto di Farmacologia e Terapia Sperimentale 1987, Univ. di Torino.

26. Block, E. S. The chemistry of garlic and onions. *Scientific American,* 1985, 252, 114–119.

27. Stoll, A., & Seebeck, E. Chemical investigations on Alliin, the specific principle of garlic. *Adv. Enzymol.,* 11, 377–400.

28. Iberl, B., et al. Quantitative determination of allicin and alliin from garlic by HPLC. *Planta Medica,* 1990, 56, 320–326.

29. Lawson, L. D., et al. Identification and HPLC quantitation of the sulphides and dialk(en)yl thiosulfinates in commercial garlic products. *Planta Medica,* 1991, 57, 363–370.

30. Iberl, B., et al. Products of allicin transformation: ajoenes and dithiins, characterization and their determination by HPLC. *Planta medica,* 1990, 56, 202–11.

31. Bordia, A. Effects of garlic on blood lipids in patient with coronary heart disease. *Am. J. Clin. Nutr.,* 1981, 34, 2100–2103.

32. Ernst, E., et al. Garlic and blood lipids. *Brit. Med. J.,* 1985, 291, 139.

33. Harenberg, J., et al. Effect of dried garlic on blood coagulation, fibrinolysis, platelet aggregation and serum cholesterol levels in patients with hyperlipoproteinemia. *Atherosclerosis*, 1988, 74, 247–249.

34. Fulder, S. Garlic and the prevention of cardiovascular disease. *Cardiology in practice*, 1989, 30, 34–35.

35. Vorberg, G., & Schneider, B. Therapy with garlic: results of a placebo-controlled double-blind study. *Brit. J. Clin. Pract.*, 1990, 44 (suppl.69), 7–11.

36. Brosche, T., et al. The effect of garlic preparation on the composition of plasma lipoproteins and erythrocytes membranes in geriatric subjects. *Brit. J. Clin. Pract.*, 1990, 44 (suppl.69), 12–19.

37. Mader, F. H. Treatment of hyperlipidemia with garlic powder tablets-Evidence from the German Association of General Practitioners' multicentric placebo-controlled double-blind study. *Arzneim. Forsch./Drug Res.*, 1990, 40, 1111–1116.

38. Jung, F., et al. Influence of garlic powder on cutaneous microcirculation: a randomized placebo-controlled double-blind crossover study in apparently healthy subjects. *Brit. J. Clin. Pract.*, 1990, 44 (suppl. 69), 30–35.

39. Kiesewetter, H., et al. Effects of garlic on blood fluidity and fibrinolytic activity: a randomized placebo-controlled double-blind study. *Brit, J. Clin. Pract.*, 1990, 44 (suppl. 69), 24–29.

40. Kiesewetter, H., et al. Effect of garlic on thrombocyte aggregation, microcirculation and other risk factors. *Intern. J. Clin. Pharmacol. Ther. Toxicol.*, 1991, 29, 151–155.

41. Mansell, P. & Reckless, J.P.D. Garlic, Effects on serum lipids, blood pressure, coagulation, platelet aggregation and vasodilatation. *Brit. Med. J.*, 1991, 303, 379–380.

42. Apitz-Castro, R., et al. Effect of ajoene, the major antiplatelet compound from garlic on platelet thrombosis formation. *Thromb. Res.*, 1992, 68(2), 145–155.

43. Adesh, K., et al. Can garlic reduce levels of serum lipids—a controlled clinical study. *The American Journal of Medicine*, 1993, 94, 632–635.

44. Warshafsky, S., et al. Effect of garlic on total serum cholesterol. A meta-analysis. *The Annals of Internal Medicine*, 1993, 119(7), 599–605.

45. Phelps, S. & Harris, W. S. Garlic supplementation and lipoprotein oxidation susceptibility. *Lipids*, 1993, 28, 475–477.

46. Yu, W. C., et al. Allium vegetables and reduced risk of stomach cancer. *J. of National Cancer Institute*, 1989, 81, 162–164.

47. Wargovich, M. J., et al. Chemoprevention of N-Nitrosomethyl-benzya-

mine-induced esophageal cancer in rats by the naturally occurring thioether diallysulfide. *Cancer Research,* 1988, 48, 6872–6875.

48. Han, N., et al. Effect of allicin on anti-oxidant enzymes in mice. *Ying Yang XueBao,* 1992, 14(1), 107–108.

49. Horie, T., et al. Identified diallylpolysulfides from an aged garlic extract which protects the membranes from lipid peroxidation. *Planta Medica,* 1992, 58, 468–469.

50. Weisberger, A. S., & Pensky, J. Tumor inhibition by a sulhydryl-blocking agent related to an active principle of garlic (*Allium sativum*). *Cancer Research,* 1958, 18, 1301–1318.

51. Scharfenberg, K., et al. The cytotoxic effect of ajoene, a natural product from garlic, investigated with different cell lines. *Cancer Letters,* 1990, 53, 103–108.

52. Hadjiolov, D., et al. Effect of diallylsulfide on aristolochic acid-induced fore-stomach carcinogenesis in rats. *Carcinogenesis,* 1993, 14, 407–410.

53. Nagabhushan, M., et al. *Cancer Letters,* 1992, 66(3), 207–216.

54. Divivedi, C., et al. *Pharm. Res.,* 1992, 9, 1668–1670.

55. British Herbal Medicine Association. *British Herbal Pharmacopeia* Vol. 1, 1990 and *British Herbal Compendium,* Vol. 1, 1992.

GINKGO BILOBA

The Amazing 200-Million-Year-Old Healer

Frank Murray

THE FULL-SPECTRUM HEALER

The ornamental ginkgo tree, decorating city streets and parks, is now known to possess a wide range of therapeutic powers and to act as a powerful scavenger of free radicals, harmful particles that impair immune system function. Frank Murray details studies showing ginkgo extract's curative effects in cases of Alzheimer's disease, headaches, circulatory disorders, hemorrhoids, eye problems, ringing in the ears and hearing difficulties and asthma—even its ability to promote the success of organ transplants.

FOREWORD

It is always a rare pleasure, as well as an education, to read the writings of Frank Murray, a long-time health/nutrition writer-editor and a consummate professional.

I have been following his prolific publications—books and articles—for almost 25 years and have been amply rewarded by his work, which is always at the cutting edge of world research pertinent to nutrition and health, imparting information helpful to me in my medical practice and, of course, to my patients.

Gingko biloba is no exception. And Murray has chosen one of the foremost and most helpful herbs for his subject.

The release of this information at this time is most appropriate, because, in recent years, there has been a virtual explosion of interest in and use of herbs in prevention and healing, as opposed to drugs—some of them harmful, some of them habituating.

Herbs are natural products that act as food and medicines, as stated in the Old Testament, Genesis 1:29:

". . . Behold, I have given you every herb-bearing seed which is upon the face of the earth, and every tree which is the fruit of a tree yielding seed. To you, it shall be meat."

Few herbs offer more for health and well-being than *Ginkgo biloba*, derived mainly from leaves of ginkgo trees, many of which live beyond 1000 years. The ginkgo tree appeared on earth as long ago as the Permian Age, 225 to 280 million years ago.

This work is the most comprehensive, best-documented and reader-friendly treatment of *Ginkgo biloba* that I have ever seen and so will be helpful to my readers.

It deals with a great range of medical disorders for which this herb has been shown to be useful: Alzheimer's disease, asthma, circulatory disorders, eye ailments, headaches, hemorrhoids, impotency and, among others, tinnitus (ringing or other incessant noises in the ear). Rock-solid research adds factuality and credibility to *Ginkgo biloba*—particularly that in relation to preventing and/or coping with Alzheimer's disease.

Another absorbing aspect of this work is the information that *Ginkgo biloba* ranks high as an antioxidant, efficient at snuffing out free radicals, which damage or kill healthy cells and thus contribute to our premature aging.

Of special interest to middle-aged men and, of course, to the women with whom they relate sexually, is the section on impotency, the inability to attain or maintain an erection, which many males encounter during the latter years of their lives.

As explained, *Ginkgo biloba* can often correct this embarrassing and often ego-devastating disorder. For decades, it was believed that impotency was caused by emotional and psychological problems. Today, authorities claim that impaired blood circulation in the male sex organ, concurrent with this condition in other parts of the body, is the major cause for this condition—and one of *Ginkgo biloba*'s major health-giving abilities is to improve blood circulation, sometimes dramatically.

Stephen Langer, M.D.
Berkeley, California

THE "LIVING FOSSIL"

A native of southeastern China, and a popular ornamental tree in many parts of the world, ginkgo biloba is a member of the Ginkgoales family, which dates from the Permian Period of the Paleozoic Era between 225 and 280 million years ago. It is the last surviving member of that family and is regarded as a living fossil, since it cannot be found in the wild.

Ginkgo (pronounced GIHNG-koh), also known as the maidenhair tree, is a stately deciduous tree 100 feet or more in height, with a trunk that can extend to eight feet in diameter. It was widely distributed over the temperate regions of both the Northern and Southern Hemisphere during the time of the dinosaurs.

Collier's Encyclopedia says of it:

It seems to have survived the glacial era only in the Orient and has been planted throughout China and Japan for hundreds of years. There are magnificent specimens, reputed to be over a thousand years old, in the grounds of Buddhist temples. The tree is now widely planted as an ornamental in mild climates throughout the world. In the United States it is grown as far north as the Great Lakes, thriving well, for example, in the public parks of New York City and as a street tree in Washington, D. C.[1]

The fan-shaped leathery leaves of the ginkgo, from two to three inches across and the source of the tree's medicinal wonders, are not found on any other flowering plant, although they somewhat resemble the leaflets of the maidenhair fern. Since the two share several common features, ginkgo is sometimes referred to as the "maidenhair tree," and botanists believe that it is a missing link between flowering plants and ferns.

"The exact ancestry of the Ginkgo is uncertain, but it is thought to have originated from seed ferns of the orders Cordaitales or Cycadofilicales, both of which are extinct groups of gymnosperms," according to the *Academic American Encyclopedia.*[2] "Abundant fossil remains of ginkgo date from the Permian age, over 200 million years ago. Many species of this tree apparently developed rapidly after that time, reaching peak distribution and abundance in the Jurassic Period, about 130 million years ago, when several different genera of ginkgoes and about 50 species of the genus *Ginkgo* were evolving. The group declined until, at present, it is represented by only a single genus and species, which includes several cultivated varieties."

The word *ginkgo* is derived from the Japanese *ginkgo* and the Chinese *yinhsing,* which translates as "silver apricot." The leaves of the tree are divided into two lobes, hence *biloba.*

The fissured bark of the ginkgo is grayish and deeply furrowed on older trees and has a corky texture. The leaves, generally divided into two lobes by a central notch, range from dull gray-green to yellow-green during the summer. They turn golden yellow in the autumn and eventually fall off.

There are both male and female ginkgo trees. Male flowers look something like catkins (a cat's tail) and are borne on separate trees from the female flowers. The male flowers produce free-swimming reproductive cells, which is characteristic of ferns and cycads (tropical plants such as palms), but not of gnetums or conifers (cone-bearing plants). The male cells are delivered to female trees by the wind.

Female trees produce paired ovules which, when fertilized, develop into yellowish, plumlike seeds about one inch long. The seed consists of a large silvery nut surrounded by a fleshy outer covering and, when ripe, smells something like rancid butter.

The kernels from the female trees, called ginkgo, are sold in China, Japan and other countries in Southeast Asia. When roasted, they are considered a delicacy.

An authoritative book on Chinese medicinal herbs says of these kernels: "A bonus is that [they are] believed to aid digestion, besides being reputed to have the ability to expel intestinal worms. The leaves are placed between the pages of books, since ancient times in Japan, to protect them from insects. The seed coat has also been used as an insecticide."[3]

Since male ginkgo trees do not produce the foul-smelling seeds, they are generally preferred as ornamentals, so it is important to know the sex of the ginkgo tree you are planting. The large, hard kernel of the fruit from the female tree can cause pedestrians to slip and fall. If clothing is stained by the juice, it generally has to be thrown away, since washing will not remove the odor. And the juice can also cause a skin irritation almost as unpleasant as poison ivy.

Because of their stately appearance, however, male ginkgo trees have been popular ornamentals since they were discovered in China's Chekiang Province. The ginkgo tree was reportedly brought to Europe from Japan in 1727, where it was planted in the Botanic Garden in Utrecht, Holland. It is thought to have been brought to the United States in 1784 and planted in John Burtram's garden in Philadelphia. The ginkgo tree is often seen in parks and gardens in London, and is widely distributed in New York City.

Ginkgo wood is soft and white and has little commercial value, although it is sometimes used for firewood and handcrafting.

Although traditional Chinese texts, such as *A Barefoot Doctor's Manual,* refer to the medicinal properties of ginkgo seeds, seedcoats and leaves, it is the extract from the leaves that is of the greatest interest to modern-day chemists and herbalists. The *Manual* refers to a decoction made from the leaves and suggests that the seeds can be pan-fried for eating. Ginkgo is variously referred to in Chinese herbals as *kung-sun shu, fei-o-hsieh* (flying-moth leaf), *fu chi-chia* (Buddha's fingernails), *ya-chiao-pan* (duck-foot) and *ling-yen.*[4]

Extracts of ginkgo leaves are widely recommended in Asian and European medicine, and account for annual sales of about $500 million.

The leaves of the ginkgo tree are converted into a standardized preparation, such as EGb 761, GBE 24 and other formulations in Europe and the Far East. For example, EGb 761 includes 24 percent flavonoid glycosides, mostly kaempferol and quercetin glucorhamno-side esters and 6 percent of the characteristic terpenes, the ginkgolides and biloboalide. A number of other constituents make the extract water-soluble.[5] A New Zealand authority states:

> This mixture of biologically-active natural products gives the whole extract a complex range of activity; for example, the flavonoids act as free radical scavengers and the terpenes, particularly Ginkgolide B, are potent inhibitors of platelet-activating factor (PAF). Both free radical formation and PAF can disrupt vascular membranes, resulting in increased vascular permeability which in turn is associated with the impairment of cerebral blood flow seen with aging. As well as limiting membrane damage, ginkgo biloba extract appears to affect other factors which contribute to cerebral insufficiency, including disruption of vascular tone, altered cerebral-metabolism and disturbances in neurotransmitters and their receptors.[5]

Although the processing of the leaves is a closely guarded trade secret, the general approach is to collect the leaves in the fall, when they are turning from green to yellow. The yellow color signifies that the flavonoids are present in the leaves.

After the leaves have been harvested, they are dried in specially controlled warehouses where the air temperature remains constant. The leaves are first raked to eliminate twigs, branches, stalks and other foreign matter that might compromise the purity of the final extract. Pressed into bales and kept at a constant temperature and humidity to prevent the accumulation of moisture and fermentation, the leaves are then sent to an extraction plant.

At the plant, the leaves are pulverized and mixed with organic solvents, such as a water-acetone mixture, to extricate the chemical components in the plant. This mixture is heated and further refined to ensure purity. The procedure has been refined so that the flavonoids make up a precise 24 percent concentration, which is said to be the optimum for obtaining the therapeutic effects of ginkgo.

The flavonglycosides, which are part of the bioflavonoid family, are flavonoid molecules that are unique to ginkgo.

In addition to kaempferol and quercetin, ginkgo also contains these flavonoids: sciadopitysin, luteolin, amentoflavone, isorhamnetin, ginkgetin, delphidenon, isoginkgetin, procyanidin, bilobetin and prodelphinidin.

The chemical mixture also contains two other chemical groups, namely, terpene lactones (ginkgolides A, B and C and bilobalide), and minor organic acids such as hydroxykynurenic acid, pyrocatchuic acid, kynurenic acid, vanillic acid and hydroxybenzoic acid.

Although thousands of ginkgo trees are being grown in the Far East, Europe and the United States to satisfy the growing demands for this medicinal extract, researchers at Harvard University have succeeded in synthesizing one of its most potent constituents, thereby making it even more available to researchers and scientists. No doubt this will contribute to an even greater admiration for ginkgo and its therapeutic possibilities. Credit for the discovery goes to Dr. Elias J. Corey, professor of chemistry at Harvard, and his colleagues. The potent molecule is so complex that other laboratories had given up trying to synthesize it, *The New York Times* reported on March 1, 1988:[6]

> Chemists and botanists said last week that the first total laboratory synthesis of the compound, ginkgolide B, could eventually lead to its widespread use in treating asthma, toxic shock, Alzheimer's disease and various circulatory disorders. The ginkgo compound is also being studied as a possibly safer substitute for drugs now given to recipients of transplanted organs to prevent the body from rejecting them.

Ginkgo supplements have been available over-the-counter in health food stores for several years, but the Food and Drug Administration has not yet approved for medicinal purposes the various ginkgo-derived drugs that are available in other countries.

Ginkgo has been a staple of Chinese herbal medicine for thousands of years, being recommended for coughs, asthma and acute allergic inflammations. It is one of the components of an elixir called Soma, which is a traditional Hindu medicine.

Dr. Pierre Braquet, a researcher at the Institut Henri Beaufour in Paris, France, lauded the discovery. A leading authority on ginkgo constituents, Dr. Braquet had previously established the most likely process for the therapeutic action of Ginkgolide B. This substance apparently works by interfering with a chemical in the body referred to as PAF (platelet activating factor). It has been implicated in asthma, graft rejection and such immune disorders as toxic shock syndrome.

The Times also reported that "British researchers have reported positive results in tests of Ginkgolide B in treating people with asthma and allergic inflammations. Animal studies by other scientists indicate that the substance might be effective in regulating blood pressure, treating kidney disorders and counteracting a number of toxins."[6]

In addition to making ginkgolide B in the laboratory, Dr. Corey and his graduate student, Wei-guo Su, also isolated another ginkgolide, bilobalide.

The ability to make these chemicals in the laboratory is a significant step forward, since it will help scientists to evaluate the specific health benefits of each ginkgolide compound and make it easier for drug companies to obtain large amounts of the most promising substances. At the present time, ginkgolides are obtained by extraction from ginkgo leaves, a time-consuming process that yields rather small amounts of the compounds from a large number of trees.[7]

ALZHEIMER'S DISEASE

When it was first described by Alois Alzheimer (1864–1915), a German neurologist, in 1907, Alzheimer's disease was considered a rare disorder. The progressive, degenerative disease attacks the brain and results in impaired memory, thinking and behavior.

Today, Alzheimer's is regarded as the most common cause of dementia. However, dementia is not a disease per se but a group of symptoms that characterize certain diseases and conditions. In Alzheimer's, the dementia includes a decline in intellectual function that is severe enough to interfere with the ability to perform routine activities.

The second most common form of dementia is referred to as multi-infarct dementia, which is caused by vascular disease and strokes. Other causes of dementia include Huntington's disease (chorea), Parkinson's disease, Pick's disease and Creutzfeldt-Jacob disease.

A number of conditions have dementialike symptoms, such as depression, drug reactions, thyroid disorders, nutritional deficiencies, brain tumors, head injuries, alcoholism, infections (meningitis, syphilis and AIDS) and hydrocephalus (a buildup of water on the brain).

An Alzheimer's Association publication explains the special characteristics of the disease:

> Alzheimer's disease is distinguished from other forms of dementia by characteristic changes in the brain that are visible only upon microscopic examination. At autopsy, Alzheimer's disease brains show the presence of tangles of fibers (neurofibrillary tangles) and clusters of degenerating nerve endings (neurotic plaques) in areas of the brain that are important for memory and intellectual function. Another characteristic of Alzheimer's disease is the reduced production of certain brain chemicals, especially acetylcholine and somatosatin. These chemicals are necessary for normal communication between nerve cells.[1]

Scientists are still unraveling the mysteries of Alzheimer's, and there are a variety of possible causes. One form of the disease, called familial or uncommon Alzheimer's, may be caused by a defect in a single gene on Chromosome 21.

> However, for most Alzheimer's disease patients the genetic involvement is less clear. Although there does seem to be a genetic predisposition for the disease, other factors influence whether or not an individual develops Alzheimer's disease. Scientists continue to explore the importance of such things as a

slow virus, environmental toxins, such as aluminum, and other physical conditions of an individual that may interact with the genetic defect.

Alzheimer's develops over a period of time, and there are a variety of symptoms. Typical symptoms include difficulty with memory and loss of intellectual abilities, which interfere with daily work and social activities. There may be confusion, language problems, such as trouble finding the right word, poor or decreased judgment, disorientation in place and time and changes in behavior or personality. The course of the disease averages eight years from the inception of symptoms, but there have been cases lasting as long as 25 years. In severe cases, the patients are unable to care for themselves.

When studies were initiated in the 1970s, it was believed that 2.5 million Americans suffered from the disease, according to the National Institute on Aging. However, a more recent study suggests that these figures represent only the tip of the iceberg.[2]

Scientists began to revise upward the estimates of the number of Alzheimer's patients following a study reported on in the *Journal of the American Medical Association* in 1989. Denis Evans, M.D. and his colleagues at Brigham and Women's Hospital in Boston, Massachusetts, reported on their findings of the prevalence of dementia in a community in East Boston. The researchers found that 10.3 percent of the people over age 65 had what they called "probable" Alzheimer's disease.[3]

In 1982, Dr. Evans and his colleagues began studying older people living in East Boston, a typical working-class community. Some 3,800 residents over 65 participated in the study. The methodology included a questionnaire concerning medical and social problems, a memory test and, for 476 volunteers, a comprehensive medical evaluation to rule out the presence of health problems other than Alzheimer's.

Dr. Evans and his team were surprised to find that the prevalence of Alzheimer's rose more rapidly with age than had previously been suspected. As an example, for the seniors between 65 and 74, 3 percent had probable Alzheimer's disease, compared to 18.7 percent in the 74- to 84-year-old age group and 47.2 percent in those over 85. This last figure for those 85 and older is almost double previous estimates.

Dr. Zaven Khachaturian, associate director for Neuroscience and Neuropsychology of Aging at the National Institute of Aging, commenting on the study, said:

Given Dr. Evans's data, coupled with Census Bureau estimates for the numbers of people 85 and older, the actual number of Alzheimer's cases in this country might be close to 4 million. Since the numbers of people over 85 are growing faster than any other segment of the U. S. population, there could be as many as 14 million Americans with Alzheimer's disease by the middle of the 21st century. Also, the prospects are very good that medical advances and changes in lifestyle will result in an even greater proportion of people living to extreme old age than the census data predicts, meaning even higher numbers of Alzheimer's patients in the next century.

There are two forms of Alzheimer's disease, namely, a presenile form with onset as early as age 40 and a senile form with the onset after 60. The former is classed as familial, while the latter, much more common, is considered sporadic.

A 1988 article in *Nutrition Today* explains:

The presenile form is established as familial, expressed as an autosomal dominant with a genetic defect on Chromosome 21, close to, but not identified with, genes for amloid beta-protein precursor and superoxide dismutase (SOD). Persons with this form of the disease become very severely demented before death, which usually occurs within seven years. The senile form . . . is considered sporadic. Since the individual is older at onset, death usually occurs in about three years. There may be a genetic predisposition, but the disease is strongly influenced by environmental factors, that are as yet unidentified.[4]

The brain, which is the main organ affected by Alzheimer's, consists of three major divisions, namely, the cerebrum, cerebellum and brainstem. The cerebrum, or cerebral cortex, is divided into areas with sensory function, motor function and integrative function. The latter are referred to as association areas. One such area integrates information from cortical areas receiving sensations of touch, hearing and vision, while others are considered to be sites of typically human thought processes.

> Alzheimer's disease typically affects not only the cortex but also several of these areas. . . . Each of these areas has different cell populations and organization, but all contain large and small neurons, glial cells, perikarya and neuropil, like the central cortex.

Numerous studies have shown the efficacy of using *Ginkgo biloba* extract to improve the mental acuity of geriatric patients. For example, W. V. Weitbrecht and W. Jansen, of Nuremberg, Germany, conducted a double-blind study involving 40 patients, ages 60 to 80, who had been diagnosed with primary degenerative dementia. During the three-month study, one group of 20 received either *Ginkgo biloba* extract (120 mg/day), while the other group was given a placebo.[5.]

The researchers reported that those receiving the ginkgo extract were more alert, scored higher on psychometric tests and had a more positive outlook than the controls. The *Ginkgo biloba* extract (GBE) group experienced a "significant improvement," compared with no gain for the placebo group.

At the Whittington Hospital in London, researchers examined the benefits of *Ginkgo biloba* extract on 31 patients over the age of 50 with signs of memory impairment, reported Donald J. Brown, N.D., in the May 1992 issue of *Let's Live*.[7] The study, which lasted six months, was originally published in *Current Medical Research and Opinion*.

In the double-blind study, half of the volunteers were given 40 milligrams of *Ginkgo biloba* extract three times daily, while the other half remained on a placebo. Psychometric tests were evaluated at the beginning of the study and after 12 and 24 weeks of treatments.

The results were encouraging, Dr. Brown said:

The patients who received GBE showed significantly superior improvement compared to those given a placebo. Besides demonstrating that Ginkgo extract has a beneficial effect on mild to moderate memory loss of organic origin, the study revealed that electroencephalogram (EEG) measurements in the GBE group indicated improved brain function. This supports other research that has shown GBE increases the rate of information transmission by nerve cells.

In 1975, French researchers studied the potential benefits of *Ginkgo biloba* extract in a group of 60 patients (55 females and 5 males), who had been diagnosed with cerebrovascular insufficiency, and 30 female patients who served as controls and given ergot alkaloid derivatives.[8] Pretrial examinations determined the extent of dizziness, headaches, movability, sensory manifestations, and so on, as well as typical psychometric tests.

Following the tests, the researchers determined that there was a 79 percent improvement in the GBE group, compared with 21 percent on the placebo. The trial group received 120 mg/day of GBE for three months.

Patients with cerebrovascular insufficiency showed a 92 percent improvement after being given GBE, contrasted with 44 percent improvement in the placebo group, according to a 1982 study.[9] During this one-month study, 50 patients (30 women and 20 men) were randomly assigned to the GBE group or a placebo group. The volunteers ranged in age from 45 to 74. The supplement group received 120 mg/day of GBE.

The treatment group began to show signs of improvement after 12 days, the researchers said. In the controls, it took 30 days before any change was noticeable. The study evaluated various psychological and neurological tests, as well as such symptoms as ringing in the ears, headache, vertigo and so forth.

A German researcher reported that *Ginkgo biloba* extract offers considerable promise in the treatment of Alzheimer's disease.[10] He added that; although there is a significant reduction in glucose consumption in patients with the degenerative type of dementia, there is a loss of cortical neurons, as well as a reduction in some subcortical structures, and a loss of the acetylcholine-synthesizing enzyme choline acetyltransferase, which causes a significant reduction in acetylcholine synthesis. Also involved are other transmitters such as serotonin.

"As reported by I. Hindmarch in a double-blind crossover study, including eight healthy female volunteers in an acute and ascending trial, one hour after 600 mg of GBE, there was a significant improvement of the short term memory which was not seen at the doses of 120 mg and 240 mg," Dr. Funfgeld said.[10,11]

He referred to a study involving double-blind trial using GBE versus a placebo. There were 166 patients with a mean age of 82.1 years. During the one-year study, 80 volunteers received GBE and 86 patients took a placebo. Following the study, the GBE group, which had been evaluated with the Geriatric Clinical Evaluation Scale, improved 17.1 percent, contrasted with 7.8 percent in the controls.[10,12]

In a study by Dr. Funfgeld, a 74-year-old man suffering from Parkinson's disease, memory loss, lack of energy and occasional delirious states was given infusions of 200 mg ginkgo extract daily for 10 days. Dr. Funfgeld found that the patient was more alert and had more drive following the experiment.[10,13]

"No doubt this new technique opens up big advantages in the clinical and therapeutic field. Without doubt more trials in different conditions and stages of dementias with different dosages are necessary, but, even with our present knowledge, the ginkgo biloba extract could be included in the list of therapeutics established by C. A. Bagne, et al. in 1986."[10,14]

Dr. Funfgeld and his colleagues also reported that *Ginkgo biloba* extract appears to delay mental deterioration during the early stages of Alzheimer's disease. In fact, GBE might help to reverse some of the disabilities associated with Alzheimer's and help the patient to maintain a normal life without having to be hospitalized.[15]

D. M. Warburton of the University of Reading in England reported in 1989 that from a general review of the pharmacological, psychopharmacological and clinical studies performed with *Ginkgo biloba* extract, the supplement seems to be effective in patients with vascular disorders, in all types of dementia and even in patients suffering from cognitive disorders secondary to depression, notably because of its beneficial effects on mood.[16]

"Of special concern are people who are just beginning to experience deterioration in their cognitive function," Dr. Warburton said. "Ginkgo biloba extract might delay deterioration and enable these subjects to maintain a normal life and escape institutionalization. In addition, GBE appears to be a safe drug, being well tolerated, even in doses many times higher than those usually recommended."

HEADACHES

In addition to being a symptom of emotional stress, headaches can be due to an infectious disease, teeth and mouth disorders, eye problems, colds and sinusitis, anemia, gastrointestinal disorders, very high blood pressure, a head injury, natural gas poisoning, a sensitivity to monosodium glutamate (MSG), among others.[1] Allergies and brain disorders are apparently only rarely causes of headaches.

In a 1975 study, GBE was given to patients suffering from migraine headaches. The results of an open trial were very good, with improvement or almost a total cure in 80 percent of the cases, the researcher said.[1,2] For patients with other types of headaches, the results were not as definitive.

The results of a double-blind study confirmed the effectiveness of using GBE to treat migraine headaches. Since these volunteers had suffered from migraines for a considerable time and had not had sufficient relief from other therapies, the researcher concluded that *Ginkgo biloba* extract should be considered an effective supplement against migraine.

Another researcher reported in 1978 that GBE is useful in treating some patients suffering from migraines.[3]

ORGAN TRANSPLANTS

Although the use of donated human organs has increased the lifespan and quality of life for thousands of people, there are never enough organs to go around. Almost every hospital has a number of candidates waiting for various organs to become available.

Because of the demand for organs, scientists have turned to animal donors. One of the most publicized cases, in the summer of 1992, involved transplanting a baboon liver into a 35-year-old male, whose liver had failed because of a hepatitis B infection. The unidentified patient lived for 10 weeks after the surgical procedure at the University of Pittsburgh Medical Center in Pennsylvania.

The liver looked "almost normal" after 70 days of use, and an autopsy found no signs of rejection. Death was attributed to an intracranial hemorrhaging of unknown cause, Thomas Starzl, M.D. wrote in *Medical Tribune*. It was then reported that the patient had been terminally ill and was HIV-positive, although there were no signs of AIDS. The medical center plans to go ahead with four more baboon-to-human liver transplants.[1]

One of the most promising uses of the ginkgolides may be as a less toxic alternative to the immunosuppressive drug cyclosporin during organ transplants, according to Dr. Richard W. Ramwell of Georgetown University Medical School in Washington, D.C.[2]

Also known as cyclosporine, cyclosporin A and Sandimmune, cyclosporin is a powerful immunosuppressive agent used annually by tens of thousands of patients undergoing liver, bone marrow, heart or kidney transplants. In other words, it is used to reduce the body's natural immunity in those receiving organ transplants.

The Complete Drug Reference explains cyclosporin's action and the problems it presents:

> When a patient receives an organ transplant, the body's white blood cells will try to get rid of (reject) the transplanted organ. Cyclosporine (cyclosporin) works by preventing the white blood cells from doing this. Cyclosporine is a very strong medi-

cine. It may cause side effects that could be very serious, such as high blood pressure and kidney and liver problems. It may also reduce the body's ability to fight infections. It is available only with a doctor's prescription as capsules and an oral solution as well as a parenteral injection in the United States and Canada.[3]

In addition to the side effects mentioned, the drug can also cause unwanted hair growth, so finding some way to avoid the toxicity of the drug is very important. In addition, many transplant patients must take cyclosporin for the rest of their lives.

In experimental heart transplants using different strains of laboratory rats, Dr. Ramwell and surgery professor Marine Foegh, director of transplantation research at Georgetown University Medical School, found that ginkgolide B prolonged the survival of grafted hearts in the recipient rats. Without the ginkgo extract, the animals' immune systems would have quickly rejected their new hearts. As a result of this experiment, Dr. Ramwell is confident that the ginkgo chemical may also be useful for human transplant surgery.

In addition, he says, other animal studies suggest that ginkgolide B might be effective in regulating blood pressure, treating kidney disorders and various forms of shock, reducing inflammation, treating eye diseases and serving as an antidote for a number of toxins.[2]

Dr. Pierre Braquet, a French researcher, has determined that the ginkgolides apparently work by interfering with a single chemical in the body called platelet activating factor, or PAF. It has been implicated as a cause of graft rejection among other things.

"Research for specific antagonists, or blockers, of PAF has thus been undertaken actively in recent years," Dr. Braquet said. "Ginkgolide B is a promising lead."[4]

ASTHMA

A condition that often develops in childhood, asthma is a lung disease in which "twitchy," overactive bronchial tubes narrow, swell and be-

come clogged with mucus. During an attack, the asthmatic has difficulty inhaling fresh air and exhaling spent air, and this often creates
a wheezing or whistling sound. The patient is also likely to cough
uncontrollably, have a tightness in the chest and be short of breath.
Gasping for oxygen leaves the patient anxious and fatigued.

Most people with asthma are allergic to one or more substances.
The most likely candidates are dust and mold, animals and birds,
foods such as eggs and milk, pollen and a variety of drugs, especially
those related to penicillin and related antibiotics.

Modern Chinese pharmacopoeias still list fruit and leaf extracts of
Ginkgo biloba as being beneficial in treating chronic bronchitis and
asthma, according to noted French researcher F. V. De-Feudis.[1] In
animal tests at least, bronchial constriction has been inhibited in the
presence of platelet-activating factor (PAF)-antagonistic ginkgolides
in these extracts.

Writing in *Let's Live,* Donald J. Brown, N.D. discusses the ability
of ginkgolides A, B and C to inhibit PAF, and notes that research
regarding PAF-induced disease focuses on bronchial asthma and suggests that PAF plays a central role in the creation of long-term airway
hypersensitivity and bronchial constriction noted in asthma.[2]

He went on to say that the three ginkgolides form a mixture known
as BN 52063 and equals the natural ratio of the three components
found in the *Ginkgo biloba* extract. In a study published in *Prostaglandins* in 1987,[3] BN 52063 significantly inhibited bronchial constriction
in asthmatic patients for up to six hours after they were administered
an asthma-causing allergen. Several other studies have confirmed
these results and suggest a therapeutic role for GBE in the management of asthma.

"I have had particular success with a liquid form of GBE in my
pediatric asthma cases," Dr. Brown writes. "My observations have
included a reduction in the severity and frequency of asthma attacks
and a marked reduction in the need for bronchodilating medication."

TINNITUS AND HEARING LOSS

An estimated 8.5 million Americans are afflicted with hearing loss. Of this number, 71,000 may be totally deaf, while about 235,000 experience a severe hearing problem bordering on deafness. Another 8 million have a variety of hearing handicaps, with about a million American children reporting various stages of hearing impairment.

According to *The People's Medical Manual,* you should be concerned about a possible hearing problem if you (1) hear better some days than others; (2) often fail to catch words or phrases; (3) find yourself unable to follow conversations in a group; (4) find you can better understand what a person is saying when you are facing him; (5) frequently feel that your family and friends mumble instead of speaking clearly; (6) have a running ear, or pain or irritation in the ear; (7) suffer from dizziness, loss of balance or head noises.[1]

Tinnitus or ringing in the ears is a hearing problem that can range from barely audible to quite loud, the manual continued. It affects some 9 million Americans. Most people with tinnitus report a high-pitched ringing, while others experience a buzzing, hissing, roaring or other sound. The sound can be constant or intermittent.

On the condition's causes, the *Manual* notes:

Tinnitus is often caused by exposure to loud sounds. It also can be a symptom of many conditions, accompanying virus infections, allergies and blood and circulatory disorders. Some medications—such as aspirin and quinine—may cause it. Brain cancer, meningitis and head injuries can be implicated, as can diseases of the nervous system that involve the auditory nerve. Tinnitus is usually accompanied by hearing loss.

Dizziness, vertigo and hearing disturbances are frequent complaints from patients seeing ear, nose and throat specialists. Although the genesis of these ailments is often difficult to pinpoint, they are frequently attributed to involution of the cochlea (the inner ear which harbors the main organ of hearing and is also involved with the sense of balance) or labyrinth, or to a macro- or microcirculatory deficit in these organs.

A French study from 1979 explains that these hearing organs are highly sensitive to anoxia, or oxygen deprivation.[2] Consequent disequilibrium in the vestibular nuclei can result in vertigo and hearing loss.[3]

Ginkgo biloba extract has been shown in open trials to be an effective therapeutic agent in patients with dizziness, vertigo and tinnitus. The extract, administered orally in divided doses of 60 to 160 mg/day, produced resolution or marked improvement in symptoms in between 40 and 80 percent of the volunteers who were treated, compared to those getting a placebo. The extract has been especially successful in treating patients with vestibular neuronitis, or an inflammation of inner ear nerve cells.[2]

Double-blind, placebo-controlled studies showed resolution or marked symptomatic improvement in 44 to 85 percent of patients with vertigo or dizziness treated with *Ginkgo biloba* extract for one to three months. This is twice the usual rate of placebo response.

The causes of vertigo were typically seen to be underlying disorders such as Ménière's disease, vestibular neuropathy or infection or traumatic injury. GBE was also highly effective for patients with vertigo with no definable etiology.[2]

A significant improvement in tinnitus of less than one year's duration was reported for patients given GBE versus a placebo.[3,4] In fact, there was a distinct improvement in 50 percent of the patients within 70 and 119 days.

A 1979 study reported that GBE was successful in treating 60 patients—35 men and 25 women—with hearing loss and/or vertigo and tinnitus.[5] The problems were apparently related to various vascular disorders, aging of the inner ear, trauma or infection.

In the treatment group, the volunteers were given 120 mg/day of *Ginkgo biloba* extract, while the controls received 15 mg/day of nicergoline, a European drug. The researchers reported that GBE was effective by all criteria measured, especially with respect to vertigo and electronystagmography, a device used to record side-to-side movements of the eyeballs. The drug was also effective;

however, when the dosages were compared, the extract was said to be superior.

A study, which lasted three months, analyzed the potential benefits of *Ginkgo biloba* extract in 42 patients (22 women, 19 men and a 12-year-old child) with hypoacousia, a hearing impairment, and tinnitus. The complaints involved a variety of hearing losses, such as presbyacusis (hearing loss due to aging), acoustic trauma, perceptive deafness, sudden complete deafness, buzzing or whistling noises and other forms of tinnitus.[6]

The daily dose of GBE varied between 120 and 160 mg/day, depending on the extent of the problem. Of the 42 patients given GBE for an average of three months, good and very good results on tone audiometry occurred in 40 percent of the cases, while there was a failure in 21 percent, the researchers said.

"In 28 patients with tinnitus, results were 'good' and 'very good' in 82 percent of the cases, with disappearance of symptoms in 53 percent of the cases," researcher F. V. DeFeudis reported. "In 16 patients in whom poor comprehension of conversation was a special complaint, GBE led to good recovery in 13 cases. It was concluded that ginkgo biloba extract can be particularly recommended for vertigo, hearing loss and tinnitus, and that it is exceedingly well tolerated."[5]

An improvement in hearing was reported in 40 percent of the patients receiving *Ginkgo biloba* extract in a 1973 study.[7] The patients had complained of presbyacusic hearing loss and other problems associated with a circulatory deficit. Since relief was reported in many of the patients, especially those suffering from vertigo, the researcher considered GBE to be an especially useful therapy in otolaryngology.

There was an overall success rate of 85 percent when researchers treated 49 patients afflicted with vertigo and various stages of hearing loss using *Ginkgo biloba* extract.[8] They recommend the extract for neurosensory diseases of the inner ear which have such vascular origins as headaches and vertigo.

In still another study in 1979, 70 percent of the patients with various stages of vertigo and hearing loss improved with *Ginkgo biloba* extract.[9] If the patients had suffered from deafness for an extended period, the results were poor. But positive results were noted in half of the patients with presbyacusis. The improvements were remarkable, the authors of the study said, because some of the patients had experienced considerable hearing loss. For those patients who had suffered recent deafness due to head injury or sonic damage, the results were considered very good in slightly more than 60 percent of the cases. Of the 26 patients complaining of vertigo, 24 reported that they were very satisfied with the results using GBE.

IMPOTENCE

Because it is such a shock to the ego, perhaps the disorder that most men fear the most is impotence. This malfunction, which affects most men at some time in their life, is the loss of a man's ability to acquire and maintain an erection. Physicians and urologists look at both psychological and physical factors in determining a solution. However, the problem, either temporary or otherwise, can often be traced to depression, stress, fatigue, drugs and alcohol, marital discord, smoking and other factors. Impotence is not to be confused with infertility, which means that sperm are not sufficiently healthy to fertilize an egg.

During an erection, the penis becomes engorged with blood as blood vessels enlarge or dilate and allow an increased flow. This change is due to nerve stimulation, and since some nerves are ultimately controlled in brain centers, a number of drugs that affect the brain can interfere with an erection. Some drugs that can contribute to this problem are those used to treat hypertension, such as diuretics or water pills. Tranquilizers and other drugs used to treat depression can also inhibit sexual function.

Chronic alcoholism and one of its side effects, cirrhosis of the liver, can lower the amount of testosterone circulating in the bloodstream. Testosterone, the major male sex hormone, is produced in the testes and is the hormone that gives male body hair and a deeper voice, in addition to stimulating the sex drive and producing sperm.

Circulatory problems, such as arteriosclerosis, blood vessel damage resulting from diabetes, and high blood pressure may be implicated in impotence, as can chronic illness.

Problems with sexual interest and performance can also be related to diseases that inhibit the production or action of testosterone. These generally hormonal conditions include tumors of the pituitary gland or hypothalamus, which are the centers in the brain that produce and regulate hormones.

Since *Ginkgo biloba* extract has been used successfully to treat blood pressure regulation and various vascular diseases, it should come as no surprise that GBE has a beneficial application in dealing with impotence.

A 1989 study illustrates this. Sixty patients with arterial erectile dysfunction, who had not responded to papaverine injections, the drug of choice, were treated with *Ginkgo biloba* extract.[1] The study lasted 12 to 18 months, and some improvement was reported in six to eight weeks. The dosage was 60 mg/day. Following six months of therapy with GBE, 50 percent of the patients were able to sustain penile erections. About 45 percent of the remaining men noticed some improvement, especially after being given the supplement in conjunction with papaverine.

Papaverine (pa-PAV-er-een) is one of the vasodilators that physicians often prescribe to cause blood vessels to expand, thus increasing blood flow. It is not recommended for those with angina, glaucoma, heart disease, myocardial infarction, a recent stroke, and related conditions.[2] It is also not recommended for Parkinson's patients, especially for those taking levodopa, and its effectiveness can be diminished by cigarette smoking.

CIRCULATORY DISORDERS

Without a constant blood supply, human beings would not be able to live. And when this constant flow of oxygen-carrying blood is disrupted, serious health problems can develop.

Blood is dispersed through the body via its central pump, the heart. Used blood is pumped to the lungs, where it picks up oxygen and discards carbon dioxide. The blood then returns to the heart and is pumped throughout the body. This supplies all of the body's tissues with nutrients and picks up waste products before returning the blood to the heart to become reoxygenated.

The American Medical Association Family Medical Guide describes the vessels carrying the blood:

> The arteries that carry blood away from the heart have thick, muscular walls to restrain and absorb the peaks of blood pressure that occur each time your heart beats. The main artery, the aorta, has an internal diameter of about 1¼ inches. It branches into smaller arteries, then into tiny arterioles, and finally into microscopic capillaries, whose thin, porous walls permit easy exchange of nutrients and oxygen for waste products between the blood and the tissues. Gradually the capillaries merge to form venules, and they merge to form soft-walled, flexible veins, which return oxygen-depleted blood to the heart.[1]

Your circulatory system can go awry if the central pump malfunctions or problems arise within the blood vessels. As an example, there can be a weakness in an artery wall, or the hardening of an artery may make it unable to absorb increased blood pressure. Blood clots that cause blockages can form, and a variety of other disorders can develop. Some of these include hardening of the arteries (arteriosclerosis), deep-vein thrombosis, pulmonary embolism, thrombophlebitis, aneurysms, varicose veins, Raynaud's disease, acrocyanosis, Buerger's disease, cranial arthritis, arterial embolism, dry and wet gangrene, pulmonary hypertension, low blood pressure (hypertension), and even frostbite.

Stroke is also a possibility when part of the brain is damaged because of an impaired blood supply. Such a disturbance, characterized as cerebral thrombosis, cerebral embolism or cerebral hemorrhage, can result in a deterioration of both physical and mental acuity. Cerebral thrombosis is usually due to the narrowing of an artery that supplies blood to the brain, a complication of hardening of the arteries. A cerebral embolism is caused by a foreign object, or embolus, which is carried in the bloodstream and becomes wedged in a place where it inhibits blood flow to the brain. A cerebral hemorrhage simply means that an artery bursts.

A 1965 study reported that *Ginkgo biloba* extract lowered blood pressure and dilated or expanded the peripheral blood vessels, including capillaries in 10 patients with postthrombotic syndrome.[2] This did not increase capillary permeability, but it did reduce the swelling.

In 1972 the use of *Ginkgo biloba* extract was compared with other vasodilators, notably hydrogenated alkaloids of ergot, acetylcholine chloride and sodium nicotinate.[3] All patients had varying degrees of vascular disease. The research team stated that the vasodilator action of GBE is similar to the other substances but is significantly more constant.

A study in 1977 was conducted to determine the activity of GBE on cerebral blood flow in 20 patients, ages 62 to 85, who were diagnosed with cerebral circulatory insufficiency, due to age and hardening of the arteries.[4] The patients were treated orally and intramuscularly for 15 days. Because of the age and health of the volunteers, the researchers maintained low dosages of GBE and did not expect spectacular results. However, they reported that the cerebral hemodynamics was much improved in 15 of the cases.

In another 1977 study[5,6] researchers reported functional improvement in 65 percent of patients with arterial leg disease following GBE therapy. There was only a 22.5 percent response in the placebo group. Some patients in the treatment group also reported a resolution of trophic skin conditions, better circulation to the extremities and a lessening of impotence, among other things.

About two-thirds of the patients receiving GBE showed definite clinical improvement, compared with 16 percent given a placebo, when treated for a variety of peripheral vascular diseases.[5,7] After further analysis of the 1975 study, the authors reported that the supplement was 100 percent effective in patients with Grade II lower limb arteritis (inflammation of an artery). There was a 33 percent response in volunteers with Raynaud's disease (which involves fingers and toes), but there was no response in those with Grade III arteritis.

The authors went on to say that, when compared with the placebo group, GBE produced much higher rates of improvement of peripheral pain (66 vs 13 percent); intermittent claudication (64 vs 19 percent); warmth of lower limbs (64 vs 19 percent); clearing of ulcerous lesions (100 vs 0 percent); trophic changes in lesions (100 vs 25 percent); and in pain attacks in Raynaud's disease (33 vs 0 percent).

In an open comparison, GBE—160 mg/day given orally for six months—was more effective than buflomedil (600 mg/day) in 38 patients with peripheral occlusive arterial disease and was equivalent to pentoxifylline (1,200 mg/day) in another 27 patients participating in a double-blind study with respect to improving walking distance, relieving pain and increasing microcirculation.[5,8,9]

In 1984, a double-blind study tested the efficacy of GBE in two groups of patients with peripheral arterial insufficiency.[10] The study lasted six months. There was a marked improvement in walking without pain and increased blood flow to lower limbs in the treatment group. The author of the report stated that the improvement rate was not only statistically significant but clinically remarkable.

Following success with GBE in smaller trials researchers in 1967 conducted a larger study involving patients with Parkinson's disease secondary to cerebral arteriosclerosis.[11] The supplement was given either orally or by intravenous injection.

When compared with standard vasodilator therapy in 40 postsurgical patients with lower limb arterial obstruction, GBE, in another study, brought improvement in resting and walking pain. The dosage was 160 mg/day.[5,12]

Twenty-one patients with chronic arteriopathies of the lower extremities were treated with GBE in an experiment going back to 1975. The volunteers, with a mean age of 60 years, received 160 mg/day of GBE for a month, and the trial provided encouraging results.[13,14] Functional symptoms of intermittent claudication were markedly decreased and all subjects exhibited excellent tolerance to the therapy, the researchers reported.

GBE enhances blood flow not only through the large blood vessels, but also small vessels like the capillaries close to the skin. In 1992 Donald J. Brown, N.D., reported in *Let's Live* that a study at the

University of Saarland in Hamburg, Germany, revealed that GBE increases microcirculation through the capillaries of the body. The study involved 10 patients whose skin microcirculation was monitored every 30 minutes. The results showed a 57 percent increase in blood flow through the nail fold capillaries of the finger after one hour.[15,16]

Ginkgo has been shown to increase the brain's tolerance for oxygen deficiency, according to Dr. Hans Haas of the Mannheim Clinic at Heidelberg University in Germany, wrote Rob McCaleb in *Better Nutrition for Today's Living*.[17] Dr. Haas says that human clinical experiments have also shown that ginkgo extracts can cause a significant increase in blood flow in patients with cerebrovascular disease. Unlike other circulation enhancers, GBE is said to increase blood flow not only to healthy areas of the brain, but also to the disease-damaged areas.

McCaleb also cites a recent study from the Department of Geriatric Medicine, Whittington Hospital in London, confirming the improvement in cognitive function, as measured by a Digit Copying Test and a computerized classification test.

A six-month clinical trial of the extract conducted in Germany found that GBE improved the distance patients could walk without pain by 100 percent in the test group and by 30 percent for the controls. Pain is the result when circulation to the lower limbs is too weak, causing oxygen deprivation of muscles. This in turn results in an excess production of metabolic waste products and free radicals.[17]

After reviewing 20 clinical studies in ginkgo's effects, D. M. Warburton of the University of Reading in England concluded that a dose of 120 mg of standardized ginkgo extract daily was "effective in patients with vascular disorders, in all types of dementia and even in patients suffering from cognitive disorders secondary to depression because of its beneficial effects on mood," reported Mark Blumenthal in 1991 in *Better Nutrition for Today's Living*.[18] (This study is also reported in the section on Alzheimer's disease.)

Warburton's review indicates very low toxicity or side effects from using *Ginkgo biloba* extract, except for minor reversible gastric disturbances.

A more recent study in 1989 conducted at several research centers and hospitals involving 8,505 persons observed over six months reported that the total occurrence of adverse effects was 0.4 percent. All of these were minor and temporary. Once again, gastric disturbances were the most common, totaling 0.1 percent. Thus, ginkgo extracts have proven to be quite safe.

EYE DISORDERS

One of the leading causes of blindness in people over 65, macular degeneration is of unknown etiology and usually develops gradually. This eye disorder involves the macula, the area of the retina near the optic nerve at the back of the eye. The macula is responsible for fine reading vision at the center of the field of vision.

The American Medical Association Family Medical Guide explains that

> In some elderly people, the small blood vessels of the eye become constricted or narrowed and hardened. As a result, the macula does not get enough blood, and it requires a plentiful supply. This blood deficiency causes degeneration of the macula, and blurring of the central vision follows. In nearly all cases, both eyes are affected, either simultaneously or one after the other.[1]

Antioxidants such as vitamin A and vitamin C are free-radical scavengers, and have been studied as a possible deterrent to macular degeneration.[2] Since *Ginkgo biloba* extract also serves as an antioxidant and a dispersant of free radicals, this supplement has also been investigated for the treatment of macular degeneration, although on a rather modest scale.

In 1986 French researchers administered GBE, 80 mg twice daily, or a placebo, to 20 elderly patients with recently diagnosed macular degeneration.[3,4] The randomized, double-blind study lasted six months. Aside from hardening of the arteries, the seniors apparently had few other complaints.

"At study completion, funduscopic examination revealed that distant visual acuity [in the most affected eye] had improved by 2.3 diopters [a measurement of refraction power] in Ginkgo biloba recipients, whereas in placebo patients the mean increase was only 0.6 diopters. Definite clinical improvements were demonstrable in 9 of 10 GBE recipients versus 2 of 10 placebo patients and, as expected, Ginkgo biloba extract was significantly more effective overall. . . . This therapeutic trial, although including a limited number of case histories, seems to us to furnish proof of the value of GBE in the treatment of recent senile macular degeneration. In fact, after six months of treatment, a significant improvement was found in acuity of distance vision, which for the patient is obviously an essential criterion in his life relationships.

In experimental studies, especially with laboratory animals, GBE has proved to be an effective deterrent to free-radical damage to the retina of the eye. At least one study proved that GBE prevents diabetic retinopathy in alloxan-induced diabetic rats.[5] This suggests that *Ginkgo biloba* extract might also be useful in treating human beings with this disorder.

HEMORRHOIDS

It has been assumed that one in three Americans suffers from hemorrhoids or piles, which are swollen veins in the anus. Although a common side effect is rectal bleeding, the condition can be caused by more serious problems, such as cancer of the colon or rectum or ulcerative colitis. Other complaints include pain and itching, and ruptured veins which can cause bleeding.

The People's Medical Manual[1] observes:

People with chronic constipation who frequently strain to pass hard, dry stools are prone to develop piles. To reduce your chances of getting hemorrhoids, avoid straining while moving your bowels. Women may develop hemorrhoids during pregnancy, when the enlarged uterus may press on veins, interfering with the blood supply and causing irritation. Chronic coughing and jobs involving heavy lifting or long standing can predispose you to the condition.[1]

The manual says that hemorrhoids can happen when a tumor presses on veins in the rectum. Other disorders, such as liver conditions, may also be responsible. And people who are overweight are more likely to develop hemorrhoids than people with normal weight.

One of the most obvious causes of hemorrhoids is the lack of fiber in the diet. A diet that includes generous amounts of fruits, vegetables, whole grain and the like produces a large stool and quicker transit time through the gut, thus avoiding the straining that is associated with piles. Those who do not drink at least eight glasses of water daily are also prone to hemorrhoids, since liquids are required for proper digestion.

Hemorrhoids involve vascular circulation in the lower extremities, so it should come as no surprise that *Ginkgo biloba* extract has been used in proctology. A 1971 study reported noteworthy results in 36 patients who had advanced stages of hemorrhoids. There were good to very good results in 86 percent of the patients who were treated with *Ginkgo biloba* extract.[2]

Another study, this one in 1974, reported that *Ginkgo biloba* extract is very effective in treating the pain associated with rectal bleeding that is a result of inflammation.[3] There were less encouraging results with rectal fissures on the 20 patients.

Ginkgo biloba extract was also effective in treating patients who were scheduled to undergo sclerosing injections or elastic ligation for the treatment of hemorrhoids.[4] In one-third of the cases, the results were termed to be very satisfactory when receiving GBE. In 12 out of 20 patients, rectal bleeding was stopped and it was reduced considerably in four patients. There were 37 patients in the overall study.

Whether for hemorrhoids, cerebral blood flow or other vascular complaints, the efficacy of GBE has been shown in numerous world-wide studies.

FREE-RADICAL SCAVENGER

One of *Ginkgo biloba* extract's most notable attributes is its antioxidant, free-radical scavenging properties. Like vitamin A, beta carotene, vitamin C, vitamin E, selenium, and the like, GBE helps to purge the body of potentially damaging free radicals. One of the reasons is that GBE contains such bioflavonoids as quercetin, kaempferol and rutin, which enhance the actions of vitamin C.

Free radicals are highly unstable, highly reactive molecules or fragments of molecules characterized by an unimpaired free electron that is avid to grab most anything it can grab.

In *The Complete Guide to Anti-Aging Nutrients,* Sheldon Saul Hendler, M.D., Ph.D., says:

> Free radicals are typically toxic oxygen molecules that severely damage most of the molecules they grab hold of (cell membranes and fat molecules are favorite targets). It is one of the fundamental ironies of life that oxygen both sustains us and kills us. We often forget how toxic oxygen is, though we need only look around us to be reminded of it. Most of the rust and decay that we encounter is due to oxidation. Much of the "rust and decay" of the human body is due to the same thing.[1]

Dr. Hendler also notes that to protect us from the toxic forms of oxygen—such as superoxide, singlet oxygen, hydroxy radicals—which spin off as a result of various metabolic processes, plus others which enter the body via food and air pollution, or which are byproducts of radiation, viruses and the like, we depend on free-radical scavengers.

Some of these scavengers, such as superoxide dismutase and glutathione peroxidase, are enzymes that neutralize free radicals. Other scavengers include vitamin C and selenium.

If the free-radical scavengers are not present in sufficient quantity and at the right places at the right times, the free radicals can do considerable damage to cells and to the genetic program itself. A certain amount of this kind of damage occurs almost all the time in each of us. Free radicals also help promote cross-linking and may help create destructive and sometimes malignant mutations. In polyunsaturated fats, free radicals help produce aldehydes and other substances that may produce cancer and other damage. The free-radical theory of aging is probably the most useful theory we have at the present time—from the standpoint of finding practical means of delaying the effects of aging.[1]

The human body is especially vulnerable to free-radical attacks during ischemia or a lack of blood to specific organs, stated *Ginkgo Biloba Extract (EGb 761) in Perspective.*[2] With an overabundance of free radicals, the defense mechanisms are unable to nullify these foreign particles, and so peroxidation of membrane fats occurs and the damage follows. GBE, especially the flavonoid glycoside constituent, destroys these excess free radicals, the publication added.

In a series of in vitro studies, a solution of 500 mg/dl of GBE was shown to inhibit formation of the hydroxyl radical by 65 percent and adriamycyl radical generation by 50 percent. A 1988 study noted that GBE also halted lipid oxidation.[2,3]

In vitro and in vivo studies in France reported that GBE, because of its content of quercetin and kaempferol esters, is a potent free-radical scavenger.[4] In two animal studies, GBE had little effect on cardiac functional parameters, but it induced a significant decrease in the intensity of ventricular fibrillation. For human hearts, however, GBE provided effective protection against the electrocardiographic disorders induced by ischemia. For other types of diminished blood supply, the researchers noted that GBE brought a decrease in arrhythmia without any change in cardiovascular parameters.

Since a number of the in vitro and in vivo experiments have shown that GBE possesses antioxidant properties, the extract can theoretically offset many of the problems associated with excessive free-radical formation, according to F. V. DeFeudis.[5] This would include ischemia, problems associated with biological aging of tissues and those disease states that are related to ischemia and accelerated biological aging.

It is also of interest that [researchers] have purified and characterized an iron-containing SOD from Ginkgo biloba leaves. Such iron-containing SODs are found in only a few phylogenetically diverse higher plants. . . . They could possibly contribute to the antioxidant activity of intravenously-injected GBE if present in sufficient amount in this extract.

DOSAGE AND SIDE EFFECTS

In prescribing *Ginkgo biloba* extract for various health problems, researchers generally recommend a dosage of 40 mg three times daily. This is given as drops of a standardized GBE containing 40 mg/dl of extract, including 9.6 mg of flavonoid glycosides. Others have reported that the standardized extract contains 24 percent flavoglycosides.[1,2]

As reported in this chapter, other researchers have used higher dosages of *Ginkgo biloba* extract or GBE tablets. A slightly higher dosage of GBE is listed at 160 mg/day. This dosage, recommended for vertigo, tinnitus and peripheral vascular disease, can be given in divided doses, such as 80 mg twice daily or 40 mg four times each day. For these complaints, researchers have also suggested 20 to 80 mg of GBE given three times a day.

When not using the standardized GBE, it is apparently difficult to devise a dosage, since there may be extreme variations in the active constituents of the dried leaves and crude extracts. In any case, researchers recommend a standardized extract for content and activity.

There have been few side effects from taking *Ginkgo biloba* extract reported in the scientific literature. Higher dosages have sometimes produced complaints, perhaps because of the presence of various constituents that are generally removed or altered by the standard extraction process. The usual complaints include a mild gastrointestinal upset or headache. However, some people have reported severe allergic reactions from the ginkgo fruit pulp.[1]

In a 1988 study, only 33 of 8,505 patients receiving GBE experienced side effects. Nine of these patients did complain of gastrointestinal upsets.[2,3]

In other studies, several patients experienced mild nausea and heartburn.[2,4,6] And two patients given GBE suffered severe nausea and vomiting.[2,7]

Obviously, patients taking GBE for a mild to serious health problem should have their progress monitored by a physician or other professional. However, as a therapeutic aid for keeping well, many people can benefit from the daily use of over-the-counter preparations.

CONCLUSION

Few herbal remedies have been as extensively researched as has *Ginkgo biloba* extract, and the supplement seems to be one of our most useful therapies for many complaints. As reported throughout this book, GBE is an exceptional therapeutic agent for the treatment of some patients with Alzheimer's disease, asthma, impotence, tinnitus, migraine headaches, strokes, hemorrhoids, various circulatory disorders, depression and many other illnesses.

Since GBE is so compatible with other medications, it could prove to be useful in combination therapy, according to Francis V. DeFeudis.[1] As an example, 10 patients, ranging in age from 30 to 70, who suffered from painful diabetic neuropathy, experienced a significant decrease in pain on the fifth and tenth days of the study, after receiving GBE and folic acid, the B vitamin. GBE was prescribed at 87.5 mg/day, and the folic acid dosage was 3 mg/day.

Extensive clinical trials do not seem to be necessary to guarantee the safety of GBE-containing products, De Feudis says, since its efficacy has been well documented. And even if individual constituents in GBE continue to be analyzed, it is doubtful that they will be as significant as the total extract.

REFERENCES

INTRODUCTION

1. Graves, Arthur H. *Collier's Encyclopedia.* New York: Macmillan Educational Co., 1988, p. 102.
2. Glassman, Sidney F. *Academic American Encyclopedia.* Danbury, Conn.: Grolier, Inc., 1988, p. 184.
3. Chin, Wee Yeow and Keng, Hsuan. *Chinese Medicinal Herbs.* Sebastopol, Calif.: CRCS Publications, 1992, p. 90.
4. *A Barefoot Doctor's Manual.* Washington, D.C.: DHEW Publication No. (NIH) 75–695, 1974, p. 669.
5. *Ginkgo Biloba Extract (EGb 761) in Perspective.* Auckland, New Zealand: ADIS Press Limited, 1990, p. 1ff.
6. Wilford, John Noble. "Ancient Tree Yields Secrets of Potent Healing Substance," *The New York Times,* March 1, 1988, p. C3.
7. Corey, E. J., and Su, Wei-guo. "Total Synthesis of a C15 Ginkgolide—Bilobalide," *Journal of the American Chemical Society* 109:7534, 1987.

ALZHEIMER'S DISEASE

1. *Alzheimer's Disease: An Overview.* Chicago: Alzheimer's Association, 1987, unpaginated.
2. Emr, Marian. "Scientists Revise Estimates on Prevalence of Alzheimer's Disease," *National Institute on Aging News Notes,* November 9, 1989, unpaginated.
3. Evans, D. A., et al. "Clinically-Diagnosed Alzheimer's Disease: An Epidemiologic Study in a Community Population of Older Persons," *Journal of the American Medical Association,* November 10, 1989.
4. Root, Elizabeth J., Ph.D., and Longenecker, John B., Ph.D. "Nutrition, the Brain and Alzheimer's Disease," *Nutrition Today,* July/August 1988, pp. 11–18.
5. Weitbrecht, W. V., and Jansen, W. "Double-blind and Comparative (Ginkgo Biloba vs. Placebo) Therapeutic Study in Geriatric Patients

with Primary Degenerative Dementia—a Preliminary Evaluation." In "Effects of Ginkgo Biloba Extract on Organic Cerebral Impairment," A. Agnoli et al. London: Eurotext Ltd., 1985, p. 91–99.

6. Brown, Donald J., N. D. "Ginkgo Biloba—Old and New: Part II," *Let's Live*, May 1992, pp. 62–64.

7. *Current Medical Research and Opinion*, Vol. 12, No. 6, 1991. (no page nos.)

8. Moreau, P. "Un Nouveau Stimulant Circulatoire Cerebral," *Nouv. Presse Med.* 4:2401–2402, *1975.*

9. Eckman, F., and Schlag, H. "Kontrollierte Doppelblind-Studie zum Wirk-samkeitsnachweid von Tebonin forte bei Patienten mit Zerebrovaskularer Insuffizienz," *Fortschr. Med.* 100:1474–1478, 1982.

10. Funfgeld, E. W., editor. *Rokan (Ginkgo Biloba): Recent Results in Pharmacology and Clinic.* Berlin: Springer-Verlag, 1988, pp. 11–12ff; p. 49–54; p. 99; pp. 278–286.

11. Hindmarch, I. "Activite de Ginkgo Biloba sur la Memoire a Court Terme," *Presse Med.* 15:1592–1594, 1986.

12. Taillandier, J., et al. "Traitement des Troubles du Vieillissement Cerebral par L'Extrait de Ginkgo Biloba, Etude Longitudinale Multicentrique a Double Insu Face au Placebo," *Presse Med.* 15:1583–1587, 1986.

13. Funfgeld, E. W., and Stalleicken, D. "Dynamic-Brain Mapping," *TW Neurol. Psychiatr.* 2:136–142, 1987.

14. Bagne, C. A., et al. "Alzheimer's Disease: Strategies for Treatment and Research." In "Treatment Development Strategies for Alzheimer's Disease," F. Crook, et al., editors. Madison, Conn.: Mark Pawley Assn., 1986, pp. 585–636.

15. Funfgeld, E. W. "A Natural and Broad Spectrum Nootropic Substance for Treatment of SDAT—the Ginkgo Biloba Extract." In "Alzheimer's Disease and Related Disorders," Iqbak, K. et al., editors. New York: Alan Lissa, 1989, pp. 1247–1260.

16. Warburton, D. M. "Clinical Psychopharmacology of Ginkgo Biloba Extract." In *Rokan (Ginkgo Biloba): Recent Results in Pharmacology and Clinic.* Berlin: Springer-Verlag, 1988.

HEADACHES

1. DeFeudis, F. V. *Ginkgo Biloba Extract (EGb 761) Pharmacological Activities and Clinical Applications.* Paris: Elsevier, 1991, p. 142.

2. Dalet, R. "Essai du Tanakan dans les Cephalees et les Migraines," *Extr. Vie Med.* 35:2971–2973, 1975.
3. Devic, M. "Le Tanakan dans le Traitement de Fond de la Migraine," *Lyon Mediterr. Med.* 239:735–738, 1978.

ORGAN TRANSPLANTS

1. "Baboon Liver Recipient Dies," *Medical Tribune,* September 24, 1992, p. 1.
2. Amato, Ivan. "Chemists Make Age-Old Medicines from Ginkgo Trees in Laboratory," *The American Chemical Society News,* November 25, 1987. (no page nos.)
3. *The Complete Drug Reference.* Mount Vernon, N. Y.: Consumer Report Books, 1991, p. 422.

ASTHMA

1. DeFeudis, F. V. *Ginkgo Biloba Extract (EGb 761): Pharmacological Activities and Clinical Applications.* Paris: Elsevier, 1991, p. 92.
2. Brown, Donald J., N. D. "Ginkgo Biloba—Old and New: Part II," *Let's Live,* May 1992, pp. 62–64.
3. *Prostaglandins* 34(5), 1987.
4. Wilford, John Noble. "Ancient Tree Yields Secrets of Potent Healing Substance," *The New York Times,* March 1, 1988.

TINNITUS AND HEARING LOSS

1. Lewis, Howard R., and Martha E. *The People's Medical Manual.* Garden City, N.Y.: Doubleday & Co., Inc., 1986, p. 535; pp. 297–299.
2. Chesseboeuf, L., et al. "Comparative Study of Two Vasoregulators in Syndromes of Deafness and Vertigo," *Medicine du Nord et du l'Est* 5:534, 1979.
3. *Ginkgo Biloba Extract (EGb 761) in Perspective.* Auckland, New Zealand: ADIS Press Limited, 1990, p. 11ff.
4. Meyer, B. "A Multicenter Randomized Double-Blind Study of Ginkgo Biloba Extract Versus Placebo in the Treatment of Tinnitus," *Presse Med.* 15:1562–1564, 1986.
5. DeFeudis, F. V. *Ginkgo Biloba Extract (EGb 761): Pharmacological Activities and Clinical Applications.* Paris; Elsevier, 1991, p. 11ff.

6. Artieres, J. "Effets Therapeutiques du Tanakan sur les Hypoacousies et les Acouphenes," *Lyon Mediterr. Med.* 14:2503–2515, 1978.
7. De Amicis, E. "Attivita della Ginkgo Biloba nelle Otopatie da Arteriosclerosi," *Min. Med.* 64:4193, 1973.
8. Lallemant, Y. "Etude d'un Vasoregulateur d'Origine Vegetable en Therapeutique O.R.L.," *Gax. Med. France* 82:3153, 1975.
9. Natali, R. "Le Tanakan dans les Syndromes Cochleovestibulaires Relevant d'une Etiologie Vasculaire. Traitement de Long Cours," *Gaz. Med. France* 86:1381, 1979.

IMPOTENCE

1. Sikora, R. et al. "Ginkgo Biloba Extract in the Treatment of Erectile Dysfunction," *Journal of Urology* 141:188A, 1989.
2. *The Complete Drug Reference.* Mount Vernon, N.Y.: Consumer Reports Books, 1991, p. 945.

CIRCULATORY DISORDERS

1. Kunz, Jeffrey R. M., M. D., editor-in-chief. *The American Medical Association Family Medical Guide.* New York: Random House, 1982, p. 403.
2. Trormier, H., "Klinisch—Pharmakologische Untersuchungen ue ber den Effect eines Extraktes aus G. Biloba L. biem post Thrombotischen Syndrom," *Arzneim. Forsch.* 18:551, 1968.
3. Gautherie, M., et al. "Effet Vasodilatateur de l'Extrait de Ginkgo Biloba Mesure par Thermometrie et Thermographie Cutanees," *Therapie* 27:881, 1972.
4. Safi, N., and Galley, P. "Tanakan et Cerveau Senile. Etude Radiocirculographique," *Bordeaux Medical* 10:171–176, 1977.
5. *Ginkgo Biloba Extract (EGb 761) in Perspective.* Auckland, New Zealand: ADIS Press Limited, 1990, p. 14ff.
6. Courbier, R., et al. "Double-Blind, Cross-Over Study of Tanakan in Arterial Diseases of the Legs," *Mediterranee Medicale* 126:61–64, 1977.
7. Frileux, C., and Cope, R. "The Concentrated Extract of Ginkgo Biloba in Peripheral Vascular Disease," *Cahiers d'Arteriologie de Royal* 3:117–122, 1975.
8. Berndt, E. D., and Kramar, M. "Drug Treatment of Peripheral Arterial Occlusive Disease in Stage IIB," *Therapiewoche* 37:2815–2819, 1988.

9. Bohmer, D., et al. "The Treatment of PAOD (Peripheral Arterial Occlusive Disease) with Ginkgo Biloba Extract (GBE) or Pentoxyfyline," *Herz/Kreislauf* 20:5–8, 1988.

10. Bauer, U. "6-Month Double-Blind Randomised Clinical Trial of Ginkgo Biloba Extract Versus Placebo in two Parallel Groups in Patients Suffering from Peripheral Arterial Insufficiency," *Arzneim. Forsch.* 34:716, 1984.

11. Hemmer, R., and Tzavellas, O. "Zur Zerebralen Wirksamkeit eines Pflanzenpraparates aus Ginkgo Biloba," *Arzneim. Forsch.* 17:491, 1967.

12. Bastide, G., and Montsarrat, M. "Arterite des Membres Inferieurs. Interet du Traitement Medical apres Intervention Chirurgicale. Analyse Factorielle," *Gaz. Med (France)* 85:4523–4526, 1978.

13. DeFeudis, F. V. *Ginkgo Biloba Extract (EGb 761): Pharmacological Activities and Clinical Applications.* Paris: Elsevier, 1991, p. 117ff.

14. Ambrosi, C., and Bourde, C. "New Medical Treatment for Arterial Disease of the Lower Extremities: Tanakan. Clinical Trial and Liquid Crystal Study," *Gazette Medicale de France* 82(6):628–633, 1975.

15. Brown, Donald J., N. D. "Ginkgo Biloba—Old and New: Part II," *Let's Live*, May 1992, pp. 62–64.

16. *Arzneim.-Forsch. Drug Research*, Vol. 40, No. 5, 1990.

17. McCaleb, Rob. "Ginkgo Biloba: Ancient Healer," *Better Nutrition for Today's Living*, April 1992, pp. 32–37.

18. Blumenthal, Mark. "Ginkgo: A Living Fossil and Modern Medicine," *Better Nutrition for Today's Living*, February 1991, pp. 30–33.

EYE DISORDERS

1. Kunz, Jeffrey R. M., M.D., editor-in-chief. *The American Medical Association Family Medical Guide.* New York: Random House, 1982, p. 323.

2. Goldberg, Jack, et al. "Factors Associated with Age-Related Macular Degeneration," *American Journal of Epidemiology* 128(4):700–710, 1988.

3. *Ginkgo Biloba Extract (EGb 761) in Perspective.* Auckland, New Zealand: ADIS Press Limited, 1990, p. 17.

4. Lebuisson, D. A., et al. "Treatment of Senile Macular Degeneration with Ginkgo Biloba Extract: A Preliminary Double-Blind Study Versus Placebo," *Presse Med.* 15:1556–1558, 1986.

5. Doly, M. "Effect of Ginkgo Biloba Extract on the Electrophysiology of the Isolated Diabetic Rat Retina," *Presse Med.* 15:1480–1483, 1986.

HEMORRHOIDS

1. Lewis, Howard R., and Martha E. *The People's Medical Manual.* Garden City, N. Y.: Doubleday & Co., Inc., 1986, pp. 310–311.
2. Parnaud, E. "Ginkor en Proctologie Courant. A Propos de 36 Observations," *Therapeutique* 47:483, 1971.
3. Nora, J. "Place et Interet de Ginkor dans le Traitement des Affections Hemorroidaires," *Med Chir. Dig.* 3:437, 1974.
4. Soullard, J., and Conton, J. F. "Experimentation du Ginkor en Proctologie," *Sem. Hop. Paris* 54:1177, 1978.

FREE-RADICAL SCAVENGER

1. Hendler, Sheldon Saul, M.D., Ph.D. *The Complete Guide to Anti-Aging Nutrients.* New York: Simon and Schuster, 1985, pp. 32–33.
2. *Ginkgo Biloba Extract (EGb 761) in Perspective.* Auckland, New Zealand: ADIS Press Limited, 1990, p. 3.
3. Pincemail, J., and Deby, C. "The Antiradical Properties of Ginkgo Biloba Extract." In *Rokan (Ginkgo Biloba): Recent Results in Pharmacology and Clinic,* F. W. Funfgeld, editor. Berlin: Springer-Verlag, 1988, pp. 71–82.
4. Guillon, J.M, et al. "Effects of Ginkgo Biloba Extract on Two Models of Experimental Myocardial Ischemia." In *Rokan (Ginkgo Biloba),* p. 153.
5. DeFeudis, F. V. *Ginkgo Biloba Extract (EGb 761): Pharmacological Activities and Clinical Applications.* Paris: Elsevier, 1991, p. 51ff.
6. Duke, M. V., and Salin, M. L. "Purification and Characterization of an Iron-Containing Superoxide Dismutase form a Eukaryote, Ginkgo Biloba," *Arch. Biochem. Biophys.* 243:305–314, 1985.

DOSAGE

1. *Ginkgo Biloba Extract (Egb 761) in Perspective.* Auckland, New Zealand: ADIS Press Limited, 1990, p. 17.
2. Pizzorno, J. E., and Murray, M. T., editors. *A Textbook of Natural Medicine.* Seattle, Wash.: Bastyr College Publications, 1991, p. V Ginkgo 7.

POTENTIAL SIDE EFFECTS

1. Pizzorno, J. E., and Murray, M. T., editors. *A Textbook of Natural Medicine.* Seattle, Wash.: Bastyr College Publications, 1991, p. V Ginkgo 7.
2. Stalliecken, D., et al. "Continuous Observation of Cognitive Deficits. Results of a Multicentre Study Conducted on the Basis of Psychological Tests," *Therapiewoche (Suppl.* 2):1–8, 1988.
3. Dieli, G., et al. "Double-Blind Clinical Trial with Tanakan in Chronic Cerebral Insufficiency," *Lavoro Neuropshiatrico* 68:1–10, 1981.
4. Taillandier, J., et al. "Treatment of Cerebral Disorders Due to Aging with Ginkgo Biloba Extract. Longitudinal, Multicentre, Double-Blind Study Versus Placebo," *Presse. Med.* 15:1583–1587, 1986.
5. Vorberg, G., "Ginkgo Biloba Extract (GBE): A Long-Term Study of Chronic Cerebral Insufficiency in Geriatric Patients," *Clinical Trials Journal* 22:149–157, 1985.
6. Boudouresques, G., et al. "Value of Ginkgo Biloba, Extract in Cerebrovascular Pathology," *Medecine Practicienne* 598:75–78, 1975.

CONCLUSION

1. DeFeudis, F. V. *Ginkgo Biloba Extract (EGb 761): Pharmacological Activities and Clinical Applications.* Paris: Elsevier, 1991, p. 155.

PART FOUR

·◆·

SUMMARY: AS WE LIVE AND BREATHE

As long as we breathe (hopefully a long, long time) and take in oxygen, we expose ourselves to the risk of "oxidative stress." This condition means that the balance of oxidants versus antioxidants has shifted in favor of the oxidants. When the oxidants rule, the order of the day is free-radical production. The result is cell damage that contributes to the many diseases described in this book. The ultimate result of such damage is premature aging of our cells and of ourselves.

As we learned, free radicals are not all bad. Some are necessary for the body to produce energy and hormones and to fight infections. Free radicals are also part of many necessary enzymatic reactions. Too many free radicals, however, or their uncontrolled production, must be stopped. And the antioxidants must be there to do the job.

Which antioxidant is the most important? All of them! Each has a unique way to combat free radicals or acts in a special place in the body. And they work in concert. Vitamin E works in the fat-containing areas of the body, such as the membranes surrounding the cells. It sits in the cell membrane and neutralizes the free radicals. Without antioxidant protection, cell membrane fats can become rancid, undergoing the same process that happens to cooking oils and to meats left out too long. Becoming rancid will not improve your health!

Selenium works in concert with vitamin E and is part of many of the antioxidant enzymes made in the body.

Vitamin C works in the watery environments—between and inside cells. It is found in the blood plasma, lung fluid and eye fluid. It can also recycle vitamin E. After vitamin E destroys a free radical, it is inactive. Vitamin C converts it back to its antioxidant form so that it can work again. Beta-carotene is unique in that it works inside the cell, in the cell structures or organelles called the mitochondria. These are the cell's energy-producing factories. Free-radical production in the mitochondria will stop energy production and can kill the cell.

And so the evidence is in favor of the benefits of a good supply of antioxidants—a smorgasbord for your cells. They need to pick and choose from an array of all the antioxidant nutrients and get what they need, when they need it. This is the road to optimal health.

FINLAND, FRUIT FLIES AND FREE RADICALS

And what of the controversy that makes headlines such as "Finnish study shows increased cancer risk with antioxidants"? Although the solid results of more than two hundred published medical studies have reported the cancer-preventive effects of antioxidant nutrients, scare tactics still make better headlines. But unless you are a regular reader of the *New England Journal of Medicine* and actually read the article yourself, you would never learn the facts. According to several respected physicians and researchers, the study in question has credibility problems.

For one thing, the study participants were heavy smokers for over 35 years. The small doses of antioxidants would have little, if any, effect. This is especially true if some of these smokers already had cancer when the study started.

The study was done over a period of only five to eight years, hardly long enough to make strong conclusions about the outcome. According to researchers, writing the editorial in the same *New England Journal of Medicine*, the lack of a benefit over the time period of the study did not indicate that a significant benefit would not be found in substantially longer trials.

Another fact of the study was that the supplements were colored yellow with quinoline, an artificial food dye known to have cancer-causing properties. The subjects also drank alcohol, which is known to interfere with the activity of both beta-carotene and vitamin E. The vitamin E used in the study was the least active of the several forms available, and the beta-carotene dosage was one-tenth the dosage usually recommended for lung cancer prevention in smokers. The authors indicated that the finding of increased mortality may have been due to chance in spite of its statistical significance. In the first large study of the effects of aspirin on heart attack survivors, results suggested that it actually increased their risk of a second attack. But after many more trials, aspirin is now routinely given to such patients. "We have to wait and see what other tests demonstrate," says Demetrius Albanes, a leader of the Finnish study and a researcher at the U.S. National Cancer Institute.

HOW MUCH EVIDENCE IS ENOUGH?

How much evidence do we need before there is a consensus that antioxidants have a place in our diet and in our lives? The results of several large long-term studies may soon convince the skeptics. Many good studies have already yielded significant results:

1. Flavonoids: To see whether these compounds prevent cardio-vascular disease, 805 Dutch men aged 65 to 84 were followed for five years. Conclusion: flavonoid ingestion was significantly and inversely related to death from coronary heart disease (the more flavonoid, the less deaths). The relative risk of fatal coronary heart disease or first myocardial infarction among men with the highest flavonoid intake was about half that of those with the lowest intake. (Hertog, M.G.L., et al.: Dietary antioxidant flavonoids and risk of coronary heart disease: The Zutphen Elderly Study. *Lancet* 342:1007, 1993).

2. Vitamin E: At the University of Texas Southwestern Medical Center in Dallas, researchers gave 36 healthy men vitamin E and beta-carotene and observed a 40 percent reduction of oxidation of LDL, a promoter of atherogenesis (*Environmental Nutrition*, April, 1993, p.8.).

3. Antioxidants: Dr. JoAnn Manson of Brigham and Women's Hospital, Boston, reported on the large and long-term Nurses' Health Study, still in progress. Begun in 1976, the study has followed 87,245 women with questionnaires every two years. In 1980, the nurses began recording how often they ate foods containing antioxidants and whether they took vitamin supplements. Dr. Manson and her associates found that women who ate the largest amounts of vegetables had the lowest risk of stroke. Also, women who took supplements of at least 100 mg/day of vitamin E and at least 400 mg/day of vitamin C had a reduced risk of stroke, compared with those who did not take the vitamins. There was also a 22 percent lower risk of heart disease among those nurses with high intakes of beta-carotene and a 40 per-

cent lower risk of heart disease in those with high intakes (the median being 200 IU per day) of vitamin E (*New England Journal of Medicine* 1993; 328:1444–1449).

The highest reduction in stroke risk (adjusted for age and smoking history) was noted for the highest total consumption of antioxidants from both food and supplements.

4. Two studies involving more than 120,000 men and women, published in the *New England Journal of Medicine* in May 1993, showed that people who took daily vitamin E supplements of at least 100 units for two years reduced their risk of heart disease by 40 percent. The lowest tendency toward heart disease was found among those who consumed between 100 IU and 249 IU.

5. The EURAMIC study, a European multicenter case-control study on antioxidants, myocardial infarction and breast cancer, done in Finland, Germany, Israel, the Netherlands, Norway, Russia, Scotland, Spain and Switzerland, looked at the effects of vitamin E and beta-carotene in 683 men aged 35 to 70 who had suffered acute myocardial infarctions. Low adipose (fat) tissue beta-carotene concentrations were associated with a significantly increased risk of myocardial infarction, mainly in current smokers. Although no reduction of risk was attributed to the vitamin E levels, this finding was consistent with previous evidence suggesting that protection may only be seen in supplement users. This study measured only levels of vitamin E and carotene from a dietary source. The amount of E obtained from foods may be insufficient for protection against myocardial infarction.

6. A study of more than 25,000 adults in Maryland during 15 years of followup showed that serum levels of carotenoids (particularly beta-carotene) were consistently lower in persons that developed oral cancer. Those with the highest carotenoid intake had one-third the oral cancer risk of those with the lowest intake.

7. In the National Institute on Aging's Baltimore Longitudinal Study of Aging, researchers found that overall lipid profiles (LDL and HDL cholesterol levels, triglycerides) were positively affected by vitamin C in the older population group in the study. Higher vitamin

C levels were associated with lower LDL levels and higher HDL (considered most protective against heart disease).

WHO SAYS?

Are the people who believe in the benefits of antioxidants credible? First, let us hear the words of Albert Szent-Györgyi, M.D., Ph.D. Dr. Szent-Györgyi first isolated and identified ascorbic acid (vitamin C) in 1937. For this and other work in biochemistry, he received the Nobel Prize in 1937. For over 20 years he was Scientific Director of the National Foundation for Cancer Research at Woods Hole, Massachusetts. His research on vitamin C indicated an important difference between the biological action of ascorbic acid and that of other vitamins. "The other vitamins have a strong biological action only when they correct a lack, an avitaminosis, and have no striking activity once the deficiency is corrected. Ascorbic acid acts stronger the more there is of it, without reaching a sharp maximum. Ascorbic acid acts as the foundation of life . . . the more we have of it the more alive we are, a maximum being reached only with full health and vitality. An ample supply of the vitamin is especially necessary in youth when we are building our body, beginning with intrauterine life. My own personal experience shows that at the other end of life, in senescence, the need for ascorbic acid increases rather than decreases."

1. Jeffrey Blumberg, Ph.D., Professor of Nutrition and Associate Director of the USDA's Human Nutrition Research Center on Aging at Tufts University in Boston, said in an Interview (*Medical Tribune*, January 20, 1994): "Studies have suggested that the vitamin E dose that seems most protective [against LDL oxidation] is at least 100 IU. And no matter how healthy your diet is, you can't get that amount of vitamin E from your diet." Dr. Blumberg, who is Chief of the Antioxidants Research Laboratory at Tufts, takes an antioxidant supplement containing beta-carotene and vitamin E.

When asked in an interview published in *American Health* magazine (May, 1994) whether we should wait, as the FDA recommends,

for more scientific proof before allowing health claims for antioxidants, Dr. Blumberg said, "No. We can't wait until the final, un-
equivocal evidence is in. We don't have the luxury of saying, 'Maybe
in another 10 or 20 years, we'll have conducted more clinical trials
and we'll be absolutely sure.' I think when we're facing a problem
like we're facing now—a public health crisis in chronic disease—we
need to act."

2. The Washington, D.C.-based Alliance for Aging Research is an
eight-year-old nongovernmental, nonprofit group working to advance
medical research on human aging. They advise healthy adults to
sharply increase their intake of selected antioxidant nutrients. A panel
of their experts recommend that adults should consume from 250
mg to 1000 mg of vitamin C; from 100 IU to 400 IU of vitamin E;
and from 17,000 to 50,000 IU of beta-carotene each day as a means
of preventing chronic, age-related diseases. The organization's scientific panel, made up of respected scientific experts from reputable
research and academic institutions around the country, reviewed two
decades worth of research on antioxidants from over two hundred
clinical and epidemiological studies before coming up with its recommendations. According to Dr. Blumberg, one of the advisory panel
members, these ranges offer "maximum protection" from diseases
that become increasingly common with age.

3. Biochemist Earl Stadtman of the National Heart, Lung and
Blood Institute in Bethesda, Maryland, takes beta-carotene every
day—five times the Recommended Daily Allowance, and vitamins C
and E in doses dozens of times higher.

4. An article in the Tufts University Diet and Nutrition Letter
(May 1994) states: ". . . more and more evidence is coming to light
that the ability of antioxidant nutrients to fight free radicals is stronger
than anyone had imagined just a few decades ago. And that evidence
is not just in the form of results from animal research and cell studies." Examinations of some 85,000 women and 40,000 men showed
that those taking high levels of vitamin E—higher than what is available through daily food choices—had lower rates of heart disease.

5. Amy Subar, Ph.D, R.D., Dr. Gladys Block and Blossom Pat-
terson, M.A., of the National Cancer Institute reviewed 156 dietary

studies; 128 of those studies showed that a relatively high fruit and vegetable intake helped protect subjects from a wide range of cancers. They attributed the cancer-fighting effects to antioxidants.

6. Dr. Sheldon Margen, who heads the editorial board of the University of California's Berkeley Wellness Letter, was formerly reluctant to recommend supplementary vitamins on a broad scale for healthy people eating healthy diets, but has changed his mind. He and his staff no longer dispute the role which the antioxidant vitamins E, C, as well as beta-carotene, play in disease prevention. In addition to a very healthy diet—including at least five servings of fruits and vegetables daily—the Letter recommends antioxidant supplements.

7. Balz Frei, Ph.D., Assistant Professor of Nutrition and Toxicology, Harvard School of Public Health, stated that Vitamin C is able to protect LDL lipids (fats) completely from detectable oxidative damage in vitro. Vitamin E also provided considerable protection. Frei concludes that nutrient antioxidants may play an important protective role against LDL oxidation in vivo and thus may slow the progression of atherosclerosis.

8. Dr. Paul Lachance, professor of food science and nutrition at Rutgers University in New Jersey, says, "The RDAs are set only to prevent deficiencies, which has nothing to do with cancer and free-radical intervention. And in reality, the majority of Americans don't even meet these minimum levels."

9. Although Huber R. Warner, Ph.D., Director of Molecular Biology at the National Institute on Aging, says that the prescription for living longer is not as simple as taking vitamin supplements, he adds, "Supplementation with antioxidant vitamins may reduce the incidence and severity of chronic diseases by stabilizing free radical activity."

10. David Menzel, Ph.D., Chairman of the Department of Community and Environmental Medicine at the University of California, Irvine, believes that a drop in the level of vitamin E seen in humans following chronic exposure to air pollutants could be a harbinger of lung disease. One way to prevent lung disease later in life, Dr. Menzel suggests, might be to give children antioxidant vitamin supplements to counteract environmental pollutants.

11. Jean Lud Cadet, M.D., a researcher at the Neurological Institute at the Columbia University College of Physicians and Surgeons in New York City, has done research suggesting that free-radical damage from environmental pollutants is linked to the development of Parkinson's disease and other neurological disorders. Giving Parkinson's patients supplements of vitamin E (2000 to 3000 IU a day) delays the need for dopamine drug therapy and reduces anxiety and depression in these patients.

12. Allen Taylor, Ph.D., Director of the Laboratory for Nutrition and Vision Research at the USDA Human Nutrition Research Center at Tufts University, speculates that the use of antioxidants could decrease cataract surgery by one-half. Because vitamin C accumulates in the eye in direct proportion to the amount consumed, Dr. Taylor has tested the vitamin, with good results, in guinea pigs. He also found that giving humans 2 grams a day was protective. The National Eye Institute, part of the National Institutes of Health, is undertaking a long-term study to confirm Dr. Taylor's work. Results are expected in the year 2001.

13. At the Ninth Annual Meeting of the International Society for Oral Oncology, held in June 1994 at the National Institutes of Health in Bethesda, Maryland, one of the researchers, Dr. J. L. Schwarz, said, "Chemopreventive agents such as retinoids, carotenoids, tocopherols, and intracellular antioxidants such as glutathione have demonstrated the ability to inhibit oral carcinogenesis and regress established oral carcinoma in an animal model."

MORE EVIDENCE ON THE HORIZON

The following studies are in progress, but results are not expected for at least five years or more. The National Cancer Institute is running more than 40 clinical trials to assess the use of agents that could prevent cancer from developing. Among these agents are the retinoids, of which vitamin A is a member, as well as its precursor, beta-carotene. Studies include the protective effects against development of lung, skin, breast and cervical cancers. The antioxidants, including vitamin E, will be used to study effects on genetic changes or mutations and prevention of lung cancer.

In the 10-year-old Physicians Health Study, conducted at the Harvard Medical School, and one of the largest and longest running antioxidant investigations, the effects of beta-carotene supplements to prevent both cancer and heart disease are being tested on more than 22,000 male physicians. Preliminary results show that in a subgroup of 333 physicians with angina pectoris, the beta-carotene group showed a 44 percent reduction in all major coronary events (including myocardial infarction and cardiac death). A 49 percent reduction in all major vascular events (including stroke) has also been observed.

The Women's Health Study, involving some 40,000 female health professionals, is testing both beta-carotene and vitamin E.

The Health Professionals Follow-up Study, conducted through the Harvard School of Public Health, is an ongoing observation of 40,000 men aged 40 to 75 who are free of diagnosed coronary heart disease and diabetes and who do not have high blood cholesterol. Findings to date show that men in the top fifth of vitamin E intake (median intake, 419 IU per day) had a 40 percent lower risk of coronary disease than men in the lowest fifth (median intake, 6.4 IU).

The National Cancer Institute is sponsoring a study called CARET (Carotene and Retinol Efficacy Trials). The effectiveness of 30 mg of beta-carotene and 25,000 IU of vitamin A in preventing lung cancer in two high-risk groups (13,000 smokers and 4000 people exposed to asbestos) is being tested. The results are expected in 1999.

Tannins, antioxidants found in all plants, have been shown by Kansas State University cancer researcher Jean-Pierre Perchellet to slow the growth of skin cancer tumor cells. Studies are continuing in animals.

Nearly 2000 years ago, Pliny the Elder, the Roman naturalist, described the medicinal uses of milk thistle. Research today reveals that this plant contains silymarins, with strong antioxidant properties. Ginkgo, another plant antioxidant from the world's oldest tree species, has been used medicinally for at least several thousand years. Preliminary research is also being done on the antioxidant properties of bilberry, hawthorn, turmeric, savory, thyme, lemon balm, oregano and mints. (The antioxidant herbs will be discussed in a future *Nutrition Superbook* volume, *The Herbs*.)

Cosmetic researchers have found that vitamin E, besides being a skin moisturizer, may also have anti-inflammatory effects and may provide protection from the ultraviolet (UV) damage caused by sunlight. Sunlight is the most important cause of premature aging of the skin. It has been known for many years that UV light induces the production of free radicals. Vitamin E is absorbed through the skin and hair. Vitamin A is also absorbed through the skin, improving the skin's water barrier properties and helping it remain soft and plump. This makes it useful for treating dryness, heat and pollution effects. A continued vitamin A deficiency will cause acne-like blackheads, dull brittle hair and decreased skin elasticity. Beta-carotene and vitamin C also appear to protect against skin damage and dehydration caused by UV irradiation.

Breakfast cereals will soon contain more added antioxidant vitamins to make up for those destroyed in processing. Some companies have already developed antioxidant additives derived from natural sources (beta-carotene from Australian algae).

POINTS TO PONDER

• Why are there 20 to 100 times the amount of vitamin C in immune cells as in the blood?

• Human semen has eight times the vitamin C present in the blood. "Maybe it's there to protect sperm from DNA damage by oxidants," says Bruce Ames, Director of the National Institute of Environmental Health Sciences Center at the University of California, Berkeley. "Oxidation is the critical thing. Living is like getting irradiated, in some sense," said Ames. "More and more evidence is suggesting that vitamin C and E and beta-carotene are protective."

• Four out of ten Americans do not get even the daily minimum of 60 milligrams of vitamin C (the amount in one orange) from their diet. Our Paleolithic ancestors obtained about 440 milligrams daily by foraging for wild greens and fruit.

• Fewer than 10 percent of Americans currently eat the five daily servings of fruits and vegetables recommended by the National Cancer Institute.

• It was recently proved, in fruit flies, that the free-radical hypothesis of aging is valid. First proposed in 1956, the hypothesis states that old age is essentially the result of cumulative damage caused by free radicals. The fruit flies lived 30 percent longer when their levels of two antioxidant enzymes were boosted genetically. Dr. Richard Cutler, a research chemist at the National Institute on Aging's Gerontology Research Laboratory, observes that "this is really a beautiful confirmation" of the free-radical theory of aging. Of course, science is a long way from altering genes in humans to produce similar results. Dr. Cutler in a personal interview with the Editor, stated that he takes beta-carotene and believes it to be one of the most important anti-aging nutrients.

• An "optimal intake" of vitamin C, which, according to Linus Pauling would allow us to live an extra 12 to 18 years, is 3.2 to 12 grams/day. You would have to eat 45 to 170 oranges to get this amount from your diet.

• The LDL cholesterol carrier protein, if oxidized, contributes to atherosclerosis. The carrier also holds molecules of the antioxidants vitamin E, beta-carotene and coenzyme Q, assuming these nutrients are present in the diet.

• The RDA for vitamin C was not formulated based on its antioxidant properties, but only with regard to its effect in preventing scurvy.

• Dr. Meir Stampler, Associate Professor of Epidemiology at the Harvard School of Public Health, reported at an American Heart Association annual meeting in 1994 that taking vitamin E supplements of 100 IU or more every day cut the risk of heart disease in a large group of nurses by 46 percent. At a press conference, Dr. Stampler was asked if he took vitamin E. "Every day for years," he answered. When asked whether he recommended the same to others, he replied not yet and not until further studies could paint a clearer picture.

THE FUTURE

Where is antioxidant research leading us? Nature, in her generosity, has provided us with many more antioxidants than just those discussed above. Research has already begun on some of them, and new discoveries are being made every day. For example:

1. Alpha-carotene, a recently discovered member of the carotenoid family and extracted from palm oil, has been found to have significant antioxidant properties. It is believed to be 10 times more powerful than beta-carotene in helping to inhibit the production of skin, liver and lung cancer cells.

2. Other nutrients contained in plants, called phytochemicals, are complementary or similar in action to antioxidants. For example, broccoli and other cruciferous vegetables such as cauliflower and brussel sprouts contain a chemical known as sulforaphane, with confirmed cancer-fighting potential.

3. Some regions of France report low death rates from heart disease despite diets high in saturated fat. Red wine may be the protector, and it may not be the alcohol content. Red wine contains several phenolic compounds (flavonoid and nonflavonoid) with antioxidant properties. Researchers at the University of California, Davis, are finding that these compounds (catechins, flavonols, anthocyanins and soluble tannins) can protect LDL from oxidation and thus delay the onset of atherogenesis. Research is continuing.

4. Research at the Laboratory of Immunoregulation at the National Institute on AIDS, NIH, is investigating the effects of N-acetyl-L-cysteine, an antioxidant, in the suppression of the growth human immunodeficiency virus (HIV). Clinical trials using this agent, which lacks significant toxic side effects, are currently in progress.

If the newest advances in antioxidant research are exciting, then what will the continuation of this work bring? We can expect improvements in our health, especially in the *prevention* of disease and disability. This new way of thinking will be embraced not only by the public, but by the medical establishment as well. Faced with convincing statistical evidence and a better understanding of the nature of antioxidant protection, the barriers to acceptance of these ideas will fall.

The chaotic attempts to reform the health-care system may eventually cease, but whatever the outcome, prevention of disease will play a central role in holding down costs. The need to reduce health-care costs will give added momentum to antioxidant research.

We may eventually get the best of both worlds—antioxidants and good nutrition to prevent or alleviate disease and medical care if and when necessary. It has always been easier to prevent rather than treat a disease. Antioxidants will set you on this path.

How Young Are You? Good Habits, Nutrition & Antioxidants Can Slow Down Biological Aging

Jeffery S. Bland, Ph.D.

Some 60-year-olds look and act 40, and some 40-year-olds appear to be 60. The difference seems to be more a matter of how they live and what they eat than what sort of genes they inherited.

Dr. Edward Schneider, former director of the National Institutes on Aging, in an article titled "Recommended Dietary Allowances and the Health of the Elderly" (*New England Journal of Medicine*, vol. 314:157, 1986) suggested that RDAs for older individuals should be aimed at the maintenance of optimal physiological function and the prevention of age-dependent diseases and disorders. Dr. Frank Press, director of the National Academy of Sciences, agrees: "New scientific information suggests there may be a relationship between suboptimal nutrition and later-age disease."

Statements such as these are helping to focus scientific research on identifying the effects of various nutritional factors on health and on the prevention of biological aging. An individual's biological age may be different from his or her chronological age. Biological age is related to the individual's functional ability, while chronological age is age in birthdays. We can't change chronological age, but we may be able to do quite a bit to change our biological age.

ADD LIFE TO YOUR YEARS

In our own research, we have developed a comprehensive screening program to evaluate biological age and functional ability. We have found some individuals who function so poorly their biological age far exceeds their chronological age, and others whose functional vitality places them years younger than their chronological age. Genes, we are learning, are only one part in determining biological age. For most of us, biological age is related to how we eat, think and behave.

Gerontologists tell us the human life span has not changed much over the past several thousand years. It still is around 100 years, but human life *expectancy* has changed dramatically. Life expectancy, the average number of years we can expect to live, has increased approximately 20 years during this century, to more than 70 years. To reach our genetically determined life span of 100 years or more, we clearly have room to add years to our life expectancy. But it may be even more important to put added life in our years.

For many individuals, quality of life is more important than length. Biological age is a measure of quality of life; a lower biological age is associated with reduced disease risk and increased vitality.

As we age, our physiological functions typically decline. Most of us experience impairment of vision, hearing, memory, heart and lung capacity, sexuality, bones and joints. Some fortunate individuals, however, seem to defy the aging process. They remain active and robust well into their eighth or ninth decade without experiencing any significant decrease in function. Testing reveals their biological age is far below their age in birthdays.

DECLINES ARE PREVENTABLE

Nutrition plays a key role in slowing the biological aging process. As people grow older, their immune systems become less vigilant, and they are more susceptible to infectious diseases. Recently, investigators at the U.S. Department of Agriculture's Human Nutrition Research Center on Aging at Tufts University found that many declines in immune function can be prevented by improved nutrition. Dr. Jeffrey Blumberg examined the effect of vitamin E supplementation on the immune systems of healthy older adults and found that daily supplementation with 800 mg improved immune responsiveness (*American Journal of Clinical Nutrition*, vol. 52:557, 1990).

In a similar study, 97 older-aged patients in two Danish homes for the elderly participated in a nutrition supplementation program utilizing antioxidant nutrients selenium, zinc, vitamin C, beta-carotene, vitamin B6 and vitamin E. In this study, researchers from the University of Roskilde found significant improvements in the psychological scores of individuals who received vitamin supplementation compared to those who were not supplemented (*Biological Trace Element Research*, vol. 20:135, 1989).

Many people worry about losing their mental abilities as they age, and once again optimal nutrition can make a difference. Recent research from the U.S. Department of Agriculture in North Dakota found brain function and nervous system performance in older individuals are closely related to their nutritional status. Dr. Harold Sandstead and his colleagues at the USDA Research Center studied brain wave patterns in older people and found that alertness of the brain was closely correlated to vitamin B1, vitamin B2 and iron status (*American Journal of Clinical Nutrition*, vol. 52:93, 1990). The authors suggested that research on nutrition and psychological function will help us better maintain the functional integrity of the brain as we age.

The emerging theme from this research is that accelerated biological aging and reduced functional capacity are related not just to one's genes but, more importantly, to lifestyle, nutrition and environment. An individual who smokes, drinks excessive alcohol, leads a sedentary life, is under extraordinary stress, or consumes a suboptimal diet has a much higher risk for increased biological aging.

REDUCE AGING, BOOST VITALITY

Certain nutrients, when consumed at levels higher than those found in the standard American diet, can actually help reduce the rate of biological aging and improve vitality and resilience. As scientific investigators in nutrition and aging are pointing out, there is now strong evidence to suggest that even slight nutritional deficiencies can have an adverse impact on the rate of biological aging, the integrity of brain function, and the quality of daily living.

The challenge is to identify each individual's specific nutritional needs and optimize the diet based upon his or her genetic requirements in order to decrease biological age and slow the aging process.

Smog Peril Grows, Seniors at High Risk; Antioxidants Help

Crop Damage Also a Hazard; Vitamins E, C and A, Selenium, Cysteine, Glutathione, SOD Fight Free Radicals in Deadly Ozone-Oxide Pollutant Brew

The caveman faced his hazardous life armed with nature's answers but he didn't have the environmental burdens modern man has to contend with. What's a saber-toothed tiger or a cave bear compared to air, water, and food pollution? If the caveman outran the peril the danger was over, at least for the time being. Environmental peril is insidious, always present, sometimes invisible, and you can't outrun it. In fact, if you run, you invite the amorphous enemy into your lungs and eyes.

I'm referring to one major problem attacking our metropolitan areas and their inhabitants: SMOG.

Smog contains ozone and nitrogen oxides, two of the most deadly toxins known, and responsible for more human disease and death than any other toxin or pollutant. And humans are not the only victims. In the United States alone, annual crop loss from the effects of smog amounts to over $86 million, and the cost is going higher.

The Clean Air Act established a 1987 deadline for ozone levels, mandating that all communities had to reduce the amount of ozone in their air so that it would not exceed 0.12 parts per million in any 24-hour period. Now, the Environmental Protection Agency's latest estimate is that few if any of the metropolitan areas will be able to accomplish the proposed reduction.

That's bad news for all of us, and particularly for older people, to whom smog is a proven danger—and note that the percentage of seniors is increasing yearly. Natural levels of ozone do appear in the atmosphere as it diffuses down from the stratosphere; normally this amounts to about 0.01 ppm. But when we run our automobiles and pour our hydrocarbon wastes into the air, gasoline fumes and other material mix with sunlight and heat and the result is ozone at a level that threatens the health of all people subjected to high concentrations.

Los Angeles, where the term "smog" was coined about 40 years ago, is apt to be hard hit unless the wind is moving the air in the basin in which it sits. If it isn't, the ozone level frequently reads as high as 0.3 ppm. On those smog alert days nursing homes report a sharp increase in deaths among their elderly patients.

LUNGS HARMED

In high concentrations, ozone affects our pulmonary capability in a strongly negative manner, increasing our susceptibility to all forms of respiratory diseases. How much ozone must be present to bring about problems? According to the EPA, 0.3 ppm can cause a significant decrease in lung vital capacity, and even with concentrations as low as 0.24 ppm, pulmonary measurements show a decrease in operational ability. It's hard to realize that we're only dealing with fractions of one part per million, but that tiny amount is enough to do it.

The body is not completely helpless against the ozone onslaught. Ozone is an oxidant, and the body defends against dangerous oxidation with antioxidants and with enzymes. The antioxidants are mainly vitamin E (alpha-tocopherol), vitamin C (ascorbic acid), selenium, zinc, and the amino acid L-cysteine. The enzymes include superoxide dismutase (SOD) and glutathione peroxidase.

Vitamin A also plays a strong role in controlling oxidant free radicals, particularly in combination with vitamins E and C. Vitamin A appears in nature in two forms, that found in animals and fish which we know as the oil-soluble vitamin A found in cod liver oil and other fish oils, and the vegetable form called beta-carotene. Although there is some evidence that vitamin A from the animal kingdom can be stored in the body and cause possible side reactions if used in excessive amounts, beta-carotene appears to be an absolutely safe way for humans to insure adequate intake without fear.

Beta-carotene can be considered to be two molecules of vitamin A linked together. If the links remain intact there seems to be no vitamin A activity, but when they are broken through the intervention of a body enzyme, two molecules of vitamin A action are released. Since the body will separate the molecules only if there is need for vitamin A, safety is assured.

CAVEMAN'S ADVANTAGES

Since the human race has survived and left the caves for the concrete buildings we now call home, it appears that the caveman was able to obtain sufficient raw material from the food he ate to ward off the few oxidants in his environment. It is doubtful if we can do the same in our highly polluted environment without resorting to some supplemental program. Supplemental vitamin E, in particular, appears to be a leader in body protection.

Vitamin E is active against ozone and nitrogen dioxide, both present in smog and both among the most harmful of its ingredients. Animals supplemented with vitamin E are able to resist the deleterious effects much longer than animals who are deficient in vitamin E. They also live longer. When rats supplemented with E were exposed to a concentration of 1 ppm of ozone they survived for 18 days, while a control group lasted only 8 days.

It is of course prudent to keep supplementation at a reasonable and modest level, but you should be aware that vitamin E and vitamin C are among the least toxic of the vitamins. For example, vitamin E has been tested in humans at levels up to 55,000 international units for five months and 3,000 IU for up to eleven years without any reported side effects.

Therefore, at least in what are deemed to be risk areas, the low toxicity of antioxidant vitamins and their potential for defending against the oxidative stressors suggest the value of their use on a daily basis. Unless otherwise indicated, 400 IU of vitamin E and up to 1000 milligrams of vitamin C appear to be adequate protection in most cases. Certainly it would be better to eliminate the causes of ozone and nitrogen oxides but since there appears to be little chance of that in the near future, we modern cavemen have to take special precautions.

GLOSSARY &
BIBLIOGRAPHY

—◆—

GLOSSARY

Aldosterone A steroid hormone made by the adrenal gland and which acts on the kidney to regulate salt and water balance.

Amino acid The building blocks from which proteins are made.

Angiopathy Vascular disease

Angiotensin A protein in the blood that causes the release of aldosterone from the adrenal gland and can also raise blood pressure.

Anion A molecule with a negative charge.

Antioxidant Substance made in the body or found in food, that neutralizes the harmful effects of free radicals.

Arteriopathy Arterial disease

Azo dye A yellow dye used in food products. It is very reactive with cell membranes and causes free-radical damage.

BCNU A drug used for treating cancer.

Beta blocker A heart medicine used to treat angina and high blood pressure.

Carcinogen A cancer-causing substance

Cardiac index The cardiac output per square meter of body surface area.

Cardiac output The volume of blood ejected from the heart per minute.

Catalyst A substance that causes a chemical reaction to go faster, but is not itself changed during the reaction.

Catecholamine A group of substances in the body that function mainly as neurotransmitters.

Chymotrypsin An enzyme from the pancreas that helps digest proteins.

Citric acid cycle A complex metabolic cycle which produces energy for body reactions, also called the Krebs cycle.

Croton oil A cancer-promoting substance.

Crucifers A family of plants that includes cabbage, collard greens, cauliflower, broccoli and others.

Dehydroascorbate An oxidized form of ascorbic acid (vitamin C).

Denaturation Changes in a protein brought about by heat or chemical reactions that interfere with its action.

Diastolic Blood pressure when the ventricles of the heart are relaxing and filling.

DMBA A carcinogen.

DNA Deoxyribonucleic acid, the genetic material of the cell that controls heredity and directs cellular processes.

DPPH A type of free radical.

Duodenal Pertaining to the first portion of the small intestine.

Electron A particle that, when paired, keeps molecules stable.

Electron transport chain A system of energy production and transport found in the mitochondria of the cell.

Embolism A blood clot that is stuck in an artery.

Empiric Results based on experience or observation.

Enzyme A compound that helps reactions occur in the body without entering into the reaction itself. It is a reusable catalyst that controls a reaction.

Epidemiological Study of the characteristics of populations of people.

Epigastric Referring to the upper central region of the abdomen.

FAD Flavin adenine dinucleotide—a molecule derived from the B vitamin riboflavin that takes part in many oxidation-reduction reactions in the body.

FASEB Federation of American Societies for Experimental Biology.

Fatty acid The chemical building blocks from which fats and oils are made.

Fibrinolytic Dissolving a blood clot.

Free radical Highly reactive chemical particle produced during normal body oxidation of foods or as a result of environmental pollutants.

Gluconeogenesis A process that takes place in the liver whereby glucose is made from proteins.

Glycosuria The presence of high amounts of glucose in the urine.

Heterozygous A genetic term where only one copy of a gene is present and where the gene characteristic may not be expressed.

Histamine A substance found in body cells that, when released, causes inflammation or allergic symptoms.

Histidine decarboxylase The enzyme that helps produce histamine.

Homozygote A genetic term indicating that there are two copies of a gene and a greater chance that the gene will be expressed.

Hyperglycemia An excess of glucose (sugar) in the blood.

Hyperlipidemic Having an abnormally high concentration of fats in the blood.

Hypoglycemia Low blood glucose (sugar).

In vitro Conducting experiments in the laboratory as opposed to in a live animal or human.

In vivo Conducting an experiment in a live animal or human.

Inotropic effect Affecting the force or energy of muscular contractions. (The heart is a muscle.)

Interferon A protein made in the body or produced in the laboratory from human cells. It is used as a treatment for some types of cancer.

Isoprene A structural unit in a molecule.

IU International units; a standard unit of measurement used to measure nutrients including vitamin A, vitamin E and beta-carotene.

Lipoproteins Complex substances made of proteins, lipids and cholesterol. According to their density when separated by ultracentrifugation, a distinction is made between the low-density (LDL) and the high-density (HDL) lipoproteins.

Macrophage An immune system cell that scavenges bacterial and other foreign material in the blood and tissues.

Macular Degeneration A pigmentary disturbance in the macular region of the eye, bringing a loss of central visual acuity.

Malondialdehyde A product of free radical damage that can destroy cells.

MCA A carcinogen.

mcg Microgram—a metric unit of measurement, 1/1,000,000 of a gram.

Metabolism The sum of all the chemical and physical changes that take place within the body and enable its continued growth and functioning.

Metabolite A substance that takes part in the process of metabolism in the body.

mg Milligram—a metric unit of measurement, 1/1000 of a gram.

Microsomes A part of the cell membrane that takes part in the production of proteins.

Mitochondria Structures inside a cell that are the location of the cell's energy production machinery.

Molecule Building blocks in nature such as oxygen, glucose, fatty acids, amino acids and DNA.

Mucopolysaccharide Carbohydrates that act as support structures in connective tissue in the body.

Mucosa A mucous membrane, such as that lining the mouth or stomach.

Mutagenic Causing alterations in genetic material.

Myelin A substance made of protein and lipid (fat) that protects the nerves, especially in the brain.

Myocardial Pertaining to the heart muscle.

NAD Nicotinamide adenine dinucleotide—a molecule derived from the B vitamin niacin and important in the energy transport processes in the body.

NCI National Cancer Institute.

Neurotransmitter A chemical substance which causes the transmission of nerve impulses at nerve junctions (synapses).

Normolipidemic Having a normal level of fats in the blood.

Oxidant A substance that attacks a molecule and produces a free radical.

Oxidation The process of removing an electron from a molecule and creating a free radical.

Oxidative phosphorylation A process taking place in the mitochondria of the cell that contributes to energy production.

Peroxidation A type of oxidation that results in the formation of peroxides in body tissues.

Phospholipids A fat or lipid containing phosphorus found in high quantities in the brain.

Placebo A substance that is ineffective but may relieve a medical condition because the patient believes it will do so.

Plasma The straw-colored fluid in which blood cells are suspended in the cardiovascular system.

Polyunsaturated fat A fat usually found in vegetables or marine (fish) oils.

Prospective study A study that is ongoing and looks at what people are doing now and predicts what they will do in the future.

Prostaglandin A hormonelike substance found in many parts of the body which regulates many metabolic processes.

Proteolytic The property of a substance that breaks down proteins.

Reducing agent (Reductant)—the electron donor in an oxidation-reduction reaction.

Retinopathy Disease of the retina.

Retrospective study A study that looks at past behavior of people.

RNA Ribonucleic acid, the genetic material in the cell that regulates protein production.

Saturated fat A "hard" fat, usually from animal sources and solid at room temperature.

Scorbutogenic Causing the condition of scurvy (vitamin C or ascorbic acid deficiency).

Spasmolytic Relaxing smooth muscles.

Stroke volume The volume of blood ejected from the heart with each beat.

Systolic Blood pressure when the ventricles of the heart are contracting.

Telangiectasia Dilatation of the superficial blood vessels.

Teratogenic Causing malformations in a fetus.

Thermogenic Producing heat.

Thyroxin One of the hormones made and secreted by the thyroid gland.

T Lymphocytes Mononuclear white blood cells having the property of destroying target cells.

Tumorigenic A substance causing a tumor.

Unsaturated fat A fat that is liquid (oil) at room temperature and usually found in vegetable and marine oils.

BIBLIOGRAPHY

Barilla, Jean, M.S. A Radical Way of LIfe. *The Challenge of the Cancer Federation.* Moreno Valley, Calif. Spring, 1993.

Barilla, Jean, M.S. Free radicals, aging tied. *Mobile Press Register*, Mobile, Ala. January 30, 1985.

Becker, Gail L., R.D. *The Antioxidant Pocket Counter.* New York: Times Books (Random House), 1993.

Borek, Carmia, Ph.D. Maximize Your Health-Span with Antioxidants: The Baby-Boomer's Guide, July 1995.

Kardinaal, A.F.M., Kok, F.J., Ringstad, J., et al. Antioxidants in adipose tissue and risk of myocardial infarction: The EURAMIC Study. *Lancet* 342(8884):1279–1384, 1993.

Lin, David J. *Free Radicals and Disease Prevention. What You Must Know.* New Canaan, Conn.: Keats Publishing Inc., 1993.

Pauling, Linus. *How to Live Longer and Feel Better.* New York: W. H. Freeman and Co., 1986.

Szent-Györgyi, Albert. *The Living State and Cancer.* New York and Basel: Marcel Dekker, 1978.

APPENDICES

APPENDIX A

◄●►

More About Free Radicals

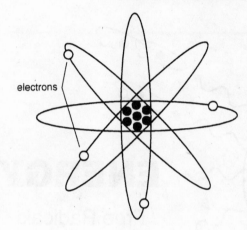

Molecules such as oxygen, fatty acids, amino acids, glucose and DNA are held together by electrons.

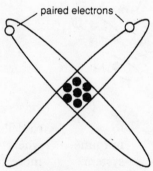

Stable molecules have paired electrons.

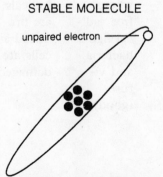

An unpaired electron produces an unstable molecule—a reactive free radical. It will take an electron from a nearby stable molecule and a destructive chain reaction will occur. Antioxidants stop this process.

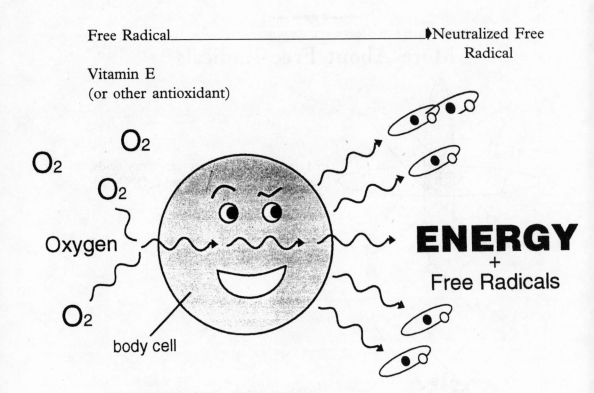

Free Radical _____ ▸Neutralized Free Radical

Vitamin E
(or other antioxidant)

O_2

O_2

O_2

O_2

Oxygen

O_2

body cell

ENERGY
+
Free Radicals

Free radicals are a natural by-product of the energy-producing reactions in the body. But some free radicals can cause damage. Antioxidants prevent this damage.

to immune system where free radical fights bacteria and viruses (good)

to cells where more free radicals are produced as cells are damaged

Free Radicals Shouldn't Be Free!

Minute Molecules Can Wreak Havoc

Most of us are aware that certain bacteria, viruses, fungi, and parasites can destroy health if allowed to multiply within us. We also know that the only protection we have is the body's natural defenses . . . white blood cells, macrophages, antibodies, lymphatic tissue and the thymus gland.

However, a radically different adversary in the battle to maintain health has been uncovered . . . substances called free radicals.

For over 30 years, scientists and medical researchers have substantially increased their knowledge of free radicals and their roles in disease. Many consider free radical processes the major common denominator in the cause and progression of numerous disease conditions, conditions which before seemed unrelated. Today, free radicals are one of the most exciting areas of research, perhaps because natural defenses against these harmful substances are very simple nutrients and enzymes, the antioxidants.

Simply described, free radicals are molecules with electrons which are unpaired. Molecules are basic building blocks in nature, such as oxygen, fatty acids, amino acids, glucose and DNA. Molecules are held together by electrons. Stable molecules have electrons that are in pairs, like a buddy system. But if a molecule has an electron which does not have a partner, it becomes unstable and reactive . . . a free radical. It will steal an electron from a stable molecule.

Once the stable molecule loses an electron, it becomes another free radical. This second free radical will steal an electron from a third molecule, and a destructive cycle begins. Each time a molecule loses an electron, it is damaged and will damage another molecule.

WHERE DO THEY COME FROM?

Free radicals come from three sources. First, our bodies form free radicals every moment. Living cells need energy to live. This energy comes from reactions involving various substances and oxygen. During this process, intermediates of oxygen are formed, including superoxide and hydroxyl radicals. Exercise, illness, and certain medications increase oxygen-related reactions in our bodies, consequently increasing the number of free radicals formed.

Moreover, our immune systems specifically produce free radicals to destroy bacteria and viruses. When we are invaded by harmful microorganisms and our immune system works overtime, tremendous amounts of free radicals are produced to try to overcome the infection. During these times, controlling the flood of free radicals is vital to protect healthy tissues from damage.

TOXIC ENVIRONMENT

Free radicals also come from the environment. Air pollution, tobacco smoke, excessive radiation, toxic waste and runoff, herbicides, and pesticides all form free radicals, which we inhale or ingest. For instance, ozone is an extremely reactive air pollutant resulting from vehicle exhaust. When we breathe in ozone, it forms free radicals in our lung tissue. Moreover, since blood is constantly being pumped to the lungs for oxygen, ozone-induced free radicals may involve blood cells, diminishing the oxygen supply.

Many of the health woes of the past few decades are directly related to the increasing use of dangerous chemicals and technologies, leading to vastly more free radical production than was the case a few generations ago. Hopefully, the "green movement" toward cleaning and preserving our environment will result in tremendous reduction of free radical sources in the environment, substantially decreasing chronic and acute diseases. Earth will treat us well if we treat her well.

DAVID J. LIN

Antioxidant Nutrients May Act As Armor Against Free-Radical Damage, Cancer

Supplements May Also Alleviate Side Effects of Traditional Toxic Drugs

A revolution in the concept of treating disease is on the horizon that will help displace the dependence upon toxic drugs. Instead, many physicians are turning to natural, safe substances, such as the antioxidant nutrients beta-carotene, vitamin C, vitamin E, and selenium as the body of scientific evidence continues to substantiate the effectiveness of such therapies.

Let's look at the etiology of cancer. Cancer is the uncontrolled growth and multiplication of cells, resulting in their consuming all available nutrients until healthy cells are starved to death. A cancerous cell is simply a once-normal cell which can't stop growing and multiplying. Researchers believe much of the cause of this behavior lies on a genetic level.

A normal cell contains genes which tell it when to stop growing. If these genes are mutated, such as by free-radical destruction, then the "stop" instruction is lost, and the cell will continue to grow without limitation. The situation is similar to someone removing a stop sign so that cars continue through an intersection without concern or caution, with the potential for devastation.

Another scenario may be that free radicals turn on a gene which overrides any other gene's instruction to stop growing, like someone short-circuiting a traffic light to always be green. Again, the cell receives no instruction to stop growing and will continue devouring nutrients.

The cancerous cell keeps growing and then multiplies. Now, there are two wildly growing cells, which eventually multiply to form 4 cancer cells, then 8, 16, 32 and very quickly, millions and billions. More and more nutrients are demanded by the voracious metabolism of these cells, producing enormous amounts of free radicals which then destroy surrounding tissues. Soon, not enough nutrients are available and the body starves to death.

EARLY STAGES

In the early stages of cancer, the immune system tries to contain the proliferating mass by surrounding it with a tough, protective net. Hopefully, the cancer will thus be controlled. However, free radicals can destroy the protective net, allowing the cancerous mass to continue growing.

Ironically, some of the modern treatments for cancer use drugs or radiation to destroy cancerous cells which in turn generate huge amounts of free radicals. Unfortunately, this barrage of free radicals will indiscriminately destroy healthy cells as well. As a result, the patient under this treatment may experience profound side effects, such as the loss of hair, weight, energy, immunity, and mental alertness. Some have commented that in certain cases, chemotherapy and radiotherapy may be more deadly to the patient than the original cancer!

Hopefully, with a clearer understanding of how cancer starts and progresses, medical researchers will be able to help patients more effectively. Already, the use of the free-radical fighter nutrients or antioxidants has been found to alleviate many of the toxic side effects which occur during chemotherapy. Prevention is better than cure. Antioxidants may help substantially reduce the risk of developing cancer and other degenerative diseases.

Yet, just as no miracle drug will ever cure all disease, so no miracle nutrient will. Health depends upon much more than a simple formula. Antioxidants may help provide many healthy benefits but will never replace health-supportive diets and lifestyles.

DAVID J. LIN

———— • ————

Free Radical–Fighting Foods

TOP SOURCES OF ANTIOXIDANTS

BETA CAROTENE

Carrots (and juice)
Sweet potatoes
Pumpkin
Cantaloupe
Leafy greens (spinach, kale, mustard, collard, swiss chard)
Winter squash
Fresh or dried apricots
mangoes and persimmon
Broccoli

VITAMIN C

Melons (especially **cantaloupe**)
Citrus fruits and juices (oranges and grapefruits)
Red and green peppers
Leafy greens (mustard, turnip, kale, collard)
Strawberries
Papaya, kiwi, **mangoes**
Cruciferous vegetables (**broccoli**, cauliflower, brussels sprouts, kohlrabi, cabbage)
Tomatoes and tomato juice
Sweet potatoes, with skin
Blackberries and raspberries

VITAMIN E

Seeds
Nuts and peanut butter
Vegetable oils
Wheat germ
Leafy greens (fresh spinach, kale, collard)
fish and shellfish
avocados
mangoes
whole grain products

SELENIUM

Cashews
Halibut
Meat
Oysters
Salmon
Scallops
Tuna
Eggs
Garlic

Foods in bold type are the best sources.

APPENDIX C

———◦———

Disorders Associated with
Free Radical Damage

Adverse drug reactions
Alcohol-induced liver damage
Arthritic tissue damage
Cancer
Cardiac toxicity from adriamycin
Cataracts
Coronary heart disease
Diabetic cataracts
Immune hypersensitivity
Inflammatory bowel disorders
Neurological degeneration
Red blood cell damage
Traumatic inflammation

Adapted from: Bland, J., Ph.D. The Nutritional Effects of Free Radical Pathology. In: *A Year in Nutritional Medicine*. New Canaan, Conn.: Keats Publishing, Inc. 1986.

APPENDIX D

———◆———

Recommended Amounts of Antioxidants
including dietary sources and supplements

Antioxidant	U.S. RDA	Recommended Preventive Amount per day
Vitamin A	5,000 IU	12,500 IU[1]–25,000 IU[2]
Vitamin C	60 mg	1,000 mg[1]–18,000 mg[2]
Vitamin E	30 IU (20 mg)	300,800 IU[1]–1600 IU[2] (133–533 mg)
Beta-carotene	no RDA* established	15 mg[2]

*U.S. Department of Agriculture suggested diet provides 5–6 mg/day.

1. Becker, Gail L., R.D. *The Pocket Antioxidant Counter.* New York: Times Books (Random House) 1993.

2. Pauling, Linus *How to Live Longer and Feel Better*, New York: W.H. Freeman and Co., 1986.

APPENDIX E

———◆———

Antioxidant Food Values

Food	Beta-carotene (I.U.)	Vitamin A (I.U.)	Vitamin C (mg)	Vitamin E (mg)
FRUITS				
Apple, fresh + skin, (1 med.)	tr	73	8	1
Apricots, fresh (3 med.)	1	1,109	11	1
Banana, fresh (1 med.)	tr	92	10	tr
Blueberries, fresh	tr	145	19	1
Cantaloupe, fresh, (½ med.)	8	12,688	195	1
Cherries, fresh, sweet, (½ cup)	tr	155	5	tr
Grapes, fresh (½ cup)	tr	58	9	tr
Grapefruit, fresh (1 med.)	tr	361	100	1
Kiwi fruit, fresh (1 med.)	tr	133	74	1
Mango, fresh (1 med)	5	8,061	57	2
Orange, fresh (1 med.)	tr	269	70	tr
Peach, fresh (1 med.)	tr	465	6	1
Pear, fresh (1 med.)	tr	33	7	1
Plum, fresh (1 med.)	tr	213	6	tr
Strawberries, fresh/frozen, (1 cup)	tr	40	84	tr
Watermelon, fresh (1 slice)	1	1,764	46	0
VEGETABLES				
Artichokes, cooked (1 cup)	tr	149	8	tr
Asparagus, fresh/frozen, cooked (1 cup)	tr	736	22	1
Broccoli, fresh/frozen, cooked (½ cup)	4	1,740	37	1
Carrots, fresh/frozen, cooked (½ cup)	11	19,152	2	1
raw (½ cup)	5	8,511	5	tr
Cauliflower, fresh/frozen, cooked (½ cup)	tr	20	28	tr

Food	Beta-carotene (I.U.)	Vitamin A (I.U.)	Vitamin C (mg)	Vitamin E (mg)
Cucumber, raw (½ cup)	tr	23	2	tr
Green beans, fresh cooked (½ cup)	tr	356	6	tr
Lettuce, raw (1 cup)	tr	182	2	tr
Pepper, green, raw (½ cup)	tr	316	45	tr
Pumpkin, cooked, canned (½ cup)	16	27,016	5	1
Spinach, fresh/frozen, cooked, (½ cup)	4	7,395	12	2
Tomato, raw (1 cup)	1	1,122	34	1
canned (1 cup)	1	1,450	36	3
juice (1 cup)	1	1,349	44	0
Carrot juice (1 cup)	36	63,347	21	1
Vegetable juice cocktail (1 cup)	2	2,831	67	0

For a complete listing see Becker, Gail L., R.D., *The Antioxidant Pocket Counter*. New York: Times Books (Random House), 1993.

For additional information on antioxidants please contact:

Bronson Pharmaceuticals
1945 Craig Rd. P.O. Box 46903
St. Louis, Missouri 63146
1–800–235–3200
(mail order nutritionals, physician's newsletter)

Carlson Laboratories
15 College Drive
Arlington Heights, Ill. 60004
1–800–323–4141
(Retail stores, literature)

Solgar Vitamin and Herb Company
500 Willow Tree Road
Leonia, New Jersey 07605
201–944–2311
(Retail stores, literature)

Henkel Corporation
P.O. Box 2016
LaGrange, IL 60525
(Literature on antioxidants)

ABOUT THE AUTHORS

The Nutrition Superbooks are based on material previously published in Keats Publishing's Good Health Guide series and in its newspaper *Health News & Review* (now *Health News Naturally*). Here are brief biographical sketches of the contributors to this volume.

Jeffrey Bland, Ph.D. is a promoter of good health—whether he is teaching, practicing, lecturing or writing, he is actively committed to the idea that the relationship between health and lifestyle when properly revised leads to longer, healthier lives and more productive contributions to the survival of our species. With a Ph.D. in biochemistry, he is former Director of the Laboratory for Nutritional Supplement Analysis at the Linus Pauling Institute, President of the Northwest Academy of Preventive Medicine, and founder and President of HealthComm, Inc. of Gig Harbor, Washington. He is a dedicated advocate of healthful common sense and lectures to physicians, dentists and other scientists.

Jack Challen is one of the more active writers on health and nutrition topics today. His articles and interviews with the leading orthomolecular nutrition specialists such as Linus Pauling, Ph.D., Drs. Wilfrid E. Shute and Abram Hoffer, among others, appear regularly in *Let's LIVE, The Health Quarterly* and general consumer and professional publications. Mr. Challen wrote *Spirulina*, a Good Health Guide.

William H. Lee, R.Ph., Ph.D. practiced pharmacy and had his doctorate in nutrition in addition to a Master Herbalist's degree. He wrote for many popular, professional and trade magazines on a variety of health-related subjects, was the nutrition columnist for *American Druggist* magazine and lectured frequently to lay and professional meetings.

David Lin has written about and illustrated the complex subject of free radical biochemistry in his book *Free Radicals and Disease Prevention: What You Must Know* and in articles in *Health News & Review.*

Len Mervyn, Ph.D. is a chartered chemist and fellow of the Royal Institute of Chemistry in England. He taught at Ewell College of Advanced Technology in Surrey before becoming technical director of Booker Health Foods Ltd. Dr. Mervyn's work with vitamin B12 earned him awards from the New York Academy of Sciences and from the University of Pavia in Italy. He has written many books on biochemistry and nutrition including *Minerals and Your Health* and *Chelated Mineral Nutrition in Plants, Animals and Man.*

J. Auguste Mockle, D.Pharm. is a graduate of the University of Montreal Faculty of Pharmacy, and received his Doctor of Pharmacy degree from the University of Paris for his research on medicinal plants.

Dr. Mockle has for many years taught pharmacognosy, and has performed medicinal plant research at the University of Montreal Faculty of Pharmacy. He is now a consultant on medicinal plants and phytomedicines.

A graduate of Southern Methodist University, where he received the Sigma Delta Chi Outstanding Graduate Award, **Frank Murray** is the editor of *Better Nutrition for Today's Living*, a monthly consumer magazine with a circulation of 470,000. He is the author or coauthor of 28 books on health and nutrition, including *Happy Feet* and the recent *Big Family Guide to All the Minerals.*

Richard A. Passwater, Ph.D. is one of the most called upon authorities for information relating to preventive health care. A noted biochemist, he is credited with popularizing the term *supernutrition,* largely as a result of having written two bestsellers on the subject— *Supernutrition: Megavitamin Revolution* and *Supernutrition for Healthy Hearts.* His other books include *Easy No-Flab Diet, Cancer Prevention* *and Nutritional Therapies, Selenium as Food and Medicine, Trace Elements, Hair Analysis and Nutrition* (with Elmer M. Cranton, M.D.).

William H. Pryor, Ph.D. is the Thomas & David Boyd Professor in the Departments of Chemistry and Biochemistry and in the Institute for Environmental Studies at Louisiana State University, and is Director of the Biodynamics Institutes at LSU. He has been awarded more 14 national and international medals and honors, including a National Institutes of Health MERIT Award. He is the author of more than 500 articles and author or editor of more than 20 books and co-Editor-in-Chief of the journal *Free Radical Biology and Medicine.*

Jean Barilla (Editor) is a medical writer, lecturer and health consultant. She became interested in the effects of antioxidants during her Master's degree research in Biology at New York University. She completed two years of medical school as part of a graduate program in biochemistry and has taught vitamin metabolism to medical students. Her writing appears in medical journals, medical-legal textbooks, magazines and newspapers. She writes and edits educational materials for physicians, health care personnel and the general public.

Index

Abuirmeileh, N., 169
adenosine triphosphate (ATP),
    218–220
Adiamycin, anti-cancer drug, 45
adriamycin (chemotherapy drug),
    coenzyme Q-10 and,
    237–238
aging, 25–26, 37–38
    antioxidants slow, 338–340
    coenzyme Q-10 slows, 220
    vitamin C slows, 74, 85
air pollution
    antioxidants and, 341–342
    vitamin C and, 93
alcoholics and vitamin C, 94
allergies
    antioxidants and, 32
    ginkgo and, 298
    pycnogenol and, 206
    vitamin C and, 92
allicin, garlic ingredient, 274
Allium sativum: *See* garlic
alpha tocopherol: *See* vitamin E
alpha-carotene, 69–70, 336
    food sources of, 72
    suppresses cancer growth, 70
Alvares, Olav, 89, 90
Alzheimer's disease
    causes of, 289–290
    gingko treats, 271, 288–295
*American Medical Association Family
    Medical Guide*, 304, 308
Ames, S.A., 123, 124
anascorbemia, rebound scurvy, 82;
    See also scurvy
Anastasi, John, 28
Anderson, Ronald, 37
anemia
    Mediterranean, 116
    vitamin E treats, 114–117

angina pectoris, coenzyme Q-10
    and, 223–224
antibiotics, vitamin C enhances, 84
antioxidant combinations, 25
antioxidants, 5–46; *See also* beta-
    carotene, bilberry, garlic,
    ginkgo, pycnogenol, selenium,
    vitamin A, vitamin C,
    vitamin E
    benefits of, 334–335
    cancer and, 360–361
    food sources of, 361–362
    free radicals and, 357–358
    information sources, 367
    medical research review, 327–334
arthritis
    ginkgo and, 297–298
    pycnogenol and, 208
    selenium and, 159–161
    vitamin C and, 93
    vitamin E and, 30–31, 132
atherosclerosis; *See also* heart disease
    pycnogenol and, 191–192
    selenium and, 157–158
    vitamin E and, 108–114
athletic performance, coenzyme
    Q-10 and, 238–239
Azizi, E., 112

babies, premature
    blindness in, 117–118
    low vitamin E levels, 115
    vitamin E supplementation, 118
bacterial infection, vitamin E
    prevents, 121
Barboriak, Joseph, 111
Barrett, M., 107
Baumann, C.A., 17
Baumann, Joachim, 188
Bell, Duncan, 205

Benditt, Earl, 27
beta-blockers, coenzyme Q-10 and, 225, 229
beta-carotene, 14
　cancer protection, 8, 43–44, 49–68
　daily requirement of, 64–65
　excess of, 51
　Finnish smokers and, 71, 326
　food sources of, 64–66, 361, 365–366
　recommended dosage, 33, 364
　stroke risk and, 192
　vitamin A and, 50–53
　vitamin A conversion, 51
bilberry, 272–273
　blood circulation and, 272–273
　eyesight and, 272–273
　night vision and, 272–273
　safety of, 273
　varicose veins and, 273
bilirubinemia, 115
Binder, H.J., 101
bioflavonoids, 181, 244–265
　classifications of, 181
　clinical research, 248–252
　diabetic cataract and, 252–254
　duodenal ulcers and, 252
　food sources of, 246, 256
　heart disease and, 327
　natural versus synthetic, 257–258
　need for, 249
　nutritional controversy, 254–257
　vitamin C and, 249–250, 256, 258–260, 263–265
Bjelke, E., 11, 22, 57
Bjorksten, Johan, 154
blindness, diabetic, pycnogenol prevents, 207
Bliznakov, E.Z., 220
blood circulation
　bilberry improves, 272–273
　ginkgo improves, 269–271, 303–308
blood clotting
　garlic prevents, 274
　ginkgo prevents, 275

selenium prevents, 158
blood pressure; See also hyptertension
　antioxidants for, 40
　vitamin C and, 35–37
Blumberg, Jeffrey, 71, 329, 339
bowel tolerance, vitamin C and, 80–81
Boxer, L.A., 121
brain function
　ginkgo for, 288–295
　pycnogenol improves, 204–205
Braquet, Pierre, 288, 297
breast cancer; See also cancer
　selenium treatment, 36, 150–151
　vitamin E and, 120
breast disease, cystic, 119–121
Breslow, Lester, 21
Brewer, Bryan, 108
Brin, M., 124
bronchial constriction, ginkgo and, 298
Brown, Donald, 292, 298
Bunce, Edwin, 131
Burk, Dean, 22
Butturini, U., 110

Cadet, Jean, 332
Cameron, Ewan, 20, 86, 87, 98
cancer
　alpha-carotene suppresses, 70
　antioxidants and, 8–9, 360–361
　beta-carotene and, 8, 43–44, 49–68
　carotenoids and, 35–36
　progression of, 12–13
　protection from, 42–46
　pycnogenol therapy, 208
　selenium and, 8, 140–153
　vitamin A and, 9, 35, 43–44, 49–68, 62
　vitamin C and, 8, 19–25, 86–88
　vitamin E and, 8, 19, 36, 132
Cancer and Its Nutritional Therapies, 25, 58, 152

capillaries
  bioflavonoids and, 250
  ginkgo and, 270
Carbone, Paul, 56
carcinogens used in animal tests, 17
cardiomyopathy, coenzyme Q-10
    and, 225
cardiovacular disease, coenzyme
    Q-10 deficiency and, 222–223
Carlson, Susan, 127
carotenoids
  cancer and, 35–36
  family of, 50
Cartier, Jacques, 178
catalase, defined, 8
cataracts, 31–32, 38
  diabetic, bioflavonoids and,
    252–254
  vitamin C and, 41
  vitamin E and, 131
Cataract Breakthrough, 32
catechin, 181
Cathcart, Robert, 79, 83, 84
cervical cancer, vitamins A and E
    and, 132; *See also* cancer
chemotherapy
  coenzyme Q-10 and, 237–238
  vitamin A and, 60–61
Cheraskin, Emanuel, 89
cholesterol; see also HDL and LDL
  garlic and, 166, 168–169, 170,
    274
  vitamin C and, 90–92
  vitamin E and, 108–109
Chope, A.C., 21
Chopra, Dharam, 57
Chretien, Paul, 23
Chu, E.W., 55
Chytill, Frank, 10
circulatory disorders; *See also* heart
    disease
  coenzyme Q10 and, 223–224
  gingko and, 269–270, 303–308
Clark, Larry, 147, 149
Clayton, C.G., 17
coenzyme Q-10, 215–244
  anti-aging benefits of, 231–232

  athletic performance and,
    238–239
  chemotherapy and, 237–238
  defined, 218, 220
  diabetes and, 235–237
  heart disease and, 223–224
  immune system and, 239–240
  need for, 221–222
  periodontal disease and, 232,
    234–235
  safety of, 225, 241–242
  weight loss and, 238–239
Cohen, Martin, 56
colds, common
  cause of, 77–78
  preventing, 79–80, 99
  vitamin C prevents, 74
collagen, vitamin C's effect on, 85
colon cancer and vitamin A
    deficiency, 57; *See also*
    cancer
Combs, Gerald, 149
Comfort, Alex, 26
*Complete Guide to Anti-Aging
    Nutrition*, 311
Comstock, George, 34
Cone, M.T., 56
congestive heart failure, coenzyme
    Q-10 prevents, 224–225; *See
    also* heart disease
Connor, William, 71
Cooper, M. Robert, 24
Corash, L., 116
Corey, Elias, 287, 288
Cornwall, D., 106
Crary, E., 159
Cutler, Richard, 37
cyclosporin, immune suppressor,
    296–297
cystic breast disease, vitamin E
    and, 119–121
cystic fibrosis, vitamin E deficiency
    and, 101

d-alpha tocopherol acetate (natural
    vitamin E), 110

Davies, R.E., 55
De-Feudis, F., 298
DeChatelet, Lawrence, 24
detoxification, coenzyme Q-10 and,
    232–233
Deucher, W.G., 21
diabetes
    cataract, bioflavonoids and,
        252–254
    coenzyme Q-10 and, 235–237
    pycnogenol and, 207
    vitamin E and, 132
Dierenfeld, Ellen, 134
DiMascio, Paolo, 70
dl-alpha tocopherol, 122–123
DMBA, carcinogen, 170
Doll, Richard, 14, 44, 59
Donaldson, R., 152
drug addiction and vitamin C, 94
Duarte, Alex, 33
Duke, James, 171

edema, pycnogenol and, 200
elephants, vitamin E treatment for,
    134
Ellis, John, 251
endothelium-dependent relaxation
    factor (EDRF), xii
enzymes, defined, 217
epicatechin (bioflavonoid), 247–248
Esterbauer, Hermann, 191
Evans, Denis, 290, 291
exercise increases vitamin E
    requirement, 131–132
eyesight
    bilberry and, 272–273
    ginkgo and, 308–309
    pycnogenol and, 208

Fahn, Stanley, 37
Faucett, J., 29
Feigen, George, 24
Feine-Haake, G., 200
Finland, beta-carotene research in,
    71, 326

fluid retention, pycnogenol and, 200
Folkers, Karl, 217, 220, 235
Fox, Arnold, 163
free radicals, 6, 27, 102, 137, 177,
    184–186, 357–358
    damage, disorders associated
        with, 7–8, 363
    free-radical pathology, 43
    ginkgo and, 270, 311–313
    rancidity and, 34
    selenium removes, 163–164
    superoxide radicals, 102
Frei, Balz, 331
Fridovich, Irwin, xi
Frost, Doug, 15
Fruchart, J.C., 36
Fujimaki, Y., 54
Funfgeld, E., 294
Furchgott, Robert, xii

garlic, 165–171, 273–276
    aged extracts, 169–170
    consumption, cancer and, 170
    garlic therapy, 169–170
    preparations of, 273
    recommended dosage, 274,
        313–314
    safety of, 275, 276
germanium, mineral in garlic, 166
ginkgo, 269–271, 275–276,
    281–321
    active ingredients of, 286–287
    allergies and, 298
    bronchial constriction and, 298
    circulation and, 269–270
    circulatory disorders and,
        303–308
    clinical trials, 292–295
    eye disorders and, 308–309
    free radical scavenger, 311–313
    free radicals and, 270
    hearing loss and, 299–302
    hemorrhoids and, 309–311
    history of plant, 283–286
    impotence and, 302–303
    processing of, 286

ginkgo (*Cont.*)
  recommended dosage, 271
  safety of, 271, 308
  side effects of, 314
  tinnitus and, 299–302
  vertigo and, 300
ginkgolides, 288
  ginkgolide B, 297
glutathione, defined, 8
Godwin, K., 153
Goerner, A. and M., 54
Goth and Littman, 22
Grey, Fred, 192
Grey, K. Friedrich, 37
Griffin, A. Clark, 18
Gross, S.J., 115
gums, bleeding, 89; *See also*
  periodontal disease
Gunby, P., 118
Gurewich, Victor, 171
Gwebu, E.T., 106

Haas, Hans, 307
Haeger, K., 101
Harman, Denham, xii, 26
Harr, J.R., 18
Hatam, L., 110
headaches, ginkgo and, 295
The Healing Factor: Vitamin C
  Against Disease, 76
hearing loss, ginkgo and, 299–302
heart disease, 27–30
  antioxidant therapy, 192–194
  antioxidants protect against, xiii
  coenzyme Q-10 and, 223–228
  death rates and selenium, 155,
    156
  garlic and, 166
  ginkgo for, 269–270
  heart attack prevention, 113
  ischemic, 162
  protection from, 39–41
  pycnogenol and, 190–191
  selenium deficiency and,
    153–154, 155, 157
  selenium therapy, 162

vitamin C and, 90–92
vitamin E and, 35, 104–108, 192
Hemila, Harri, 99
hemolytic anemia, vitamin E and,
  114
hemorrhoids
  ginkgo and, 309–311
  vitamin C and, 94
Hendler, Sheldon, 311
Hennekens, Charles, 63
herbology, history of, 266–269
Hermann, W.J., 29, 110
herpes simplex, vitamin C and, 84
hesperidin (bioflavonoid), 246–247,
  264
Hess, John, 131
high-density lipoproteins (HDL),
  29, 109–110, 112, 120, 171
Hill, Donald, 56, 57
Hittner, Helen, 118
Hoffer, Abram, 93, 98
Hoon, David, 170
Horvath, Paula, 147
Horwitt, M.K., 123, 124
Howard, Donald R., 111
Huber, L, 21
Huggins, Hal, 89
hyaluronidase, "spreading factor"
  enzyme, 85
Hyaluronidase and Cancer, 22
hyperoxy fatty acids, 106–107
hypertension (high blood pressure)
  antioxidants for, 40
  coenzyme Q-10 and, 228
  garlic therapy, 169, 274
  vitamin C and, 35–37
hyperthyroidism
  coenzyme Q-10 levels and, 227
  heart failure, coenzyme Q-10
    and, 227

Ignarro, Louis, xii
illness and rancidity of fats, 34
immune system
  coenzyme Q-10 and, 239–240
  vitamin E enhances, 121, 131

impotence, ginkgo and, 302–303
inflammatory disease, pycnogenol
    treats, 206, 208
injury
    pycnogenol and inflammation,
        206–207
    vitamin C treats, 92
interferon, 78
intermittent claudication, vitamin E
    and, 101
Ip, Clement, 147
Irie, Reiko, 170

Jaakkola, Kaarlo, 162
Jacques, Paul F., 38, 40
Johnson, J.E., 55

Kalokerinos, Archie, 92
Kanofsky, J. and P., 113
Kaufman, David, 56
Kayden, H., 110
Kennes, Bernard, 25
Keshan disease, 154–155
Khachaturian, Zaven, 291
Koh, Eunsook, 36
Korsan-Bengsten, K., 28
Krebs (citric acid) cycle enzyme
    system, 221
Kritchevsky, David, 40
Kyolic garlic, 167

Lachance, Paul, 331
Lane, Bernard, 57
Langer, Stephen, 227
Langsjoen, Per, 226
Lasnitzki, I., 55
leukemia, selenium treatment, 151
leukocytes, role of, 78
leukopenia, carrot overdose, 67–68
Levine, Stephen, 32
Lewin, Sherry, 77, 91
Leydhecker, H., 207
Lin, Robert, 169
Lind, James, 75, 245

lipoproteins, vitamin E and, 109;
    See also HDL and LDL
lipoxygenase, 106, 107
Liu, Jimzhou, 169
London, R.S., 119
longevity
    coenzyme Q-10 and, 222, 230
    nutrition and, 230–232
low-density lipoprotein (LDL), 28,
    36, 109–110, 166, 171
lung cancer; See also cancer
    vitamin A and, 57
    vitamin E and, 132
lutein, carotene, 69
lycopene, powerful carotene, 69, 70

Machlin, L., 124
Malmgren, R.A., 55
Manson, JoAnn, 39, 192, 327
Margen, Sheldon, 331
Marletta, Michael, xii
Masquelier, Jacques, 179, 187, 202
Maugh, T.H., 56
Maynard, G., 207
McCaleb, Rob, 307
McCall, Charles, 24
McConnel, K., 151
McCord, Joe, xi
McCormick, W.J., 22
medicinal plants, history of,
    266–269
Mediterranean anemia, vitamin E
    and, 116
melanoma, garlic prevents, 170–171
memory, ginkgo improves, 271
menopause, vitamin E and, 132
Menzel, David, 331
Mickle, Donald, 40
migraine headache, ginkgo and, 295
Milner, John, 149, 169
Miniero, R., 116
mitochondria (fuel cells), 231
mitral valve prolapse, coenzyme Q-
    10 and, 227
Modan, B., 60
mononucleosis, vitamin C and, 83

Moore, Julie Ann, 157
Mori, S., 54
Morishige, Fukumi, 83, 98
Morkin, Eugene, 226
mulberry heart disease, 153
Murad, S., 85
Murakoshi, Michiaki, 69
Murata, Akira, 83

Natta, C.L., 117
Nettesheim, P., 56, 57
Neuquinon (coenzyme Q-10), 227
neurological abnormalities, vitamin
    E deficiency, 132
Newberne, Paul, 10, 57
night vision, bilberry and, 272–273
nitric oxide, xii
Noiva, Robert, 157
Nurses' Health Study, 327
Nutritional Influences on Illness, 170

O'Neill, Molly, 171
O'Regan, S., 107
Ochsner, Alton, 105, 113
Oliver, Michael, 40
Ong, David, 10
organ transplants, ginkgo and,
    296–297
Osileski, Odutola, 36
Osmond, Humphry, 93
oxalic acid, 259
oxygen, singlet, 63

Packer, Lester, 131
Padwa, Albert, 63
Papaverine, vasodilator, 303
Parkinson's disease, 37
    ginkgo and, 294
    vitamin E and, 132
Passeri, M., 110
Passwater, Richard A., 5
Pauling, Linus, 20, 45, 73–74, 78,
    79, 85, 98–99, 245
People's Medical Manual, 299, 309

periodontal disease
    coenzyme Q-10 and, 232,
        234–235
    vitamin C and, 89
Petro, R., 59, 60, 62
phospholipids, 102
phototherapy treatment of anemia
    in babies, 115
phytochemicals, 336
phytomedicine, 269
Pierson, Herbert, 171
pine bark, source of pycnogenol,
    179–180
plant drugs, history of, 266–269
Plant Bioflavonoids in Biology and
    Medicine, 182
platelet-activating factor (PAF), 298
Plotkin, George, 10
poisoning, vitamin C protects
    against, 93
polymorphonuclear leukocytes
    (PMNs), 89
polyunsaturated fatty acids
    (PUFA), 102
Port, Curtis, 57
premenstrual syndrome (PMS),
    vitamin E prevents, 132
procyanidins, 181
prostacyclin, 106, 108, 158
prostaglandin X, 28
    prostaglandin, defined, 28, 105,
        166
protoporphyria, skin disease, beta-
    carotene treatment of, 67
Pryor, William, xi, 7
pycnogenol, 175–214
    benefits of, 213
    brain function and, 204–205
    discovery of, 178
    edema and, 200
    effects of, 176–178
    eyesight and, 207–208
    free radical scavenger, 177
    heart disease and, 190–191
    recommended dosage, 210
    safety of, 186, 209–210
    sources of, 178–179, 214

pycnogenol (*cont.*)
  stroke protection, 205
  tumor inhibition, 208
  use as sunscreen, 203
  vericose veins and, 200

quercetin (bioflavonoid), 247–248
Quereshi, Asaf, 169
Quillen, Patrick, 131

radiation, vitamin C and, 74, 93
Ramwell, Richard, 296, 297
rancidity, 34–35
Rath, Matthias, 98
red blood cell disorders, vitamin E
  and, 115
retinoids, 12; defined, 13
retinol, 52
rheumatoid arthritis
  selenium levels and, 160
  vitamin E improves, 132
  rheumatoid factor titer (RFT),
  161
Roberts, H.J., 113
Rogers, Adrianne, 57
rutin (bioflavonoid), 246–247, 264

Saffioti, Umberto, 10, 55
Sakula, Alex, 57
Salonen, Jukka, 148, 157
Sanstead, Harold, 340
scar tissue, vitamin C with E
  prevents, 92
Schiavon, R., 158
schizophrenia, vitamin C helps, 93
Schlegel, J.U., 22
Schneider, Edward, 338
Schrauzer, Gerhard, 15
Schwartz, J., 332
scurvy
  Canadian explorers and, 178
  rebound, 82
  vitamin C and, 75
Seifter, Eli, 14, 56, 57, 60

Selatoc, veterinary drug, 154
selenium, 14–19, 136–164
  cancer and, 8, 15, 16, 36,
  150–153
  coenzyme Q-10 and, 233
  deficiency, 30, 31, 44
  deficiency in animals, 153–154
  food sources of, 362
  garlic source of, 165–166
  heart disease and, 153–154, 155,
  157, 162
  Keshan disease treatment,
  155–156
  recommended dosage, 33
  removes free radicals, 163–164
  review of research, 138–139,
  141–149
  vitamin E and, 29–30, 31
Selenium as Food and Medicine, 15,
  161
Shamberger, Raymond, 14, 55,
  154, 163
Shapiro, H.M., 101
Shaw, Charles, 19
Shekelle, Richard, 62
Shih, Tzu-Wen, 56
shock, vitamin C prevents, 93
Shute, Evan and Wilfrid, 29,
  127–129, 130, 133
sickle-cell anemia, vitamin E
  improves, 116–117, 132
Siegel, Ivens, 90
singlet oxygen, 63
skin health, pycnogenol and,
  201–203
smog, antioxidants and, 341–342
smokers, vitamin A protects, 57
Spittle-Leslie, Constance, 90
Sporn, Michael, 11, 14, 56, 59
Stadtman, Earl, 330
Stamler, Jeremiah, 62
Stead, N.W., 158
Steiner, Manfred, 28
Stone, Irwin, 21, 76, 78
stress, vitamin C reduces, 93
stroke
  beta-carotene and, 192

pycnogenol and, 205
Su, Wei-guo, 288
Subar, Amy, 330
succinate dehydrogenase-CoQ10
   reductase, 221
Sudden Infant Death Syndrome
   (SIDS), vitamin C prevents,
   74, 91–92
Supernutrition for Healthy Hearts,
   28, 183
superoxide dismutase (SOD), xi, 8,
   31, 159, 313
superoxide radicals, 102
surgery, vitamin C and, 83
Swarm, Richard, 57
synthetic vs. natural vitamin E,
   123–124, 127
Szczeklik, A., 108
Sze, Lan, 170
Szent-Györgyi, Albert, 75, 176,
   245, 263, 329

Tannenbaum, Steven, xii
Tappel, Al, 26, 138
Taylor, Allen, 332
Tehniger, T.F., 23
Telsem, veterinary drug, 154
thrombosis, 112
   vitamin E protects against, 104
thromboxane, 106
tinnitus, ginkgo and, 299–302
A Treatise of the Scurvy, 75
Trout, David, 36
Tsao, Constance, 259

ubiquinone (coenzyme Q-10), 217,
   220
ulcers, duodinal, and bioflavonoids,
   252
Urethan, cancer drug, 54

Vaccinium myrtillus: See bilberry
varicose veins

bilberry improves, 273
   pycnogenol treats, 200, 202
Vecchi, M., 124
vertigo, ginkgo and, 300
viral infections, bioflavonoids and,
   250
vitamers, 52
vitamin A
   beta-carotene and, 50–53
   biological role of, 52–53
   cancer and, 35
   cancer protection, 8
   chemotherapy and, 60–61
   content on labels misleading, 65
   deficiency and cancer, 10–11, 43
   dosage recommended, 33,
      64–65, 364
   food sources of, 362, 365–366
   immune system and, 9–13
   International Units, 52
   levels and cancer, 62
   palminate, 52
   research, history of, 53–56
   symptoms of deficiency, 67
   symptoms of toxicity, 67
   toxicity of, 13
vitamin C, 73–99
   air pollution and, 93
   allergies and, 92
   animals that do not manufacture,
      76
   antibiotics and, 84
   bioflavonoids and, 249–250, 256,
      258–260, 263–265
   biological role of, 75–76
   bowel tolerance and dosage,
      80–81
   cancer and, 8, 19–25, 45–46,
      86–88
   cold prevention, 79–80, 99
   collagen production and, 22
   conditions treated, 92–94
   depletion, symptoms of, 83
   discovery of, 75
   dosage, recommended, 33,
      76–77, 79, 80–81, 98–99,
      364

vitamin C (*Cont.*)
    food sources of, 361, 365–366
    heart disease and, 40
    high blood pressure and, 35–37
    injuries and, 92
    pain reduction and, 22
    periodontal diseases and, 89
    rebound scurvy and, 82
    safety of, 95
    scar tissue and, 92
    scurvy and, 75
    shock and, 93
    Sudden Infant Death Syndrome
        (SIDS) and, 74, 91–92
*Vitamin C: Its Molecular Biology and
    Medical Potential*, 77
Vitamin C and the Common Cold, 74
vitamin E, xiii, 100–135
    benefits of, 129
    cancer and, 8, 19, 35, 36
    contradictory studies on, 113–114
    deficiency, symptoms of, 103, 132
    deficiency in captive animals, 134
    dosage, recommended, 33, 133, 364
    food sources of, 128, 365–366
    forms of, 122–123
    heart disease and, 28–30, 35, 40,
        113
    potency, 122–123
    selenium, 29–30, 31
    supplementation, 128–129
    synthetic vs. natural, 123–124
vitamin P, defined, 245
von Euler, B., 50, 54

Wald, Nicholas, 58

Warburton, D., 295, 307
Ward, K., 29
Ware, Charles, 160
Warner, Huber, 331
Wattenberg, Lee, 18
Weed, Earl, 225
Weg, Ruth, 99
weight loss, coenzyme Q-10 and,
    238–239
Weil, Andrew, 268
Weiner, Michael, 71
Weiser, H., 124
Wells, Ibert, 157
Wendt, Von, 21
Werbach, Melvyn, 170
White, David, 191, 206
Wilkinson, Edward, 234
Willet, W.C., 141
Willis, Charles, 154
Wilson, Christine, 16, 44
Wilson, R.B., 110
Wolbach, D.S.B., 11, 54
Wolf, George, 62

Yau, Terrence, 131
Yokata, F., 111
Yonemoto, Robert, 23
Yu, Shu-Yu, 146

zeaxanthin, carotene, 70
Ziegler, Regina, 35
Zisblatt, Martin, 56
Zloch, Z., 246
zoo animals, vitamin E levels in, 134